Accession no.
36134197

KW-221-521

WITHDRAWN

Reducing saturated fats in foods

© Woodhead Publishing Limited, 2011

Related titles:

Improving the fat content of foods
(ISBN 978-1-85573-965-9)
Dietary fats have long been recognised as having a major impact on health, negative in the case of consumers' excessive intake of saturated fatty acids, positive in the case of increasing consumers' intake of long chain n-3 polyunsaturated fatty acids (PUFAs). However, progress in ensuring that consumers achieve a nutritionally optimal fat intake has been slow. This important book reviews the range of steps needed to improve the fat content of foods whilst maintaining sensory quality.

Modifying lipids for use in food
(ISBN 978-1-85573-971-0)
Any oil or fat should have the optimum physical, chemical, and nutritional properties dictated by its end use. Modification of natural fats and oils is therefore important to improve the quality of lipids for use in foods. When lipids are modified, though, compromises have to be made as the physical, chemical and nutritional properties of lipids are not always mutually compatible and this provides an important challenge for food technologists. Edited by an eminent specialist, this collection shows how these challenges have been met in the past, how they are being met today, and how they may be met in the future.

Reducing salt in foods: practical strategies
(ISBN 978-1-84569-018-2)
Eating too much salt is a significant risk factor in developing high blood pressure, a condition often described as a 'silent killer' as those living with it are much more likely to develop heart disease or suffer a stroke. A high proportion of consumers eat more than the recommended daily level of salt each day and consumers are increasingly looking for ways to lower their salt intake: therefore reducing the level of salt in food products is a priority for many in the food industry. Written by a distinguished team of international authors, this collection covers key themes such as the health effects of excessive salt intake and the influence of salt on the quality of foods and offers practical strategies for reducing and replacing salt in food products.

Details of these books and a complete list of Woodhead's titles can be obtained by:

- visiting our web site at www.woodheadpublishing.com
- contacting Customer Services (e-mail: sales@woodheadpublishing.com; fax: +44 (0) 1223 832819; tel.: +44 (0) 1223 499140 ext. 130; address: Woodhead Publishing Limited, 80 High Street, Sawston, Cambridge CB22 3HJ, UK)

If you would like to receive information on forthcoming titles, please send your address details to: Francis Dodds (address, tel. and fax as above; e-mail: francis. dodds@woodheadpublishing.com). Please confirm which subject areas you are interested in.

© Woodhead Publishing Limited, 2011

Woodhead Publishing Series in Food Science, Technology and Nutrition:
Number 221

Reducing saturated
fats in foods

Edited by
Geoff Talbot

LIS - LIBRARY

Date	Fund
19-6-13	U-che

Order No.

2412093

University of Chester

WOODHEAD
PUBLISHING

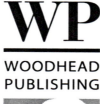

Oxford   Cambridge   Philadelphia   New Delhi

© Woodhead Publishing Limited, 2011

Published by Woodhead Publishing Limited,
80 High Street, Sawston, Cambridge CB22 3HJ, UK
www.woodheadpublishing.com

Woodhead Publishing, 1518 Walnut Street, Suite 1100, Philadelphia, PA 19102–3406, USA

Woodhead Publishing India Private Limited, G-2, Vardaan House, 7/28 Ansari Road,
Daryaganj, New Delhi – 110002, India
www.woodheadpublishingindia.com

First published 2011, Woodhead Publishing Limited
© Woodhead Publishing Limited, 2011; Chapter 7 © W. G. Morley, 2011
The authors have asserted their moral rights.

This book contains information obtained from authentic and highly regarded sources.
Reprinted material is quoted with permission, and sources are indicated. Reasonable
efforts have been made to publish reliable data and information, but the authors and the
publishers cannot assume responsibility for the validity of all materials. Neither the
authors nor the publishers, nor anyone else associated with this publication, shall be
liable for any loss, damage or liability directly or indirectly caused or alleged to be caused by
this book.
    Neither this book nor any part may be reproduced or transmitted in any form or by
any means, electronic or mechanical, including photocopying, microfilming and recording,
or by any information storage or retrieval system, without permission in writing from
Woodhead Publishing Limited.
    The consent of Woodhead Publishing Limited does not extend to copying for general
distribution, for promotion, for creating new works, or for resale. Specific permission
must be obtained in writing from Woodhead Publishing Limited for such copying.

Trademark notice: Product or corporate names may be trademarks or registered trademarks,
and are used only for identification and explanation, without intent to infringe.

British Library Cataloguing in Publication Data
A catalogue record for this book is available from the British Library.

ISBN 978-1-84569-740-2 (print)
ISBN 978-0-85709-247-2 (online)
ISSN 2042-8049 Woodhead Publishing Series in Food Science, Technology and Nutrition (print)
ISSN 2042-8057 Woodhead Publishing Series in Food Science, Technology and Nutrition (online)

The publisher's policy is to use permanent paper from mills that operate a sustainable forestry
policy, and which has been manufactured from pulp which is processed using acid-free and
elemental chlorine-free practices. Furthermore, the publisher ensures that the text paper and
cover board used have met acceptable environmental accreditation standards.

Typeset by RefineCatch Limited, Bungay, Suffolk

Contents

Contributor contact details.. *xi*

Woodhead Publishing Series in Food Science, Technology
and Nutrition .... *xv*

Part I   Saturated fats in foods: functional and nutritional aspects

1 Saturated fats in foods and strategies for their replacement:
   an introduction **3**
   G. Talbot, The Fat Consultant, UK
   1.1   Background to the need to reduce saturated fats 3
   1.2   Chemistry and structure of fatty acids and triglycerides 5
   1.3   Saturated fat and fatty acid consumption in the EU,
          US and UK.. 10
   1.4   Opposing views on effects of saturates on cardiovascular
          disease.. 15
   1.5   Replacements for saturates 18
   1.6   Areas not covered by specific chapters in this book................. 22
   1.7   Future trends 25
   1.8   Sources of further information and advice 26
   1.9   References.. 26

2 The functional attributes that fats bring to food............................. **29**
   E. H. A. de Hoog, R. M. A. J. Ruijschop, S. P. Pyett and P. M. T. de Kok,
   NIZO Food Research B.V., The Netherlands
   2.1   Introduction... 29
   2.2   Perception of fat.. 30
   2.3   Role of fat in the texture of foods 33

© Woodhead Publishing Limited, 2011

2.4   Engineering fat to tailor appetite 38
2.5   Consequences for strategies to reduce fat.................... 41
2.6   Future trends 42
2.7   Sources of further information and advice 43
2.8   Acknowledgements... 43
2.9   References.. 43

3 Sources of saturated and other dietary fats................. **47**
G. Talbot, The Fat Consultant, UK
3.1   Introduction... 47
3.2   Vegetable oils rich in saturated fats 48
3.3   Mammalian milk fats 61
3.4   Animal carcass fats.. 65
3.5   Hydrogenated fats 67
3.6   The *trans* effect 69
3.7   Future trends 73
3.8   Sources of further information and advice 74
3.9   References.. 74

4 Health aspects of saturated fatty acids......................... **77**
J. I. Pedersen, University of Oslo, Norway and B. Kirkhus,
Nofima – Food, Fisheries and Aquacultural Research, Norway
4.1   Introduction... 77
4.2   Atherosclerosis as the basis for cardiovascular
        diseases (CVD) 78
4.3   Effects of individual fatty acids on plasma total cholesterol,
        LDL cholesterol, HDL cholesterol and triglycerides
        (VLDL).. 81
4.4   Effects of fatty acids on other biomarkers related to
        coronary heart disease (CHD) 84
4.5   Evidence linking LDL cholesterol to the development of
        atherosclerosis and CHD 85
4.6   Effects of saturated fatty acids (SFA) on disease states
        related to CVD 88
4.7   Cancer 90
4.8   Dietary recommendations related to SFA 90
4.9   Trends in consumption of SFA as related to trends in
        mortality and incidence of CVD................................. 92
4.10   Conclusion 93
4.11   References.. 93

5 Chronic disease risk associated with different dietary
    saturated fatty acids... **98**
D. I. Givens and K. E. Kliem, University of Reading, UK
5.1   Introduction... 98

© Woodhead Publishing Limited, 2011

5.2   Key dietary saturated fatty acids...   99
5.3   Chronic disease risk differences between different saturated
       fatty acids...   100
5.4   The 'stearic acid' effect – chronic disease risk effects of
       stearic acid   105
5.5   Future trends   106
5.6   Sources of further information and advice   108
5.7   References...   108

6 Nutritional characteristics of palm oil   112
  P. Khosla, Wayne State University, USA and K. Sundram,
  Malaysian Palm Oil Council, Malaysia
6.1   Introduction..   112
6.2   Serum cholesterol, lipoproteins and dietary fatty acids.............   113
6.3   Effects of palm olein as part of a low-fat healthy diet...............   115
6.4   Effects of dietary fatty acids on LDL-C/HDL-C ratios   117
6.5   Palm oil minor components...   120
6.6   Conclusion and future trends..   122
6.7   Sources of further information and advice   124
6.8   References...   124

Part II   Food reformulation to reduce saturated fats

7 Reducing saturated fat using emulsion technology.........................   131
  W. G. Morley, Leatherhead Food Research, UK
7.1   Introduction..   131
7.2   Fat composition   134
7.3   Emulsion droplets   138
7.4   Phase structuring and emulsions..   141
7.5   Fat replacers...   146
7.6   Processing...   150
7.7   Applications..   151
7.8   Future trends   152
7.9   Sources of further information and advice   153
7.10   References...   154

8 Diacylglycerol oils: nutritional aspects and applications
  in foods   158
  O. M. Lai, Universiti Putra Malaysia, Malaysia and S.-K. Lo,
  Sime Darby Research Sdn. Bhd., Malaysia
8.1   Introduction..   158
8.2   Digestion, absorption and metabolism of DAG   161
8.3   Production process patents   164
8.4   Product application patents...   167

© Woodhead Publishing Limited, 2011

8.5   Regulatory status 172
8.6   Future trends 173
8.7   Source of further information 174
8.8   References... 174

9 Saturated fat reduction in milk and dairy products **179**
   E. S. Komorowski, Dairy UK, UK
   9.1   Introduction.. 179
   9.2   Milk... 182
   9.3   Cheese.. 184
   9.4   Butter and spreadable fats.. 187
   9.5   Reducing the saturated content of milk fat through feed........... 189
   9.6   Future trends 190
   9.7   Sources of further information and advice 190
   9.8   References... 191

10 Saturated fat reduction in butchered meat................................ **195**
   K. R. Matthews, Agriculture and Horticulture Development Board, UK
   10.1   Introduction.. 195
   10.2   Animal production 196
   10.3   Preparation of cuts 203
   10.4   In the kitchen and on the plate 204
   10.5   Effect on meat quality.. 205
   10.6   Future trends 207
   10.7   Conclusions... 207
   10.8   Sources of further information and advice 208
   10.9   References.. 208

11 Saturated fat reduction in processed meat products **210**
   S. Barbut, University of Guelph, Canada
   11.1   Introduction... 210
   11.2   Ground-meat products (burgers)............................... 212
   11.3   Sausages – coarse-ground (e.g. cooked salami,
           breakfast sausage)... 215
   11.4   Sausages – emulsion-type products (e.g. bologna,
           frankfurters) 218
   11.5   Sausages – dry fermented (e.g. summer sausage, dry salami).... 225
   11.6   Prepared and coated meat products (e.g. nuggets, pies)............ 227
   11.7   Future trends 229
   11.8   Sources of further information................................. 229
   11.9   References.. 230

12 Altering animal diet to reduce saturated fat in meat and milk **234**
   A. P. Moloney, Teagasc, Ireland
   12.1   Introduction.. 234

© Woodhead Publishing Limited, 2011

12.2 The fat content of meat and milk................................... 237
12.3 Dietary effects on the fat content and fatty acid composition
      of meat 238
12.4 Dietary effects on the fat content and fatty acid composition
      of milk... 249
12.5 Influence of 'additives' on saturated fatty acids in meat and milk.. 255
12.6 Future trends 258
12.7 Sources of further information and advice 259
12.8 References.. 260

13 Reducing saturated fat in savoury snacks and fried foods **266**
*A. M. Kita, Wrocław University of Environmental and Life
Sciences, Poland*
13.1 Introduction.. 266
13.2 Frying oils... 267
13.3 Effects of frying oils and frying parameters on the quality
      of fried foods.. 268
13.4 Innovating technologies in frying and their impact on the
      quality of fried foods 274
13.5 Changes in savoury snacks 277
13.6 Future trends 279
13.7 Sources of further information and advice 279
13.8 References.. 279

14 Saturated fat reduction in biscuits **283**
G. Atkinson, AarhusKarlshamn UK Ltd, UK
14.1 Introduction.. 283
14.2 Types of fat used in biscuits................................... 284
14.3 The technology of biscuits...................................... 285
14.4 Techniques for saturates reduction 289
14.5 Future trends 299
14.6 Sources of further information and advice 299
14.7 References.. 299

15 Saturated fat reduction in pastry **301**
B. de Cindio and F. R. Lupi, University of Calabria, Italy
15.1 Introduction.. 301
15.2 The dough/fat matching process in pastry 304
15.3 Process rheological modeling 308
15.4 Margarine and shortenings for reducing saturated fats.......... 311
15.5 Conclusions.. 314
15.6 Future trends 315
15.7 Sources of further information and advice 315
15.8 Acknowledgements... 316
15.9 References... 316

© Woodhead Publishing Limited, 2011

16 Reducing saturated fat in chocolate, compound coatings and filled confectionery products... **318**
G. Talbot, The Fat Consultant, UK
16.1   Introduction.. 318
16.2   Chocolate 321
16.3   Compound coatings 333
16.4   Filled confectionery products 341
16.5   Future trends 346
16.6   Sources of further information and advice 347
16.7   References.. 347

17 Saturated fat reduction in ice cream **350**
J. Underdown and P. J. Quail, Unilever R&D, UK and K. W. Smith, Fat Science Consulting Ltd, UK
17.1   Introduction.. 350
17.2   Basic components and processing of ice cream 352
17.3   Sources of fat and saturated fat in ice cream products 353
17.4   The function of fat in ice cream.............................. 354
17.5   Properties of fats used in current ice cream products 358
17.6   Challenges associated with saturated fatty acid (SFA) reduction 359
17.7   Future trends 365
17.8   References.. 366

18 Saturated fat reduction in sauces **370**
P. Smith, Cargill R&D Centre Europe, Belgium
18.1   Introduction.. 370
18.2   Sensory properties of sauces................................... 371
18.3   Product lifetime 373
18.4   Conclusions.. 375
18.5   Future trends 375
18.6   Sources of further information and advice 376
18.7   References.. 376

Index *379*

© Woodhead Publishing Limited, 2011

Contributor contact details

(* = main contact)

Editor and chapters 1, 3 and 16

G. Talbot
The Fat Consultant
Suite 250
St Loyes House
20 St Loyes Street
Bedford
MK40 1ZL
UK

E-mail: geoff@thefatconsultant.co.uk

Chapter 2

E. H. A. de Hoog*, R. M. A. J.
  Ruijschop, S. P. Pyett and P. M. T.
  de Kok
NIZO Food Research B.V.
P.O. Box 20
6710 BA Ede
The Netherlands

E-mail: els.de.hoog@nizo.nl

Chapter 4

J. I. Pedersen*
Institute of Basic Medical Sciences
Department of Nutrition
University of Oslo
P.O. Box 1046 Blindern
0316 Oslo
Norway

E-mail: j.i.pedersen@medisin.uio.no

B. Kirkhus
Nofima – Food, Fisheries and
  Aquacultural Research
1430 Ås
Norway

Chapter 5

D. I. Givens* and K. E. Kliem
Animal Science Research Group
School of Agriculture, Policy and
  Development
University of Reading
Earley Gate
Reading
RG6 6AR
UK

E-mail: d.i.givens@reading.ac.uk
        k.e.kliem@reading.ac.uk

© Woodhead Publishing Limited, 2011

Chapter 6

P. Khosla*
Department of Nutrition and Food
    Science
Wayne State University
Detroit
MI 48202
USA

E-mail: pkhosla@sun.science.
    wayne.edu

K. Sundram
Malaysian Palm Oil Council
Selangor Darul Ehsan
Malaysia

Institute of Bioscience
Universiti Putra Malaysia
43400 UPM
Serdang
Selangor
Malaysia

E-mail: omlai@biotech.upm.edu.my

S.-K. Lo
Sime Darby Research Sdn. Bhd.
R & D Centre-Downstream
Lot 2664, Jalan Pulau Carey
42960 Pulau Carey, Selangor
Malaysia

E-mail: lo.seong.koon@simedarby.com

Chapter 7

W. G. Morley
Leatherhead Food Research
Randalls Road
Leatherhead
Surrey
KT22 7RY
UK

E-mail: WMorley@LeatherheadFood.
    com

Chapter 8

O. M. Lai*
Dept. of Bioprocess Technology
Faculty of Biotechnology &
    Biomolecular Sciences
Universiti Putra Malaysia
43400 UPM
Serdang
Selangor
Malaysia

Chapter 9

E. S. Komorowski
Dairy UK
93 Baker Street
London
W1U 6QQ
UK

E-mail: ekomorowski@dairyUK.org

Chapter 10

K. R. Matthews
Agriculture and Horticulture
    Development Board
Stoneleigh Park
Kenilworth
Warwickshire
CV8 2TL
UK

E-mail: kim.matthews@eblex.org.uk

© Woodhead Publishing Limited, 2011

Chapter 11

S. Barbut
Food Science Department
University of Guelph
Guelph
Ontario
Canada
N1G 2W1

E-mail: sbarbut@uoguelph.ca

Chapter 12

A. P. Moloney
Teagasc
Animal and Grassland Research and
    Innovation Centre
Grange
Dunsany
Co. Meath
Ireland

E-mail: aidan.moloney@teagasc.ie

Chapter 13

A. M. Kita
Department of Food Storage and
Technology
Faculty of Food Science
Wrocław University of Environmental
    and Life Sciences
C.K. Norwida 25
50-375 Wrocław
Poland

E-mail: agnieszka.kita@wnoz.up.
    wroc.pl

Chapter 14

G. Atkinson
AarhusKarlshamn UK Ltd
King George Dock
Hull
HU9 5PX
UK

E-mail: gary.atkinson@aak.com

Chapter 15

B. de Cindio* and F. R. Lupi
University of Calabria
Dept. of Engineering Modeling
Laboratory of Rheology and Food
    Engineering
Via P. Bucci Cubo 39c
I-87036 Arcavacata di Rende (CS)
Italy

E-mail: bruno.decindio@unical.it
    francesca.lupi@unical.it

Chapter 17

J. Underdown* and P. J. Quail
Unilever R&D
Colworth Science Park
Sharnbrook
Bedford
MK44 1LQ
UK

E-mail: jeff.underdown@unilever.com
    patricia.quail@unilever.com

K. W. Smith
Fat Science Consulting Ltd
16 Arundel Drive
Bedford
MK41 8HP
UK

E-mail: kevin.w.smith@fatscience.co.uk

© Woodhead Publishing Limited, 2011

Chapter 18

P. Smith
Cargill R&D Centre Europe
Havenstraat 84
B1800 Vilvoorde
Belgium

E-mail: paul_smith@cargill.com

© Woodhead Publishing Limited, 2011

Woodhead Publishing Series in Food Science, Technology and Nutrition

1   Chilled foods: a comprehensive guide *Edited by C. Dennis and M. Stringer*
2   Yoghurt: science and technology *A. Y. Tamime and R. K. Robinson*
3   Food processing technology: principles and practice *P. J. Fellows*
4   Bender's dictionary of nutrition and food technology Sixth edition *D. A. Bender*
5   Determination of veterinary residues in food *Edited by N. T. Crosby*
6   Food contaminants: sources and surveillance *Edited by C. Creaser and R. Purchase*
7   Nitrates and nitrites in food and water *Edited by M. J. Hill*
8   Pesticide chemistry and bioscience: the food-environment challenge *Edited by G. T. Brooks and T. Roberts*
9   Pesticides: developments, impacts and controls *Edited by G. A. Best and A. D. Ruthven*
10 Dietary fibre: chemical and biological aspects *Edited by D. A. T. Southgate, K. W. Waldron, I. T. Johnson and G. R. Fenwick*
11 Vitamins and minerals in health and nutrition *M. Tolonen*
12 Technology of biscuits, crackers and cookies Second edition *D. Manley*
13 Instrumentation and sensors for the food industry *Edited by E. Kress-Rogers*
14 Food and cancer prevention: chemical and biological aspects *Edited by K. W. Waldron, I. T. Johnson and G. R. Fenwick*
15 Food colloids: proteins, lipids and polysaccharides *Edited by E. Dickinson and B. Bergenstahl*
16 Food emulsions and foams *Edited by E. Dickinson*
17 Maillard reactions in chemistry, food and health *Edited by T. P. Labuza, V. Monnier, J. Baynes and J. O'Brien*
18 The Maillard reaction in foods and medicine *Edited by J. O'Brien, H. E. Nursten, M. J. Crabbe and J. M. Ames*
19 Encapsulation and controlled release *Edited by D. R. Karsa and R. A. Stephenson*
20 Flavours and fragrances *Edited by A. D. Swift*
21 Feta and related cheeses *Edited by A. Y. Tamime and R. K. Robinson*

© Woodhead Publishing Limited, 2011

22   **Biochemistry of milk products** *Edited by A. T. Andrews and J. R. Varley*
23   **Physical properties of foods and food processing systems** *M. J. Lewis*
24   **Food irradiation: a reference guide** *V. M. Wilkinson and G. Gould*
25   **Kent's technology of cereals: an introduction for students of food science and agriculture Fourth edition** *N. L. Kent and A. D. Evers*
26   **Biosensors for food analysis** *Edited by A. O. Scott*
27   **Separation processes in the food and biotechnology industries: principles and applications** *Edited by A.S. Grandison and M. J. Lewis*
28   **Handbook of indices of food quality and authenticity** *R.S. Singhal, P. K. Kulkarni and D. V. Rege*
29   **Principles and practices for the safe processing of foods** *D. A. Shapton and N. F. Shapton*
30   **Biscuit, cookie and cracker manufacturing manuals Volume 1: ingredients** *D. Manley*
31   **Biscuit, cookie and cracker manufacturing manuals Volume 2: biscuit doughs** *D. Manley*
32   **Biscuit, cookie and cracker manufacturing manuals Volume 3: biscuit dough piece forming** *D. Manley*
33   **Biscuit, cookie and cracker manufacturing manuals Volume 4: baking and cooling of biscuits** *D. Manley*
34   **Biscuit, cookie and cracker manufacturing manuals Volume 5: secondary processing in biscuit manufacturing** *D. Manley*
35   **Biscuit, cookie and cracker manufacturing manuals Volume 6: biscuit packaging and storage** *D. Manley*
36   **Practical dehydration Second edition** *M. Greensmith*
37   **Lawrie's meat science Sixth edition** *R. A. Lawrie*
38   **Yoghurt: science and technology Second edition** *A. Y Tamime and R. K. Robinson*
39   **New ingredients in food processing: biochemistry and agriculture** *G. Linden and D. Lorient*
40   **Benders' dictionary of nutrition and food technology Seventh edition** *D A Bender and A. E. Bender*
41   **Technology of biscuits, crackers and cookies Third edition** *D. Manley*
42   **Food processing technology: principles and practice Second edition** *P. J. Fellows*
43   **Managing frozen foods** *Edited by C. J. Kennedy*
44   **Handbook of hydrocolloids** *Edited by G. O. Phillips and P. A. Williams*
45   **Food labelling** *Edited by J. R. Blanchfield*
46   **Cereal biotechnology** *Edited by P. C. Morris and J. H. Bryce*
47   **Food intolerance and the food industry** *Edited by T. Dean*
48   **The stability and shelf-life of food** *Edited by D. Kilcast and P. Subramaniam*
49   **Functional foods: concept to product** *Edited by G. R. Gibson and C. M. Williams*
50   **Chilled foods: a comprehensive guide Second edition** *Edited by M. Stringer and C. Dennis*
51   **HACCP in the meat industry** *Edited by M. Brown*
52   **Biscuit, cracker and cookie recipes for the food industry** *D. Manley*
53   **Cereals processing technology** *Edited by G. Owens*
54   **Baking problems solved** *S. P. Cauvain and L. S. Young*
55   **Thermal technologies in food processing** *Edited by P. Richardson*
56   **Frying: improving quality** *Edited by J. B. Rossell*
57   **Food chemical safety Volume 1: contaminants** *Edited by D. Watson*

© Woodhead Publishing Limited, 2011

58 **Making the most of HACCP: learning from others' experience** *Edited by T. Mayes and S. Mortimore*
59 **Food process modelling** *Edited by L. M. M. Tijskens, M. L. A. T. M. Hertog and B. M. Nicolaï*
60 **EU food law: a practical guide** *Edited by K. Goodburn*
61 **Extrusion cooking: technologies and applications** *Edited by R. Guy*
62 **Auditing in the food industry: from safety and quality to environmental and other audits** *Edited by M. Dillon and C. Griffith*
63 **Handbook of herbs and spices Volume 1** *Edited by K. V. Peter*
64 **Food product development: maximising success** *M. Earle, R. Earle and A. Anderson*
65 **Instrumentation and sensors for the food industry Second edition** *Edited by E. Kress-Rogers and C. J. B. Brimelow*
66 **Food chemical safety Volume 2: additives** *Edited by D. Watson*
67 **Fruit and vegetable biotechnology** *Edited by V. Valpuesta*
68 **Foodborne pathogens: hazards, risk analysis and control** *Edited by C. de W. Blackburn and P. J. McClure*
69 **Meat refrigeration** *S. J. James and C. James*
70 **Lockhart and Wiseman's crop husbandry Eighth edition** *H. J. S. Finch, A. M. Samuel and G. P. F. Lane*
71 **Safety and quality issues in fish processing** *Edited by H. A. Bremner*
72 **Minimal processing technologies in the food industries** *Edited by T. Ohlsson and N. Bengtsson*
73 **Fruit and vegetable processing: improving quality** *Edited by W. Jongen*
74 **The nutrition handbook for food processors** *Edited by C. J. K. Henry and C. Chapman*
75 **Colour in food: improving quality** *Edited by D MacDougall*
76 **Meat processing: improving quality** *Edited by J. P. Kerry, J. F. Kerry and D. A. Ledward*
77 **Microbiological risk assessment in food processing** *Edited by M. Brown and M. Stringer*
78 **Performance functional foods** *Edited by D. Watson*
79 **Functional dairy products Volume 1** *Edited by T. Mattila-Sandholm and M. Saarela*
80 **Taints and off-flavours in foods** *Edited by B. Baigrie*
81 **Yeasts in food** *Edited by T. Boekhout and V. Robert*
82 **Phytochemical functional foods** *Edited by I. T. Johnson and G. Williamson*
83 **Novel food packaging techniques** *Edited by R. Ahvenainen*
84 **Detecting pathogens in food** *Edited by T. A. McMeekin*
85 **Natural antimicrobials for the minimal processing of foods** *Edited by S. Roller*
86 **Texture in food Volume 1: semi-solid foods** *Edited by B. M. McKenna*
87 **Dairy processing: improving quality** *Edited by G Smit*
88 **Hygiene in food processing: principles and practice** *Edited by H. L. M. Lelieveld, M. A. Mostert, B. White and J. Holah*
89 **Rapid and on-line instrumentation for food quality assurance** *Edited by I. Tothill*
90 **Sausage manufacture: principles and practice** *E. Essien*
91 **Environmentally friendly food processing** *Edited by B. Mattsson and U. Sonesson*
92 **Bread making: improving quality** *Edited by S. P. Cauvain*
93 **Food preservation techniques** *Edited by P. Zeuthen and L. Bøgh-Sørensen*
94 **Food authenticity and traceability** *Edited by M. Lees*
95 **Analytical methods for food additives** *R. Wood, L. Foster, A. Damant and P. Key*

© Woodhead Publishing Limited, 2011

96 Handbook of herbs and spices Volume 2 *Edited by K. V. Peter*
97 Texture in food Volume 2: solid foods *Edited by D. Kilcast*
98 Proteins in food processing *Edited by R. Yada*
99 Detecting foreign bodies in food *Edited by M. Edwards*
100 Understanding and measuring the shelf-life of food *Edited by R. Steele*
101 Poultry meat processing and quality *Edited by G. Mead*
102 Functional foods, ageing and degenerative disease *Edited by C. Remacle and B. Reusens*
103 Mycotoxins in food: detection and control *Edited by N. Magan and M. Olsen*
104 Improving the thermal processing of foods *Edited by P. Richardson*
105 Pesticide, veterinary and other residues in food *Edited by D. Watson*
106 Starch in food: structure, functions and applications *Edited by A-C Eliasson*
107 Functional foods, cardiovascular disease and diabetes *Edited by A. Arnoldi*
108 Brewing: science and practice *D. E. Briggs, P. A. Brookes, R. Stevens and C. A. Boulton*
109 Using cereal science and technology for the benefit of consumers: proceedings of the 12th International ICC Cereal and Bread Congress, 24-26th May, 2004, Harrogate, UK *Edited by S. P. Cauvain, L. S. Young and S. Salmon*
110 Improving the safety of fresh meat *Edited by J. Sofos*
111 Understanding pathogen behaviour in food: virulence, stress response and resistance *Edited by M. Griffiths*
112 The microwave processing of foods *Edited by H. Schubert and M. Regier*
113 Food safety control in the poultry industry *Edited by G. Mead*
114 Improving the safety of fresh fruit and vegetables *Edited by W. Jongen*
115 Food, diet and obesity *Edited by D. Mela*
116 Handbook of hygiene control in the food industry *Edited by H. L. M. Lelieveld, M. A. Mostert and J. Holah*
117 Detecting allergens in food *Edited by S. Koppelman and S. Hefle*
118 Improving the fat content of foods *Edited by C. Williams and J. Buttriss*
119 Improving traceability in food processing and distribution *Edited by I. Smith and A. Furness*
120 Flavour in food *Edited by A. Voilley and P. Etievant*
121 The Chorleywood bread process *S. P. Cauvain and L. S. Young*
122 Food spoilage microorganisms *Edited by C. de W. Blackburn*
123 Emerging foodborne pathogens *Edited by Y. Motarjemi and M. Adams*
124 Bender's dictionary of nutrition and food technology Eighth edition *D. A. Bender*
125 Optimising sweet taste in foods *Edited by W. J. Spillane*
126 Brewing: new technologies *Edited by C. Bamforth*
127 Handbook of herbs and spices Volume 3 *Edited by K. V. Peter*
128 Lawrie's meat science Seventh edition *R. A. Lawrie in collaboration with D. A. Ledward*
129 Modifying lipids for use in food *Edited by F. Gunstone*
130 Meat products handbook: practical science and technology *G. Feiner*
131 Food consumption and disease risk: consumer–pathogen interactions *Edited by M. Potter*
132 Acrylamide and other hazardous compounds in heat-treated foods *Edited by K. Skog and J. Alexander*
133 Managing allergens in food *Edited by C. Mills, H. Wichers and K. Hoffman-Sommergruber*

© Woodhead Publishing Limited, 2011

134 **Microbiological analysis of red meat, poultry and eggs** *Edited by G. Mead*
135 **Maximising the value of marine by-products** *Edited by F. Shahidi*
136 **Chemical migration and food contact materials** *Edited by K. Barnes, R. Sinclair and D. Watson*
137 **Understanding consumers of food products** *Edited by L. Frewer and H. van Trijp*
138 **Reducing salt in foods: practical strategies** *Edited by D. Kilcast and F. Angus*
139 **Modelling microorganisms in food** *Edited by S. Brul, S. Van Gerwen and M. Zwietering*
140 **Tamime and Robinson's Yoghurt: science and technology Third edition** *A. Y. Tamime and R. K. Robinson*
141 **Handbook of waste management and co-product recovery in food processing: Volume 1** *Edited by K. W. Waldron*
142 **Improving the flavour of cheese** *Edited by B. Weimer*
143 **Novel food ingredients for weight control** *Edited by C. J. K. Henry*
144 **Consumer-led food product development** *Edited by H. MacFie*
145 **Functional dairy products Volume 2** *Edited by M. Saarela*
146 **Modifying flavour in food** *Edited by A. J. Taylor and J. Hort*
147 **Cheese problems solved** *Edited by P. L. H. McSweeney*
148 **Handbook of organic food safety and quality** *Edited by J. Cooper, C. Leifert and U. Niggli*
149 **Understanding and controlling the microstructure of complex foods** *Edited by D. J. McClements*
150 **Novel enzyme technology for food applications** *Edited by R. Rastall*
151 **Food preservation by pulsed electric fields: from research to application** *Edited by H. L. M. Lelieveld and S. W. H. de Haan*
152 **Technology of functional cereal products** *Edited by B. R. Hamaker*
153 **Case studies in food product development** *Edited by M. Earle and R. Earle*
154 **Delivery and controlled release of bioactives in foods and nutraceuticals** *Edited by N. Garti*
155 **Fruit and vegetable flavour: recent advances and future prospects** *Edited by B. Brückner and S. G. Wyllie*
156 **Food fortification and supplementation: technological, safety and regulatory aspects** *Edited by P. Berry Ottaway*
157 **Improving the health-promoting properties of fruit and vegetable products** *Edited by F. A. Tomás-Barberán and M. I. Gil*
158 **Improving seafood products for the consumer** *Edited by T. Børresen*
159 **In-pack processed foods: improving quality** *Edited by P. Richardson*
160 **Handbook of water and energy management in food processing** *Edited by J. Klemeš, R. Smith and J-K Kim*
161 **Environmentally compatible food packaging** *Edited by E. Chiellini*
162 **Improving farmed fish quality and safety** *Edited by Ø. Lie*
163 **Carbohydrate-active enzymes** *Edited by K-H Park*
164 **Chilled foods: a comprehensive guide Third edition** *Edited by M. Brown*
165 **Food for the ageing population** *Edited by M. M. Raats, C. P. G. M. de Groot and W. A Van Staveren*
166 **Improving the sensory and nutritional quality of fresh meat** *Edited by J. P. Kerry and D. A. Ledward*
167 **Shellfish safety and quality** *Edited by S. E. Shumway and G. E. Rodrick*
168 **Functional and speciality beverage technology** *Edited by P. Paquin*

© Woodhead Publishing Limited, 2011

169 Functional foods: principles and technology *M. Guo*
170 Endocrine-disrupting chemicals in food *Edited by I. Shaw*
171 Meals in science and practice: interdisciplinary research and business applications *Edited by H. L. Meiselman*
172 Food constituents and oral health: current status and future prospects *Edited by M. Wilson*
173 Handbook of hydrocolloids Second edition *Edited by G. O. Phillips and P. A. Williams*
174 Food processing technology: principles and practice Third edition *P. J. Fellows*
175 Science and technology of enrobed and filled chocolate, confectionery and bakery products *Edited by G. Talbot*
176 Foodborne pathogens: hazards, risk analysis and control Second edition *Edited by C. de W. Blackburn and P. J. McClure*
177 Designing functional foods: measuring and controlling food structure breakdown and absorption *Edited by D. J. McClements and E. A. Decker*
178 New technologies in aquaculture: improving production efficiency, quality and environmental management *Edited by G. Burnell and G. Allan*
179 More baking problems solved *S. P. Cauvain and L. S. Young*
180 Soft drink and fruit juice problems solved *P. Ashurst and R. Hargitt*
181 Biofilms in the food and beverage industries *Edited by P. M. Fratamico, B. A. Annous and N. W. Gunther*
182 Dairy-derived ingredients: food and neutraceutical uses *Edited by M. Corredig*
183 Handbook of waste management and co-product recovery in food processing Volume 2 *Edited by K. W. Waldron*
184 Innovations in food labelling *Edited by J. Albert*
185 Delivering performance in food supply chains *Edited by C. Mena and G. Stevens*
186 Chemical deterioration and physical instability of food and beverages *Edited by L. H. Skibsted, J. Risbo and M. L. Andersen*
187 Managing wine quality Volume 1: viticulture and wine quality *Edited by A.G. Reynolds*
188 Improving the safety and quality of milk Volume 1: milk production and processing *Edited by M. Griffiths*
189 Improving the safety and quality of milk Volume 2: improving quality in milk products *Edited by M. Griffiths*
190 Cereal grains: assessing and managing quality *Edited by C. Wrigley and I. Batey*
191 Sensory analysis for food and beverage quality control: a practical guide *Edited by D. Kilcast*
192 Managing wine quality Volume 2: oenology and wine quality *Edited by A. G. Reynolds*
193 Winemaking problems solved *Edited by C. E. Butzke*
194 Environmental assessment and management in the food industry *Edited by U. Sonesson, J. Berlin and F. Ziegler*
195 Consumer-driven innovation in food and personal care products *Edited by S.R. Jaeger and H. MacFie*
196 Tracing pathogens in the food chain *Edited by S. Brul, P.M. Fratamico and T.A. McMeekin*
197 Case studies in novel food processing technologies: innovations in processing, packaging, and predictive modelling *Edited by C. J. Doona, K Kustin and F. E. Feeherry*

© Woodhead Publishing Limited, 2011

198 **Freeze-drying of pharmaceutical and food products** *T-C Hua, B-L Liu and H Zhang*

199 **Oxidation in foods and beverages and antioxidant applications: Volume 1 Understanding mechanisms of oxidation and antioxidant activity** *Edited by E. A. Decker, R. J. Elias and D. J. McClements*

200 **Oxidation in foods and beverages and antioxidant applications: Volume 2 Management in different industry sectors** *Edited by E. A. Decker, R. J. Elias and D. J. McClements*

201 **Protective cultures, antimicrobial metabolites and bacteriophages for food and beverage biopreservation** *Edited by C. Lacroix*

202 **Separation, extraction and concentration processes in the food, beverage and nutraceutical industries** *Edited by S. S. H. Rizvi*

203 **Determining mycotoxins and mycotoxigenic fungi in food and feed** *Edited by S. De Saeger*

204 **Developing children's food products** *Edited by D. Kilcast and F. Angus*

205 **Functional foods: concept to product Second edition** *Edited by M. Saarela*

206 **Postharvest biology and technology of tropical and subtropical fruits Volume 1** *Edited by E. M. Yahia*

207 **Postharvest biology and technology of tropical and subtropical fruits Volume 2** *Edited by E. M. Yahia*

208 **Postharvest biology and technology of tropical and subtropical fruits Volume 3** *Edited by E. M. Yahia*

209 **Postharvest biology and technology of tropical and subtropical fruits Volume 4** *Edited by E. M. Yahia*

210 **Food and beverage stability and shelf life** *Edited by D. Kilcast and P. Subramaniam*

211 **Processed meats: improving safety, nutrition and quality** *Edited by J. P. Kerry and J. F. Kerry*

212 **Food chain integrity: a holistic approach to food traceability, authenticity, safety and bioterrorism prevention** *Edited by J. Hoorfar, K. Jordan, F. Butler and R. Prugger*

213 **Improving the safety and quality of eggs and egg products Volume 1** *Edited by Y. Nys, M. Bain and F. Van Immerseel*

214 **Improving the safety and quality of eggs and egg products Volume 2** *Edited by Y. Nys, M. Bain and F. Van Immerseel*

215 **Feed and fodder contamination: effects on livestock and food safety** *Edited by J. Fink-Gremmels*

216 **Hygiene in the design, construction and renovation of food processing factories** *Edited by H. L. M. Lelieveld and J. Holah*

217 **Technology of biscuits, crackers and cookies Fourth edition** *Edited by D. Manley*

218 **Nanotechnology in the food, beverage and nutraceutical industries** *Edited by Q. Huang*

219 **Rice quality** *K. R. Bhattacharya*

220 **Meat, poultry and seafood packaging** *Edited by J. P. Kerry*

221 **Reducing saturated fats in foods** *Edited by G. Talbot*

222 **Handbook of food proteins** *Edited by G. O. Phillips and P. A. Williams*

223 **Lifetime nutritional influences on cognition, behaviour and psychiatric illness** *Edited by D. Benton*

© Woodhead Publishing Limited, 2011

Part I

Saturated fats in foods: functional and nutritional aspects

© Woodhead Publishing Limited, 2011

1

Saturated fats in foods and strategies for their replacement: an introduction

G. Talbot, The Fat Consultant, UK

Abstract: This book as a whole is concerned with the reduction of saturated fats in foods. The background to this, both in terms of the clinical nutritional studies backing up the need for such reductions to be made and the sources of saturated fats in the diet, are discussed in the first part of the book. The second part of the book deals with ways of reducing saturates in those food categories that contribute the most saturates to the diet. This opening chapter sets the scene for the rest of the book by outlining the background as to why we should be reducing saturated fat intake, but also giving some details of the opposite view. For those unfamiliar with the chemistry of fats and fatty acids a brief introduction to this is given. The chapter then goes on to give some information on the usage of some of the more common 'saturated' fats (palm oil, palm kernel oil, coconut oil, butterfat and lard) over the past 15 years in the EU, US and UK. The chapter also discusses what the various options are in terms of the materials that could be used to replace saturates, before concluding with a brief examination of some food categories that are not considered in their own right in later separate chapters – foods such as cakes and doughnuts, ready meals and non-chocolate confectionery.

Key words: saturated fat, chemistry of fats, usage of oils, fat replacers, cakes, doughnuts, ready meals, toffees.

1.1 Background to the need to reduce saturated fats

The World Health Organization (2003) has recommended a daily intake of total fat comprising between 15% and 30% of dietary energy. In the same report the WHO recommends that less than 10% of daily energy should come from saturated fats. The UK Food Standards Agency (2008) published its Saturated Fat and Energy Intake Programme and recommended that saturated fat consumption should be reduced from a level of about 13.3% of dietary energy (from the National Diet and Nutrition Survey (HMSO, 2002)) to a level of 11% of dietary

© Woodhead Publishing Limited, 2011

energy, a reduction of about 20%. The reason for this is the effects that saturated fatty acids are considered to have on blood cholesterol levels which, in turn, are considered to affect the risk of developing cardiovascular diseases such as coronary heart disease and strokes.

There have been numerous publications showing the effects of saturated fat on blood cholesterol and references to many of these are made in subsequent chapters. One of the most commonly quoted is a meta-analysis of 60 controlled trials carried out by Mensink *et al.* (2003). In this paper, the authors show that different saturated fatty acids have different effects on total blood cholesterol levels when used to replace 1% carbohydrate (see Fig. 1.1). Within the range of what might be considered long-chain saturates (i.e. C12:0 up to C18:0) there is the suggestion that the longer the chain length the lower is the increase of total cholesterol in the blood, suggesting that stearic acid has a relatively neutral effect compared with lauric acid, which raises blood cholesterol levels significantly. As with many aspects of clinical nutrition, things are not always as clear-cut as they seem and delving deeper into this meta-analysis it becomes clear that much of the increase in cholesterol in the blood from lauric acid is high-density lipoprotein (HDL) cholesterol, the so-called 'good' cholesterol. This, and other studies, will be considered in more detail in section 1.4 of this chapter and reviewed in considerably greater detail in later chapters.

Although both the World Health Organization and the UK Foods Standards Agency are calling for reductions in saturated fat in the diet, considerable reductions have already been made between 1986/87 and 2002 in the UK (Table 1.1). In that 15-year period total energy from fat has reduced from about 40.4% down to about 35.4%, a reduction of over 12%. Almost all of this reduction has been to saturated fats (down from 16.8% to 13.3% of energy) and *trans* fats (down from 2.2% to 1.2% of energy). This reduction in energy from saturates is already one of 20%, but a further 20% reduction is now being called for.

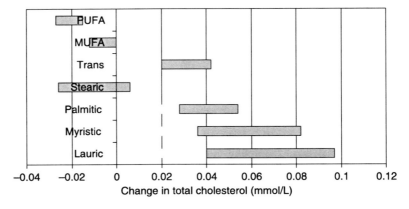

Fig. 1.1   Effect of different fatty acids in changing total cholesterol levels (1% replacement of carbohydrate) (Source: Mensink *et al.*, 2003).

© Woodhead Publishing Limited, 2011

Table 1.1   Changes in UK energy intake from fat between 1986/87 and 2002

Type of fat	Men		Women	
	1986/87	2002	1986/87	2002
Total	40.4	35.8	40.3	34.9
Saturated	16.5	13.4	17.0	13.2
trans	2.2	1.2	2.1	1.2
cis monounsaturated	12.4	12.1	12.2	11.5
cis n-3 polyunsaturated	0.8	1.0	0.8	1.0
cis n-6 polyunsaturated	5.4	5.4	5.3	5.3

Source: Talbot, 2006.

One of the main questions that this book will address is how and where such a reduction can be made. Before trying to answer that, though, it is useful to look at where most of the saturated fat in our diet comes from. Chapter 3 will look at the animal and vegetable sources of saturated fats but, in terms of food groups, we can see from Table 1.2 that, in the UK (HMSO, 2002), 24% of saturates were from a milk (dairy) source, 22% were from meat and meat products, 18% were from cereal-based products (i.e. bakery and baked products) and 11% were from fat spreads (including butter). Three-quarters of our intake was from these four broad food groups. Other groups contributing lesser, but still significant, levels were potatoes and savoury snacks (7% of total saturates) and chocolate confectionery (5% of total saturates). Not surprisingly, these are the areas that this book will concentrate on.

1.2   Chemistry and structure of fatty acids and triglycerides

Fats are triesters of the trihydric alcohol, glycerol, and hence are known as triacylglycerols (TAGs) or, more commonly, triglycerides (TGs). Glycerol forms the backbone to the structure but it is the three fatty acids that are esterified to it that give fats both their functional and nutritional characteristics. All fatty acids are hydrocarbon chains with a methyl (CH_3) group at one end and a carboxylic acid (COOH) group at the other. It is the carboxylic acid group that links to the glycerol backbone, reacting with the alcohol group of the glycerol to produce an ester linkage. Saturated fatty acids contain no carbon–carbon double bonds within the fatty acid chain and have a straight, linear structure (albeit with small 'zig-zags' moving from one carbon atom to the next) (Fig. 1.2). The structures of the most commonly occurring saturated fatty acids, lauric (C12:0), myristic (C14:0), palmitic (C16:0) and stearic (C18:0) are shown in this diagram. Because they have this straight linear structure, triglycerides that contain significant amounts of saturated fatty acids can crystallize together in a closer crystal structure (because the straight chains can get physically closer together). This gives the fat a thermodynamically more stable structure which results in a higher melting point. Thus, fats containing higher levels of saturates tend to be more solid at ambient temperatures than fats containing higher levels of unsaturates.

© Woodhead Publishing Limited, 2011

Table 1.2   Contribution of food groups to total and saturated fat intake (in the UK, 2002)

Food group	Contribution to daily total fat intake (%)	Contribution to daily energy intake from total fat (%)	Contribution to daily saturated fat intake (%)	Contribution to daily energy intake from saturated fat (%)	Saturate intake as % of total fat intake
Cereals and cereal products:	19	6.4	18	2.3	36%
Pizza	2	0.7	2	0.3	43%
White bread	2	0.7	1	0.1	14%
Biscuits	3	1.0	4	0.5	50%
Buns, cakes and pastries	4	1.3	4	0.5	38%
Milk and milk products:	14	4.7	24	3.0	64%
Whole milk	3	1.0	4	0.5	50%
Semi-skimmed milk	3	1.0	5	0.6	60%
Cheese (incl. cottage cheese)	6	2.0	10	1.3	65%
Eggs and egg dishes	4	1.3	3	0.4	31%
Fat spreads:	12	4.0	11	1.4	35%
Butter	4	1.3	6	0.8	62%
Margarines	1	0.3	1	0.1	33%
Reduced fat spreads	5	1.7	3	0.4	24%
Low fat spreads	1	0.3	1	0.1	33%
Meat and meat products:	23	7.7	22	2.8	36%
Bacon and ham	2	0.7	2	0.3	43%
Beef, veal and dishes	3	1.0	4	0.5	50%
Lamb and dishes	1	0.3	1	0.1	33%
Pork and dishes	1	0.3	1	0.1	33%
Coated chicken and turkey	1	0.3	1	0.1	33%
Chicken, turkey and dishes	4	1.3	3	0.4	31%
Burgers and kebabs	2	0.7	2	0.3	43%
Sausages	3	1.0	3	0.4	40%
Meat pies and pastries	4	1.3	4	0.5	38%
Other meat and meat products	1	0.3	1	0.1	33%
Fish and fish dishes:	3	1.0	2	0.3	30%
Coated and or fried white fish	2	0.7	1	0.1	14%
Oily fish	1	0.3	1	0.1	33%

© Woodhead Publishing Limited, 2011

Vegetables (excl. potatoes)	4	1.3	2	0.3	23%
Potatoes and savoury snacks:	10	3.4	7	0.9	26%
Chips	5	1.7	3	0.4	24%
Other fried or roast potatoes	1	0.3	0	0.0	0%
Savoury snacks	3	1.0	3	0.4	40%
Fruit and nuts	2	0.7	1	0.1	14%
Sugars, preserves and confectionery:	3	1.0	5	0.6	60%
Chocolate confectionery	3	1.0	5	0.6	60%
Drinks	0	0.0	1	0.1	
Miscellaneous	5	1.7	3	0.4	57%

Source: from Talbot (2006) and sourced from HMSO (2002).

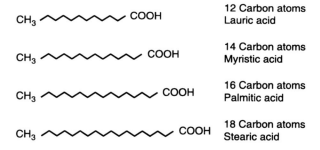

Fig. 1.2   Saturated fatty acid structures.

Unsaturated fatty acids, on the other hand, generally have a more bent structure (Fig. 1.3). Unsaturated fatty acids contain one or more carbon–carbon double bonds within the fatty acid chain. In naturally occurring vegetable oils these are almost exclusively in the *cis* configuration. This means that the carbon–carbon chains leading into and away from the two carbon atoms associated with the double bond are on the same side of the double bond as each other. This results in a bend in the chain. Figure 1.3 shows the most commonly occurring *cis*-monounsaturated fatty acid, oleic acid (C18:1). This has 18 carbon atoms in the chain and the double bond occurs between the ninth and tenth carbon atom (counting from the carboxylic acid end of the chain). Adding another *cis* double bond three carbon atoms along (i.e. between the 12th and 13th carbon atoms) gives linoleic acid (C18:2), and adding another *cis* double bond between the 15th and 16th carbon atoms gives linolenic acid (C18:3). As well, of course, as counting the position of the double

© Woodhead Publishing Limited, 2011

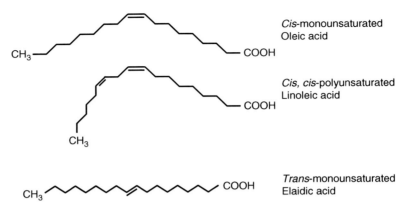

Fig. 1.3   Unsaturated fatty acid structures.

bond from the carboxylic acid end of the fatty acid chain it is possible to count it from the other end, the methyl group end. This results in the now well-known 'omega' nomenclature. If we count from the methyl group end of the chain then the first double bond to be encountered in linolenic acid is after the third carbon atom and so this is known as an omega-3 fatty acid. Similarly, linoleic acid is an omega-6 fatty acid and oleic acid is an omega-9 fatty acid.

The bent structures of these fatty acids are such that a crystal structure with a lower thermodynamic stability is produced which gives these *cis* unsaturated fatty acids a lower melting point and, indeed, they are all liquid at 20°C, whereas the four saturated fatty acids referred to earlier all have melting points well above 20°C.

There is, however, a fourth fatty acid structure shown in Fig. 1.3, that of a *trans* unsaturated fatty acid. The example shown does, like oleic acid, consist of 18 carbon atoms and has a double bond between the ninth and tenth carbon atoms but its configuration is different. In this case, instead of the chain leading into and away from the double bond being on the *same* side of the chain as each other, now they are on *opposite* sides – hence the term, *trans* fatty acid. The example shown is elaidic acid (C18:1*t*). It is clear from the diagram that *trans* fatty acids have a much straighter chain structure, more akin to that of saturates, than do the corresponding *cis* fatty acids. This means that they too can pack more closely together and therefore give a thermodynamically more stable and, hence, higher melting crystal structure. This, too, makes them highly functional in terms of giving structure and texture to those food products that require these attributes. However, they have a major drawback, one that has only been discovered in the past couple of decades, and that is that they increase blood cholesterol levels even more than do saturates. Not only that but, whereas saturates increase both 'good' HDL cholesterol and 'bad' low-density lipoprotein (LDL) cholesterol levels, *trans* fatty acids decrease the 'good' HDL cholesterol and increase the 'bad' LDL cholesterol.

© Woodhead Publishing Limited, 2011

Trans fatty acids have three main origins. They are found naturally in the milk and meat of ruminant animals such as cattle and sheep at levels, typically, of about 5% of the total fat. They can be produced if fats are heated to very high temperatures (usually in excess of those used in the deodorization of oils). They are produced from the partial hydrogenation of oils and fats. Historically this was the source of the greatest amount of *trans* fatty acids in the diet. Because of the need to reduce *trans* fatty acid intake significantly, the elimination of partially hydrogenated oils from foods has been the main way in which this has been achieved. Over the past decade, partially hydrogenated, *trans*-containing fats have been almost eliminated from processed foods and food service in the Western world. In some countries fats are still hydrogenated, but this is now generally a complete hydrogenation in which all unsaturates are converted to saturates giving what is, in effect, a fat that is 100% saturated. Such fats have, despite their high level of saturates, considerable functionality and this will be referred to in a number of later chapters. This does, however, lead into one of the 'side effects' of removing partially hydrogenated oils from the food chain and that is that, to maintain functionalities such as structure and texture, it has often been necessary to replace the *trans* fatty acids by saturates, thus leading to an increase in saturates in the diet rather than a reduction.

Trans fatty acids from dairy sources are clearly more difficult to eliminate without removing dairy fats from the diet. As this is not something that is being proposed then we obviously need to accept that there will be a baseline of, typically, 0.5 to 1.0% of dietary energy coming from such *trans* fats. Indeed the TRANSFACT Study (Chardigny *et al.*, 2008) suggests that *trans* from natural sources can have a different effect on blood cholesterol levels than *trans* from industrially produced sources insofar as cardiovascular disease risk factors in women are concerned.

Also important, both in the functionality and metabolism of triglycerides, is the positioning of the fatty acids on the glycerol backbone. Clearly there are three positions in which a fatty acid can be found. These are generally referred to as the *sn*-1, *sn*-2 and *sn*-3 positions (Fig. 1.4). Fatty acids on the *sn*-1 and *sn*-3 positions are metabolized differently from those on the *sn*-2 position. Fats are broken down firstly into 1,2- and 2,3-diglycerides, then into 2-monoglycerides, making the fatty acid in the *sn*-2 position different metabolically from those in the *sn*-1 and *sn*-3 positions (Gortner, 1958). The position of fatty acids on the glycerol backbone also gives them different functionalities. There has been a hypothesis (Vander Wal, 1960) that, in vegetable oils and fats, the *sn*-2 position is first 'filled' with unsaturated fatty acids and that what is then left over is randomly distributed between the *sn*-1 and *sn*-3 positions. There are exceptions to this, the most common one being palm oil, which contains a significant level of palmitic acid in the *sn*-2 position. The hypothesis goes on to say that in animal fats both saturates and unsaturates are more randomly distributed across all three positions. Despite the fact that this hypothesis has been questioned (Kartha, 1968; Vlahov, 2005), it does still form a useful starting point and demonstrates the difference, for example, between cocoa butter and lard. Both have fairly similar saturated/unsaturated fat compositions, but almost all of the saturates in cocoa butter are in the *sn*-1 and

© Woodhead Publishing Limited, 2011

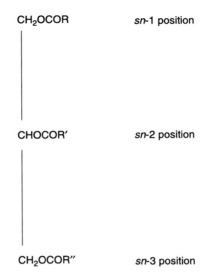

CH₂OCOR   sn-1 position

CHOCOR′   sn-2 position

CH₂OCOR″   sn-3 position

Fig. 1.4   Triglyceride structure showing *sn*-1, *sn*-2 and *sn*-3 positions.

sn-3 positions whereas a significant level of saturates in lard is in the *sn*-2 position. It is this positional distribution difference that prevents lard, for example, being used as a cocoa butter alternative.

1.3   Saturated fat and fatty acid consumption in the EU, US and UK

Oil World (1996–2010) publishes statistics annually on the movements of oilseeds, oils and oilmeal throughout the world. From this can be calculated the 'domestic disappearance' of oils and fats in each country. The domestic disappearance is defined as opening stocks + imports – exports – ending stocks. Although not all significant sources of saturated fats are included in this survey (cocoa butter and hydrogenated fats, for example, are not included), it is instructive to look at five of the main sources that are included. These are palm oil, palm kernel oil, coconut oil, butterfat and lard. The domestic disappearances of these oils between 1995 and 2009 are shown in Fig. 1.5 to 1.9. It should be noted that 'domestic disappearance' does not necessarily mean 'human consumption' because some proportions of these oils will be used for non-food uses. For example, some palm oil is now being used as biofuel; palm kernel oil and coconut oil also have uses in soaps and detergents.

1.3.1   Palm oil
The use of palm oil throughout the EU has increased year-on-year since 1995 (see Fig. 1.5) from a usage of 1.69 million tonnes in 1995 (when there were only 15 countries in the EU) up to a usage of 5.62 million tonnes in 2009 (when there were

© Woodhead Publishing Limited, 2011

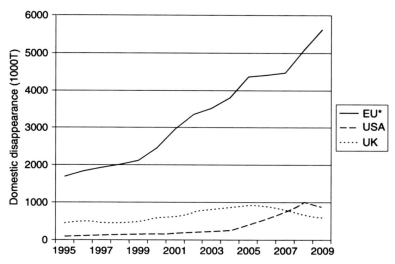

*1995–1999 – 15 countries; 2000–2004 – 25 countries; 2005–2009 – 27 countries
Drawn from data in *Oil World* (1996–2010)

Fig. 1.5   Consumption of palm oil (EU, USA, UK, 1995–2009).

27 countries in the EU). While the greater number of consumers over this time period has undoubtedly had an effect, the increase has been a relatively steady one without significant stepwise changes as the number of countries in the EU increased. Some of this increased consumption will be as a result of the use of palm oil in non-food applications but a significant proportion is also as a result of the replacement of partially hydrogenated fats in food with palm oil.

In the United Kingdom, the rate of increase of usage of palm oil has been slower but, nevertheless, significant between 1999 (473 000 tonnes) and 2005 (912 000 tonnes). Again, much of this will be due to the replacement of partially hydrogenated oils. Since 2005, however, there has been a slow decline in the UK consumption of palm oil from 912 000 tonnes in 2005 to 579 000 tonnes in 2009. Some of this will be due to manufacturers switching from palm oil to other oils in order to reduce saturated fat levels (this has been significant in the latter part of this period in both savoury snacks and biscuits). Some will also be due to concerns about sustainability and the environmental effects of increased palm oil production (despite assurances from the Roundtable for Sustainable Palm Oil and the insistence of some major users of palm oil that the oil they use is coming increasingly from sustainable sources).

Consumption of palm oil in the United States was very low up to about 1999 (consumption of 136 200 tonnes) but after 2003 increased significantly, peaking in 2008 at 989 800 tonnes. This initially very low usage of palm oil in the United States compared with Western Europe was due mainly to two things. Firstly, the use of tropical oils such as palm oil was minimal as a result of a mass press campaign in the 1980s claiming that such oils were having adverse effects on the health of the American people. Secondly, partially hydrogenated domestic oils

© Woodhead Publishing Limited, 2011

such as soyabean oil and cottonseed oil were widely used where some solid fats were needed. With the issues of *trans* fatty acids, however, in the early part of the present century the use of such partially hydrogenated oils declined and, in many areas, the easiest solution was to replace these with palm oil. Greater development has, in the meantime, come up with different solutions (for example, the interesterification of fully hydrogenated and non-hydrogenated oils) and so, as in the UK, there has since been a slight decline in consumption.

1.3.2   Palm kernel oil

The consumption of palm kernel oil in the EU has also shown a steady increase from about 317 000 tonnes in 1995 to a peak of 651 000 tonnes in 2007 (Fig. 1.6). This increase has also been mirrored in the United States. Despite the fact that palm kernel oil was also classed as a 'tropical oil' in the United States, the consumption of this oil was greater than or equal to that of palm oil up to 2004. However, some of this consumption would have been in personal care products rather than in foods for human consumption. Usage of palm kernel oil in the United Kingdom has been relatively low (less than 100 000 tonnes throughout the timescale considered) and has been in a more or less steady decline since about 1998.

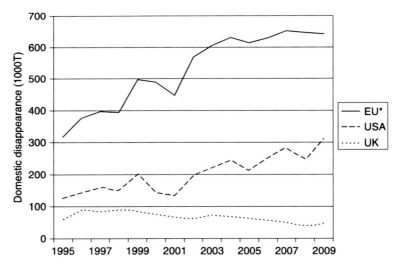

*1995–1999 – 15 countries; 2000–2004 – 25 countries; 2005–2009 – 27 countries
Drawn from data in *Oil World* (1996–2010)

Fig. 1.6   Consumption of palm kernel oil (EU, USA, UK, 1995–2009).

1.3.3   Coconut oil

Unlike palm oil and palm kernel oil, the consumption levels of coconut oil have been relatively constant over the period from 1995 to 2009 in both the EU and the United States (Fig. 1.7). There have been ups and downs from year to year (for

© Woodhead Publishing Limited, 2011

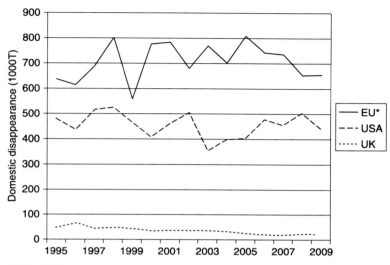

*1995–1999 – 15 countries; 2000–2004 – 25 countries; 2005–2009 – 27 countries
Drawn from data in *Oil World* (1996–2010)

Fig. 1.7   Consumption of coconut oil (EU, USA, UK, 1995–2009).

example a particularly low EU consumption in 1999) but, in general, EU consumption has been between 600 000 tonnes and 800 000 tonnes per annum and US consumption has been between 400 000 tonnes and 500 000 tonnes per annum (with only two or three years outside these ranges). Consumption in the United Kingdom has been in steady decline from 1996 (when 62 000 tonnes were used) to 2009 (when only 16 600 tonnes were used).

1.3.4   Butterfat
Butterfat is the main milk fat used in food. In the EU there was a large jump in consumption between 1999 and 2000 as a result of the increase in the number of countries represented in the EU (Fig. 1.8). Since then, consumption has been fairly constant at about 1.7 million tonnes per annum. In the United States there has been a steady increase in butterfat consumption from 1998 (404 700 tonnes) to 2009 (579 100 tonnes). Although a slight rise in UK consumption between 1998 and 2005 can be seen, in general, consumption levels in the United Kingdom have been fairly constant at about 200 000 tonnes per annum.

1.3.5   Lard
Although beef tallow has some food uses both industrially and domestically, lard is probably the more widely used animal fat in food. Consumption in the United Kingdom has been low over the time period considered but, even, within that timescale, it has been in a steady decline from 66 600 tonnes in 1995 to 18 600 tonnes in 2009 (Fig. 1.9). In contrast there has been an increase in consumption in

© Woodhead Publishing Limited, 2011

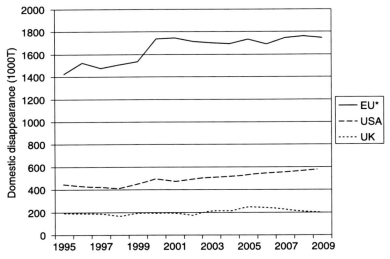

*1995–1999 – 15 countries; 2000–2004 – 25 countries; 2005–2009 – 27 countries
Drawn from data in *Oil World* (1996–2010)

Fig. 1.8   Consumption of butterfat (EU, USA, UK, 1995–2009).

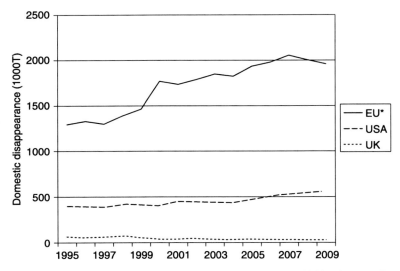

*1995–1999 – 15 countries; 2000–2004 – 25 countries; 2005–2009 – 27 countries
Drawn from data in *Oil World* (1996–2010)

Fig. 1.9   Consumption of lard (EU, USA, UK, 1995–2009).

© Woodhead Publishing Limited, 2011

the United States between 2004 and 2009, having been fairly constant to that point, while EU consumption has increased steadily from 1995 to 2007 with a large increase between 1999 and 2000 when the size of the EU increased.

1.4   Opposing views on effects of saturates on cardiovascular disease

Although the World Health Organization and many governmental agencies across the world are all agreed that intake of saturated fat should be reduced to below 10–11% of dietary energy as a means of reducing the risks of cardiovascular disease, not all of the clinical (and even anecdotal) data would support this. Much of the support for the hypothesis is based on the meta-analysis carried out by Mensink *et al.* (2003) and summarized graphically in Fig. 1.1. This study suggested that different saturated fatty acids have different effects on blood cholesterol levels (LDL-cholesterol, HDL-cholesterol and total cholesterol) and, as has already been indicated in the introduction to this chapter, that stearic acid showed a neutral effect, neither raising nor lowering the levels of any of these different types of cholesterol. This effect had already been observed some 20 years previous to this and was then linked to an observation that, after consumption of stearic acid, it was not stearic acid levels that increased in the blood but levels of oleic acid. This led to the hypothesis that stearic acid was converted into oleic acid in the body. However, Rhee *et al.* (1997) dashed that theory when they fed deuterium-labelled fatty acids and found that just over 10% of stearic acid was converted into oleic acid. Nevertheless, the neutrality of stearic acid relative to the effects of other saturated fatty acids on blood cholesterol levels remains. A more contentious area is whether palmitic acid is good or bad.

A superficial study of the results from Mensink *et al.* (2003) would suggest that palmitic acid has an adverse effect on blood cholesterol levels. However, work carried out by Judd *et al.* (2002) and summarized by McNeill (2009) casts some doubt on this – or, at least, casts doubt on the hypothesis that palmitic acid is worse than stearic acid in this respect. The rationale behind this is that there are two types of cholesterol – one is 'good' (HDL cholesterol) and one is 'bad' (LDL cholesterol). Stearic acid raises neither; palmitic acid raises both. Since increased levels of HDL cholesterol have been shown to have a protecting effect against cardiovascular disease, the rationale suggests that the increased levels of HDL cholesterol produced when palmitic acid is consumed offset the potential cardiovascular disease risk resulting from increased levels of LDL cholesterol and the total effect is one that is not significantly different from that produced from stearic acid. In their paper, Mensink *et al.* (2003) go on to say that the ratio of total:HDL cholesterol is more important than the levels of any individual type of cholesterol in predicting the risk of cardiovascular disease. Figure 1.10 shows the effect of different fatty acids on this ratio when used to replace 1% carbohydrate in the diet. The bars show the mean +/– 2 SD and those for stearic acid, palmitic acid and myristic acid all overlap. Since a significant proportion of palmitic acid

© Woodhead Publishing Limited, 2011

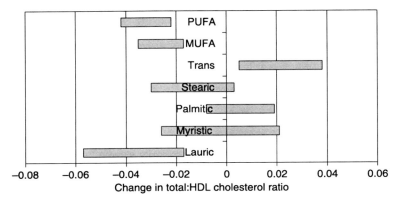

Fig. 1.10   Effect of different fatty acids in changing total:HDL cholesterol ratio (1% replacement of carbohydrate) (Source: Mensink *et al.*, 2003).

in the Western diet is now from palm oil, the effects of these different fatty acids are explored in more detail in Chapter 6.

Anecdotal evidence is often cited to cast doubts on the relationship between saturated fatty acid intake and the risk of coronary heart disease. The European Heart Network (2008) publishes statistics relating to cardiovascular disease and coronary heart disease across all European countries. The British Heart Foundation also publishes a wide range of statistics, including a series showing the percentage of energy from saturated fat country by country in Europe in 1998 (British Heart Foundation, 2010) Combining the data for saturated fat consumption across all European countries in 1998 (from British Heart Foundation, 2010) with data for deaths from coronary heart disease across the same countries for the same year (from European Heart Network, 2008), we would expect to see a direct correlation with the death rate from coronary heart disease increasing with saturated fat intake. The reality is the opposite (Fig. 1.11). The highest death rates from coronary heart disease were in Eastern European countries; the highest rates of consumption of saturated fats were in Western European countries. It is, of course, too simplistic to say that these data refute the clinical nutritional studies that show a positive relationship between saturated fatty acid intake and cardiovascular disease risk because so many other factors come into play in terms of what might have caused the death rate from coronary heart disease to be higher in Eastern Europe compared to Western Europe.

This, then, brings us back to the conclusions that may be drawn from clinical nutritional studies. The early months of 2010 saw a spate of publications studying the clinical nutrition of saturated fats. Hunter *et al.* (2010) compared the cardiovascular disease risk of dietary stearic acid with that from *trans* and other saturated and unsaturated fatty acids. They concluded that *trans* fatty acids should be reduced as much as possible and that if the product required some solid fat to be present then the use of stearic acid, compared with other saturated fatty acids,

© Woodhead Publishing Limited, 2011

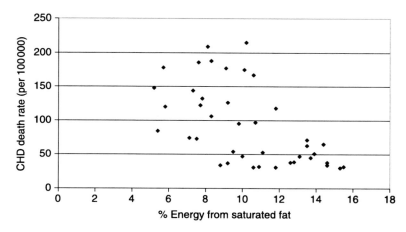

Fig. 1.11 Total energy from saturates vs. death rates from CHD in men aged under 65 (1998).

beneficially affected the levels of LDL cholesterol in the blood. If, on the other hand, there was no requirement for solid fat to be present then the use of unsaturated fats, rather than stearic acid, to replace *trans* fatty acids is preferred.

The meta-analysis of clinical data carried out by Mensink *et al.* (2003) is widely quoted (in this book as well as elsewhere) as the basis for the link between intake of saturated fats and risk of cardiovascular disease. However, a new meta-analysis by Siri-Tarino *et al.* (2010a, 2010b) says that 'there is no significant evidence for concluding that dietary saturated fat is associated with an increased risk of CHD or CVD'. Delving more deeply into the paper it is clear that they have found a relationship between the levels of saturated fat, polyunsaturated fat and carbohydrate in terms of the risk of coronary heart disease (CHD). They found that there was a lower risk of CHD if saturated fat was replaced by polyunsaturated fat and an increased risk of non-fatal CHD if it was replaced by carbohydrate. In fact 'replacement of 5% of total energy from saturated fat with polyunsaturated fat has been estimated to reduce CHD risk by 42%'. In other words, what you replace saturated fats with is just as important as actually replacing them. In their conclusion, Siri-Tarino *et al.* (2010b) say that 'more data is needed to elucidate whether CVD risks are likely to be influenced by the specific nutrients used to replace saturated fat'. This leads us into the next section of what saturates can be replaced by, but before moving on to that it is also worth mentioning a further paper from the same issue of the *American Journal of Clinical Nutrition* that the two papers from Siri-Tarino *et al.* appear in. This is from Stamler (2010) and in it he seriously questions the conclusions drawn by Siri-Tarino *et al.*, listing 12 questions resulting from the meta-analysis that are not answered by Siri-Tarino *et al.* Probably the one thing we can conclude from all of this is that the debate is far from over and that further papers will be published on the subject in the future.

© Woodhead Publishing Limited, 2011

1.5   Replacements for saturates

Before we can address the question of what saturated fats can be replaced by we need to address the question of why they are in a food in the first place. There are many reasons why fats are used in foods and, equally, there are many reasons why those fats should be saturated. To a large extent, though, these boil down to two main reasons – structure/texture and stability.

Many foods require the presence of a solid fat in order to give structure and texture to the product. Imagine, for example, a bar of chocolate made with rapeseed oil – it would have no solidity, no texture, no snap and would be very runny rather than the very solid product we are used to. The bar of chocolate needs a fat phase which is solid at room temperature and remains fairly solid at higher ambient temperatures but which then melts very sharply in the mouth. Most bakery products (pastry, biscuits, bread, cake) need to have a fat present that will either 'shorten' the dough, in the case of biscuits and pastry, or which will stabilize gas bubbles that are formed during either proving or mixing in the case of bread and cake. Again, a solid fat is needed to achieve these requirements. Take, for example, a margarine or spread based on sunflower oil or olive oil. A straight water-in-oil emulsion using these oils would be too soft to be able to be structured in a tub and so a hardstock – a high-melting triglyceride – is included in the oil phase. All of these applications require a fat that melts above ambient temperatures. The only sources of such high-melting fats are either saturated fats or partially hydrogenated fats containing *trans* fatty acids. Since the use of partial hydrogenation has been phased out in many parts of the world over the past few years because of health concerns relating to the presence of *trans* fatty acids, this has in many cases left only saturates as the means of achieving the required functionality.

When we consider the other aspect, that of stability, we are usually mainly concerned with oxidative stability, although bloom stability of chocolate can also be considered. Again, though, we come to the same conclusion – saturates and *trans* fatty acids have a greater oxidative stability than *cis* fatty acids – so we need to have a certain amount of saturates present in food to maintain its oxidative stability. In chocolate, the more unsaturated the chocolate is (either because of fats already present in the chocolate or because of migration of unsaturated oils from the centre) the softer it will be and the more prone it will be to bloom formation. Increase the level of saturated-oleic-saturated triglycerides in chocolate and the bloom resistance will increase.

There are good reasons, therefore, why saturates are present. If, however, we have to reduce them what should they be replaced with?

1.5.1   Other fatty acids

The simplest solution is to replace them with other fatty acids. If *trans* fatty acids are not permitted on health grounds, then the only alternative is to replace them with *cis* unsaturated fatty acids. These, though, are more liquid and therefore will

© Woodhead Publishing Limited, 2011

have an effect on the structure and texture of the product, particularly if it is meant to be hard (such as chocolate) but also where aeration and texture are fundamental to the acceptability of the product (cakes, pastry etc). This means that while, perhaps, some reductions can be made the degree of saturates reduction may be limited by textural changes.

In some applications – frying is a good example – the structure and solidity of the fat phase is much less important. Once an oil has been heated to a frying temperature of 180°C all structure is lost and so, from this point of view, the presence of saturates is less important. The main issue with frying oils is their oxidative stability. Partially hydrogenated oils that used to be used in frying had a very high oxidative stability. These were to a large extent replaced by palm oil or palm oleine, both of which had a lower, but still acceptable oxidative stability. The problem with them was that while they contained no *trans* fatty acids, they do contain significant levels (40–50%) of saturates. On the other hand, oils rich in *cis*-unsaturates such as rapeseed oil and sunflower oil are low in saturates but also have a low oxidative stability. In many cases a compromise has to be made between saturates level and oxidative stability, with that compromise being either to use the more expensive high-oleic sunflower oil or even a blend of that with palm oleine.

1.5.2   Fat replacers

In this context, fat replacement can mean a variety of things. It can, of course, mean replacing the fat in the product with one or other of the materials on the market that are designed to mimic and replace fats. But it can also be considered more broadly than that as a change in recipe that results in a reduction in the fat content of the product. Then, the fat replacer can be anything from air (in an aerated product sold by volume such as ice cream or tubbed mousses) through water (in a low-fat spread compared with a margarine) to sugar, flour, etc in a lower-fat baked product.

Reducing the fat content invariably leads to a change in texture in the product – biscuits and pastries become less 'short' and more 'flinty', for example. Despite this it is often instructive to look at the whole fat phase of a product and ask the question whether all of it is functional in that particular application. For example, in biscuits, palm oil was the dough fat of choice for many manufacturers when it became obvious that partially hydrogenated fats were no longer to be used. Palm oil, though, contains a broad spectrum of different types of triglyceride ranging from fully saturated, high-melting triglycerides, through triglycerides with two saturated and one unsaturated fatty acid, to triglycerides in which all three fatty acids are unsaturated. It has been observed (Talbot, 2008) that biscuits can be produced from a highly unsaturated oil such as sunflower oil but that when such an oil is used, the resulting biscuit is very oily and greasy to the touch. If a high-melting (and hence much more saturated) triglyceride is blended with the liquid oil then this greasiness disappears and a much more acceptable biscuit results. In palm oil there are these two extremes – triglycerides that are unsaturated and liquid at ambient

© Woodhead Publishing Limited, 2011

temperatures and triglycerides that are highly saturated. In addition, though, there are triglycerides that are medium-melting, too saturated to allow a saturates reduction but not saturated enough to 'structure' the system. If, though, instead of using whole palm oil as the dough fat, this middle-melting fraction were removed, leaving the low-melting unsaturated triglycerides (i.e. the 'oleine' fraction) and the high-melting saturated triglycerides (i.e. the 'stearine' or 'top' fraction) then an acceptable biscuit can be produced which is lower in both saturates and total fat.

1.5.3   Emulsion technology

Many foods contain emulsions of one kind or another. If the emulsion is of the water-in-oil type (W/O) then, theoretically, increasing the proportion of water should allow a reduction in fat content yet still give a functionally acceptable product. To some extent, in some products, this is true. The water content of a margarine can be increased from about 20% up to 40% in a reduced fat spread and even up to 60% and higher in some low-fat spreads. In their main area of use as a spread on bread then there is, arguably, little difference between them. It is when they are used as a spread on a hot product such as toast or when they are used as the fat phase in bakery products that the presence of higher levels of water becomes apparent. Even when the emulsion is of the opposite type (oil-in-water, O/W) it is possible to reduce the oil content and increase the water content either as such or in the form of so-called duplex emulsions (W/O/W), in which the initial oil phase is replaced by a W/O emulsion. The use of emulsions as a means of reducing saturates is described in more detail in Chapter 7.

1.5.4   Structured triglycerides

The term 'structured triglycerides' can mean many things. On the one hand it can mean the production of triglycerides of a specified fatty acid composition and structure; on the other it can mean the inclusion of a component within the fat phase that gives 'structure' to a more liquid, unsaturated oil. The former definition revolves around the ability of an oils and fats processor to produce specified compositions. To achieve this the industry has a number of process options to choose from and use.

One of these, hydrogenation, has been the subject of much controversy over the past decade or so because if it is not allowed to go to completion it produces *trans* fatty acids. The response to this has differed from country to country. Denmark, for example, was the first country to limit the level of industrially produced *trans* fats (as opposed to 'natural' *trans* fats found in milk and meat of ruminant animals) to a maximum of 2% in oils and fats used in food. The United States, on the other hand, introduced mandatory labeling of the *trans* fatty acid content of foods as part of the nutritional declaration. The United Kingdom has done neither but, arguably, has not needed to do either because the response of the popular media in the United Kingdom, closely followed by the response of

© Woodhead Publishing Limited, 2011

the major retailers, was to demonize the whole process of hydrogenation irrespective of whether it was partial hydrogenation producing *trans* fatty acids or complete hydrogenation producing only saturates and no *trans* fats. The result of this is that countries such as the United States can use triglycerides produced from complete hydrogenation (because there are then no longer any *trans* fatty acids present that need to be labelled) but it would be very difficult for such fats to be used in the United Kingdom, not because they are banned but because the use of 'hydrogenation' would need to be labelled. The UK consumer has been 'trained' to equate hydrogenation with *trans* even though that is not always the case.

Fractionation is another process that can be used to obtain particular groups of triglycerides and is most commonly used with palm oil and palm kernel oil, although butter fractions and coconut oil fractions are also available commercially. Possibly the most useful method for producing triglycerides of a specific structure is enzyme-catalysed interesterification. This is particularly useful for producing triglycerides of the XYX structure in which fatty acids in the outside positions are of one type of group while the acid in the middle or 2-position of the triglyceride is of a different type or group.

In terms of materials that will structure unsaturated liquid oil systems, the most commonly used is the high-melting, highly saturated triglyceride. If, however, it is necessary to reduce the level of this in order to reduce the level of saturates, then various novel structuring agents have been reported. These include, among others, organogels (Hughes *et al.*, 2009), sorbitan monostearate (Murdan *et al.*, 1999), waxes (Pernetti *et al.*, 2007), 12-hydroxystearic acid (Hughes *et al.*, 2009) and self-assembled fibre networks (Pernetti *et al.*, 2007). Many other examples of such non-saturated fat structuring agents are given in an excellent review by Wassell *et al.* (2010).

1.5.5 Diacylglycerol (DAG) oils

DAG oils are oils rich in diacylglycerols, or diglycerides. Diglycerides can be something of a two-edged sword when it comes to reducing saturates in the fat phases of food products. On the one hand, in fats such as palm oil, shea oil and cocoa butter they have the effect of slowing down crystallization and slightly softening the fat. If they are removed then the fat becomes harder but can be brought back to its original degree of hardness by the addition of an appropriate level of more unsaturated oil, thus reducing the overall degree of saturation. This is the negative side of diglycerides; more applicable is the positive side. In this they can be used to gel or structure more liquid, unsaturated fat phases (Pernetti *et al.*, 2007) or can be used as a more or less complete replacer of the triglyceride (or TAG) phase of various foods and applications. This type of use is dealt with in much more detail in Chapter 8 but a brief mention will be made here. The basis for this is twofold. The first aspect of using DAG-oils is that they are metabolized differently from normal triglycerides; the second aspect is that their physical characteristics, particularly their melting points, are such that a less saturated

DAG oil can have the same or similar physical characteristics to those of a more saturated triglyceride, thus giving considerable scope for saturates reduction.

1.6   Areas not covered by specific chapters in this book

Later chapters in this book focus on specific food sectors, specifically those that contribute the greatest levels of saturated fat to the foods we eat. What exactly are these? Assuming that consumption levels are similar across Europe and North America then we can take the United Kingdom as an example (see Table 1.2). Of the major contributors to saturated fat in the diet, milk and other dairy products, meat products, biscuits and pastries, chocolate confectionery and sauces are all covered in separate chapters. Some products, though, are not covered for various reasons – either their contribution to overall saturates intake is limited or their components are largely covered by other chapters. These will be briefly discussed here.

1.6.1   Cakes and doughnuts

Reduced fat cake products are available on the market but their scarcity could be an indication of either the difficulty of producing them or of a lack of acceptance of the product by the consumer. Reduction in the total fat content of batter-based products such as cakes can result in adverse structural changes in the end product and, because fat reduction is usually accompanied by an increase in water content, there will also be an increase in water activity. This then will have further implications for the product in terms of a reduced shelf-life and an increased possibility of mould growth. If the fat is present only for shelf-life reasons, i.e. to ensure a low water activity, rather than for any structural properties it may impart, then it might be possible to replace a more conventional bakery shortening by an oil such as rapeseed oil or sunflower oil.

The fat in a cake batter has a functionality in terms of providing a 'membrane' around the air cells and allowing them to expand during baking while still protecting them from collapse. A further function of the fat in a cake batter is to coat the flour, allowing water retention and gluten hydration to take place. The harder the fat is, the more effective it is at performing both of these functions. If these hard, largely saturates-rich fats are replaced by softer, more unsaturated fats then the quality of the cake batter could be compromised, resulting in a heavier, tougher texture in the cake. As with biscuit dough fats, cake shortenings need to have a balance between liquid and solid fats. The liquid fats are needed to provide an interface on the surface of bubbles in the cake batter but solid fats are then needed to stabilize these bubbles as they grow. Different cake batter types may well require different fat phases for optimal performance. However, carrying a wide range of bakery fats in a factory can be problematic when manufacturers prefer to consolidate their ingredients as much as possible and so, in reality, compromises are often made.

In recent years, various fat mimetics have been studied and launched as replacements of fats in cakes. One of these, N-Dulge FR® from National Starch

© Woodhead Publishing Limited, 2011

won the award for the most innovative food ingredient at Food Ingredients Europe in 2009. It is used to replace butter, margarine or bakery shortenings in a cake batter, allowing a reduction in both total fat and saturated fat of almost two-thirds. The product works in muffins and cookies as well as in cakes. Min *et al.* (2010) claim that up to 20% of bakery shortening in cakes can be replaced by steam jet-cooked buckwheat flour without any change in cake volume. They hypothesize that it mimics the use of fat because it can bind large quantities of water to give a fat-like gel. Martinez-Cervera *et al.* (2010) have studied the use of cocoa fibre at levels of 25%, 50% and 75% as a fat replacer in muffins. Apart from at the higher level of replacement (at which the muffins were considerably reduced in size), the muffins were crumblier with a more compact crumb and staled less quickly. The concept needs further development, however, because they were also perceived to have a more bitter taste and greater surface stickiness.

There are, of course, other components in cakes apart from the batter itself – components such as creams, toppings and fillings. Often creams and toppings used in and on the cake are more significant in terms of fat content than is the underlying cake. Creams can range from short-shelf-life dairy creams through buttercreams to fat-based whipped cream systems. Both dairy creams and buttercreams must, by definition, be dairy-based and so the saturated fat content is whatever level it is in the basic milk. Indeed buttercreams are defined in the EU and are subject to a minimum level of 22.5% butter with no other fat being present. This then raises the question as to whether the use of butter oleine (a more unsaturated fraction of butter) would also be classed as butter. However, while in theory this would allow a reduction in saturates there would be cost implications in switching from whole butter to a butter oleine.

As far as coatings on cakes are concerned, if they are fat-based (as opposed to a sugar-based icing) then they are generally chocolate or a chocolate-flavoured coating. These are discussed in more detail in Chapter 16.

Doughnuts are also mentioned here, mainly because they are not considered in any of the other bakery sections nor in the chapter on frying. In their basic form they are quite oil-rich because they pick up oil from the frying medium. The composition of the frying oil used is, therefore, of importance. It would be easy to suggest that this should be as low in saturates as is compatible with both the stability of the oil and the shelf-life of the doughnut. However, in practice, frying shortenings are used with doughnuts, these being oils with a slightly higher solid fat content and therefore a higher saturated fat content. The reason for this is that such oils give an improved 'hold' on things used to coat the doughnut, be these simply sugar, a glaze, or a fat-based coating. Although, depending on the oil currently used, it may still be possible to reduce saturates and keep a good product there is a limit as to how low in saturates it would be possible to go and still maintain this adhesion.

1.6.2 Ready meals

Ready meals cover such a wide range of compositions that it is difficult to categorize them in such terms. This is one reason why they not are considered as

© Woodhead Publishing Limited, 2011

an entity in their own right in a separate chapter. Another reason, though, is that they are often made up of components such as meat, pastry and sauces that are considered in separate chapters and so there would be considerable duplication. However, there are still some aspects of ready meals that can be discussed here and which are not covered elsewhere in this book.

Pasta

Fresh, dried and canned pasta products are generally low in both fat and saturates. Where there may be greater concern is in stuffed pasta products (ravioli, cannelloni and tortellini) and in layered products like lasagne. Where the filling is meat then, clearly, the comments made in the chapters on meat will apply. However, often the filling is cheese-based (for example, filled pasta products containing cheese can contain 5–9% total fat compared to 2–3% in the unfilled pasta). Although cheese is also covered in a later chapter, one of the issues with reducing the fat content of cheese is that the texture changes. This, though, would be of lesser importance in a filled pasta product and so there should be more scope for saturated fat reduction in such products.

Ethnic dishes

Many sauces are 'structured' in terms of their thickness and creaminess by saturated fats. Indeed many Asian dishes, for example, use coconut milk to give texture to dishes such as curries and dips. Inglett *et al.* (2002) investigated the possibilities of replacing coconut milk in a Thai green chicken curry with Soytrim. Soytrim is based on a 1:1 mixture of soy flour and oat bran and is made by dispersing these ingredients in boiling water and homogenizing. When 50% coconut milk was replaced by Soytrim there was no statistical difference between taste panel scores for the two types of curry, giving a significant reduction in saturated fat.

Pizzas

The total average fat content of pizzas can range typically from just over 2% to almost 15%. The lowest levels are generally found in 'healthy eating' and children's ranges; the highest levels are in pizzas with extra cheese toppings. Because, in most cases, the fat content of the base is quite low, the main source of fat and saturated fat is in the topping. A cheese and tomato-topped pizza can typically have a total fat content of 9–12% with about 40–50% of this being saturated. Meat-topped pizzas have similar total fat contents but slightly lower levels of saturates. Vegetable-topped pizzas have the lowest levels of total fat (typically 7–10%) but can have a wide range of saturates levels.

It is clear, then, that the nature of the topping is of great importance in terms of a potential reduction in saturated fat. The use of reduced-fat cheese or reduced-fat meat will give an overall reduction in saturates. Indeed, this might be one of the most ideal uses of reduced-fat cheese because in a molten form on a hot pizza some of the textural drawbacks may not be apparent.

© Woodhead Publishing Limited, 2011

Quiches
With a combination of egg and either milk or cream making up the bulk of the filling, and pastry the outside of the product, there is clearly great potential for such a product to contain a high proportion of saturated fat. Total fat contents typically range from 15% to 21% with saturates making up some 40–50% of this. Reduction in saturates content in the pastry will be considered in a later chapter but reformulation of the filling could also help in an overall saturates reduction.

Prepared sandwiches
Both the total fat and saturates content of prepared sandwiches depend on (a) the spread, (b) the dressing and (c) the filling. In some products, mayonnaise is used in place of a butter or vegetable fat-based spread. Where this mayonnaise is reduced-fat then a lower total fat content overall can be achieved. The filling also plays a great part in both total and saturated fat contents, with cheese-filled sandwiches being the highest in this respect. Egg, poultry and tuna-based sandwiches generally contain the lowest levels of total fat and saturated fat, with ham and bacon sandwiches coming somewhere in the middle.

1.6.3   Non-chocolate confectionery
Chocolate and chocolate fillings are considered in a later chapter but, in terms of non-chocolate confectionery, the main areas where fats are used are in toffees and caramels. Traditionally such products have been based on butter (which has a high level of saturates) or partially hydrogenated fats (which have a high level of *trans*). With the replacement of hydrogenated vegetable oils in these products, often by fractions of palm oil, there has been an increase in total saturates (even though this has, in many cases, been accompanied by an increase in *cis*-unsaturates). As with many foods rich in saturates, functionality is the main stumbling block in further saturates reductions. Higher unsaturates result in toffees with less ability to retain their shape and a greater propensity to flow. This then adversely affects downstream processes such as enrobing and wrapping, which are geared to the products always having the same shape, size and structure. A further factor to be taken into account is that toffee fats are often used for other functions in a confectionery or biscuit factory (as cream fats or dough fats, for example). In such cases the fat is selected for the most critical application even though perhaps a lower-saturated fat could be used for the other applications.

1.7   Future trends

For some years there was a 'certainty', based on the paper published by Mensink *et al.* (2003), that saturates raised total cholesterol levels, that stearic acid was closer to neutrality in its effects on blood cholesterol than were the next three shorter chain saturated fatty acids and that, from these results, we could infer that high intakes of saturated fats posed a health risk in terms of cardiovascular disease.

© Woodhead Publishing Limited, 2011

However, the meta-analysis by Siri-Tarino *et al.* (2010b) has cast doubts on this 'certainty' (even though there are aspects of this work that have been questioned by Stamler (2010)). This means that there will undoubtedly be further clinical studies carried out to try to make a final definition of the risk that saturates pose in terms of cardiovascular disease and to answer the points raised by Stamler.

Whether or not there is a real health risk in high intakes of saturates, food manufacturers will be under continual pressure from governments, health agencies, retailers and consumers to reduce the saturated fatty acid content of the foods they produce. In some cases they will be successful, even spectacularly successful; in others, though, for reasons of functionality, shelf-life or legislation, wholesale reductions in saturates will just not be possible. Nevertheless, in order to meet these goals, oils and fats processors will develop new, lower-saturated alternatives to some of the fats they currently supply and will also develop more 'structured' lipids to enable greater functionality for lower levels of use. Other ingredients suppliers will develop non-fat solutions as ways of reducing not just saturated fat but total fat.

1.8   Sources of further information and advice

The report written by Talbot (2006) for the Food Standards Agency in the UK, 'Independent advice on possible reductions for saturated fat in products that contribute to consumer intakes', contains a wealth of information on the background to the issues, the clinical nutrition studies carried out by that time, sections on the main food categories and what can be done in each of them, together with the industry's views on what is and what is not achievable, and ways in which the oils and fats industry can assist with new structured lipids.

Wassell *et al.* (2010) gives an excellent review of the options available in terms of components capable of replacing saturates in foods without a loss of functionality.

1.9   References

British Heart Foundation (2010). 'Percentage of energy from saturated fat by country, Europe, 1998 sourced from Ferro-Luzzi, A. (National Institute for Food and Nutrition Research)'. http://www.heartstats.org. Accessed 4 August 2010.
Chardigny, J-M, Destaillats F, Malpuech-Brugere C, Moulin J, Bauman DE, Lock AL, Barbano DM, Mensink RP, Bezelgues J-B, Chaumont P, Combe N, Cristiani I, Joffre F, German JB, Dionisi F, Boirie Y, Sebedio J-L (2008). 'Do *trans* fatty acids from industrially produced sources and from natural sources have the same effect on cardiovascular disease risk factors in healthy subjects? Results of the *trans* Fatty Acids Collaboration (TRANSFACT) study'. *Am. J. Clin. Nutr.*, **87**(3), 558–66.
European Heart Network (2008). 'European Cardiovascular Disease Statistics, 2008'. http://www.ehnheart.org/cdv-statistics.html. Accessed 4 August 2010.
Food Standards Agency (2008). 'Saturated Fat and Energy Intake Programme'. http://www.food.gov.uk/multimedia/pdfs/satfatprog.pdf. Accessed 15 July 2010.

© Woodhead Publishing Limited, 2011

Gortner WA (1958). 'The Role of Dietary Fat in Human Health'. National Academy of Sciences – National Research Council Publication No.575. Washington DC.

HMSO (2002). 'The National Diet and Nutrition Survey: adults aged 10 to 64 years'. http://www.food.gov.uk/multimedia/pdfs/ndnsprintedreport.pdf. Accessed 15 July 2010.

Hughes N, Marangoni AG, Wright AJ, Rogers MA, Rush JWE (2009). 'Potential food applications of edible oil organogels'. *Trends in Food Science and Technology.* **20** 470–80.

Hunter JE, Zhang J, Kris-Etherton PM (2010). 'Cardiovascular disease risk of dietary stearic acid compared with *trans*, other saturated, and unsaturated fatty acids: a systematic review'. *Am. J. Clin. Nutr.* **91** 46–63.

Inglett GE, Carriere CJ, Maneepun S, Boonpunt T (2002). 'Nutritional value and functional properties of a hydrocolloidal soybean and oat blend for use in Asian foods'. *J. Sci. Food Agric.* **83**, 86–92.

Judd JT, Baer DJ, Clevidence BA, Kris-Etherton P, Muesing RA, Iwane M (2002). 'Dietary *cis* and *trans* monounsaturated and saturated FA and plasma lipids and lipoproteins in men'. *Lipids* **37** 123–31.

Kartha ARS (1968). 'Some deviations from 1,3-random, 2-random distribution in natural fats'. *J.Am. Oil Chem. Soc.* **45**(2), 101–2.

Martinez-Cervera S, Salvador A, Muguerza B, Moulay L, Fiszman SM (2010). 'Cocoa fibre and its application as a fat replacer in chocolate muffins'. *LWT – Food Science and Technology* doi: 10.1016/j.lwt.2010.06.035.

McNeill GP (2009). 'Saturated fats and the risk of heart disease'. *Inform* **20**, 340–1.

Mensink RP, Zock PL, Kester AD, Katan MB (2003). Effects of dietary fatty acids and carbohydrates on the ratio of total to HDL cholesterol and on serum lipids and apolipoproteins: a meta-analysis of 60 controlled trials'. *Am. J. Clin. Nutr.* **77** 1146–55.

Min B, Lee SM, Yoo S-H, Ingletti GE, Lee S (2010). 'Functional characterization of steam-jet cooked buckwheat flour as a fat replacer in cake-baking'. *J. Sci. Food Agric.* doi 10.1002/jsfa.4072.

Murdan S, Gregoriadis G, Florence AT (1999). 'Novel sorbitan monostearate organogels'. *Journal of Pharmaceutical Sciences*, **88**, 608–14.

Oil World (1996–2010). 'EU: Consumption of Oils and Fats; US: Consumption of Oils and Fats; UK: Consumption of Oils and Fats'. ISTA Mielke GmbH.

Pernetti M, van Malssen KF, Floter E, Bot A (2007). 'Structuring of edible oils by alternatives to crystalline fat'. *Current Opinion in Colloid and Interface Science*, **12**, 221–31.

Rhee SK, Kayani AJ, Ciszek A, Brenna JT (1997). 'Desaturation and interconversion of dietary stearic and palmitic acids in human plasma and lipoproteins'. *Am. J. Clin. Nutr.* **65** 451–8.

Siri-Tarino PW, Sun Q, Hu FB, Krauss RM (2010a). 'Saturated fat, carbohydrate, and cardiovascular disease'. *Am. J. Clin. Nutr.* **91**, 502–9.

Siri-Tarino PW, Sun Q, Hu FB, Krauss RM (2010b). 'Meta-analysis of prospective cohort studies evaluating the association of saturated fat with cardiovascular disease'. *Am. J. Clin. Nutr.* **91**, 535–46.

Stamler J (2010). 'Diet-heart: a problematic revisit'. *Am. J. Clin.Nutr.* **91** 497–9.

Talbot G (2006). 'Independent advice on possible reductions for saturated fat in products that contribute to consumer intakes'. http://www.food.gov.uk/multimedia/pdfs/reductions.pdf. Accessed 18 August 2010.

Talbot G (2008). 'Reduction of Saturated Fat in Bakery Products'. Lecture given at *'Baking for a Healthier Diet'*, 17 September 2008, Campden Research Association, Chipping Campden, UK.

Vander Wal RJ (1960). 'Calculation of the Distribution of the Saturated and Unsaturated Acyl Groups in Fats, from Pancreatic Lipase Hydrolysis Data'. *J. Am. Oil Chem. Soc.* **37**(1), 18–20.

© Woodhead Publishing Limited, 2011

Vlahov G (2005). '^{13}C nuclear magnetic resonance spectroscopy to check 1,3-random, 2-random pattern of fatty acid distribution in olive oil triacylglycerols'. *Spectrosccopy*, **19**(2), 109–17.

Wassell P, Bonwick G, Smith CJ, Almiron-Roig E, Young NWG (2010). 'Towards a multidisciplinary approach to structuring in reduced saturated fat-based systems – a review'. *Int. J. Food Sci. and Technol.* **45**, 642–55.

World Health Organization (2003). 'Diet, Nutrition and the Prevention of Chronic Diseases'. *Technical Report No.916*, Geneva.

© Woodhead Publishing Limited, 2011

2

The functional attributes that fats bring to food

E. H. A. de Hoog, R. M. A. J. Ruijschop, S. P. Pyett and P. M. T. de Kok,
NIZO Food Research B.V., The Netherlands

Abstract: The functional attributes of fat in foods contribute to the overall performance and acceptance of fat-containing food products. Strategies to reduce (saturated) fat content must follow from fat functionality, including texture effects, oral breakdown, lubrication and aroma release. This chapter discusses how we perceive fat in food products, the role of fat in the properties of flavour and texture, and strategies to tailor appetites by engineering the fat in reduced-fat products.

Key words: fat perception, texture, aroma release, lubrication, fat reduction.

2.1 Introduction

Fat contributes to the texture and sensory performance of food products. First of all, how do we perceive fat? Various senses are involved in the perception of fat in foods. Section 2.2 deals with the mechanisms involved in sensation and perception, and the role of saturation of fat will be discussed. The emphasis is on taste perception. Next, in section 2.3, the role of fat in the texture of foods is discussed. Fat in foods can have different functions. Generally, incorporated fat can act as a texturizer, a lubricant or an aroma carrier. The role and combination of roles varies between different product groups, such as liquids and solids. As well as texture and flavour attributes, fat plays an important role in appetite and satiation. Strategies to enhance the sensory reward of reduced-fat foods are discussed in Section 2.4. In contrast to dietary energy intake restrictions, this strategy is expected to satisfy the consumer, preventing the frustration of having to discontinue eating a meal before being satiated or indulged and having experienced sufficient reward. We conclude in Section 2.5 by discussing the consequences of the functional attributes of fats in foods for strategies to reduce the fat.

© Woodhead Publishing Limited, 2011

2.2   Perception of fat

We rely on our senses to experience our surroundings. When experiencing food, the traditional five senses involved are sight, hearing, touch, smell and taste, a classification first attributed to Aristotle. Taste and smell form part of the chemical senses. Perception involves not only the detection of signals by our senses, but also the interpretation of these signals by our brains.

Often, our first encounter with food is through our vision. Our sight combined with our sense of smell help us decide if we should eat a food or not. We have associated the way a food should look with what we can expect as flavour and texture. The level of fat is already anticipated by the consumer within the first 200 ms after visual inspection of a product (Toepel *et al.*, 2009). Throughout our lives, we have learned which products contain more fat and we have associated them also with the way the food should look. For example, when looking at a full-fat mayonnaise we can imagine the creamy sensation that should accompany it. Low-fat mayonnaises therefore need the same appearance in colour and smoothness, in order to be attractive. Another example where first judgement by sight is performed is reported by Brown (1958), who found that bread was judged as being fresher when wrapped in cellophane than when wrapped in wax paper.

Hearing is a physical sense that can play a role during mastication and further breakdown of the food product. Although little attention has been paid to the sound a food should make, it is clear that we also have expectations of what the sound should be when biting into a potato chip as opposed to soft bread. Fat affects the breakdown of the product and hence the sound released. The sound is interpreted based on earlier experiences with similar products, and we often use it to decide if a product is well cooked or if it is old. Sanz *et al.* (2007) recorded the sound emitted during fracture of a French fry with an acoustic sensor while simulating mastication. They found correlations of the frying conditions with sound events measured and the crispness of the product. In addition, it has been shown that amplifying the sound of crisps when eating increases the freshness perception of the crisps (Zampini and Spence, 2004).

Touch is another physical sense involving the response of mechanoreceptors to tactile stimuli (Trulsson and Essick, 1997; Engelen, 2004). In the human skin, four types of nerve endings are present: Pacinian corpuscles, Meissner corpuscles, Merkel discs and Ruffini corpuscles. They provide us with information related to pressure, stretching of skin, taps on skin and vibration. Mechanoreceptors are also present in our tongue and throat, although little is known about their morphology and mechanisms of action. The mouthfeel of a food product is sensed through these mechanoreceptors. Low-fat products are often described as less 'full' or less 'creamy' or lacking 'body'. This can be partially explained by the reduction in viscosity from liquid and semi-solid products. The in-mouth viscosity, i.e. the viscosity in the mouth during oral processing, needs to be considered as well as the tribological properties, which describe the lubrication of the oral surfaces (see also section 2.3.2).

Smell is one of our chemical senses. When perceiving a smell, the aroma molecules bind to olfactory receptors located in our nose. These receptors send

© Woodhead Publishing Limited, 2011

signals that are transduced into the olfactory system in our brain. Where vision and touch are directly fed into the neural cortex of the brain, aroma-generated signals are delivered to the limbic system, which inhabits the subconscious experience of product perception. As a result, consumers can easily discuss the colour and texture of products, but have great difficulties in finding words for flavour experiences, although these aroma sensations do affect their emotional state of mind and, with that, product quality perception and appreciation. The sensations obviously start with the combination of signals derived from different olfactory receptors reacting with the specific aroma molecules, resulting in our perception of a specific smell. There are two ways the aroma molecules can reach the olfactory receptors. They can reach the receptors when inhaled at the front of our nose, i.e. smelling (ortho-nasally), or from our throat when masticating and swallowing (retro-nasally). The rate that aroma compounds are released before and after mastication will depend on the food matrix properties and their response to oral processing (speed of structure breakdown, viscosity in the mouth, temperature increase or decrease). Most particularly, the rate of diffusion due to phase inversions of emulsions in the mouth (from water droplets in oil-continuous matrix, to oil droplets in water-continuous matrix) affects the (perceived) timely aroma profile. Apart from fat affecting the availability of aroma compounds, reduction of the fat is known to change the aroma balance due to partitioning of the aroma compounds between the oil and water phases of a product. Even in those cases where aroma release (difference in timing) is not a factor significantly affecting aroma perception, one can easily understand that similar aroma formulations applied in low- or high-fat products will result in different sensory results. Also, most particularly for very low-fat products, aroma systems which are built using lipophilic compounds will easily deplete due to the low aroma buffer capacity (see section 2.3.3).

Taste is another chemical sense. The combination of taste and smell is what we define as flavour. We detect a taste when a substance gets in contact with our taste buds and interacts with a taste receptor cell. Taste cells are normally clustered in our taste buds, which are embedded in our tongue's papillae. Once a tastant reaches our taste buds, it interacts with a specific taste receptor cell and a cascade of reactions is launched. This cascade will trigger a signal that will be transduced to our brain through the nerve fibres in the tongue. There are currently five basic tastes recognized: salty, sour, sweet, bitter and umami (or savoury). For each taste there are specific receptors that will interact and recognize the taste quality. Although, in the last decade, evidence for the role of fat in gustation has been found (Mattes, 2005a), fat taste is still not accepted as a basic taste. Animal behavioural studies on rats and mice revealed that lipid preference is not abolished by the suppression of olfactory cues, textural and post-ingestive signals (Fukuwatari et al., 2003; Laugerette et al., 2007). Although the mechanism responsible for fat perception in taste cells is not fully understood yet, specific receptors such as CD36 have been located in the lingual gustatory papillae of rats. This particular receptor is known to be involved in the detection of long-chain fatty acids in the oral cavity (Fukuwatari et al., 1997; Laugerette et al., 2005). In

© Woodhead Publishing Limited, 2011

humans there is evidence that oral lipid detection occurs through taste cues, as well as through textural and olfactory cues (Mattes, 2005a). Moreover, human studies showed that fat-specific satiety appears not to be related to taste perception of oils, but rather to that of the fatty acids (Kamphuis et al., 2003). To what degree the stimulation of receptors in mouth affect overall perception and food intake behaviour is still the subject of investigation.

Dietary fat consists predominantly of triglycerides, which are made up of three fatty acids attached to a glycerol molecule. Lipases cleave triglycerides into glycerol, mono- and diglycerides and free fatty acids. So far, only free fatty acids have been shown to stimulate taste receptor cells, not the triglycerides (Kawai and Fushiki, 2003). Therefore, the presence of lingual lipase may play an important role in the gustatory detection of fat in the oral cavity. Lingual lipase is secreted from glands in the tongue, which are located in close proximity to the taste buds in the papillae. This is expected to lead to a locally increased concentration of free fatty acids near the receptors (Schiffman et al., 1998; Kawai and Fushiki, 2003). In rats Kawai and Fushiki (2003) found that lingual lipase was released continuously to generate significant amounts of free fatty acids within several seconds, which was sufficient to perceive the fatty acids. In rats and mice, lingual lipase is predominant over gastric lipase, whereas in humans gastric lipase is predominant over lingual lipase (DeNigris et al., 1988). Consequently, the release of free fatty acids in the mouth is expected to be relatively smaller in humans, which in a way is advantageous as free fatty acids are normally described to have an aversive taste when tasted in high concentrations. However, there is no conclusive evidence on the role human lingual lipase has in gustation. Currently, most emphasis has been given to chemosensory mechanisms of free fatty acids rather than the sensory consequences of the administration of triglycerides.

In commercial food products, oil is commonly present as an emulsified triglyceride mix and, apart from the small quantity of free fatty acids already present as impurities in triglyceride oils in a concentration of about 0.5 vol% (Chalé-Rush et al., 2007b), fatty acids are not directly available for the stimulation of the receptor cells. Free fatty acids, however, can be obtained by lipolysis of triglycerides by lingual lipases as discussed before. We can expect that destabilization of emulsion droplets in the mouth and further spreading or deposition of fat onto the tongue surface might improve the accessibility for lipolytic enzymes, and thus improve our chances for tasting fat. From earlier work it is known that emulsion droplets stable under quiescent conditions can become unstable under oral processing (van Aken et al., 2005), and that emulsion droplets can deposit on the tongue surface (Dresselhuis et al., 2008a).

The effect whereby one modality (e.g. aroma) affects the sensory perception of a different modality (e.g. viscosity or fatty mouthfeel) is called cross-modal interaction. This phenomenon is well documented and many examples have been reported; Weel (2004) showed that viscosity itself negatively affects aroma intensity perception even if the physical release due to enhanced viscosity was corrected for. Knoop et al. (2008) showed that taste effects (sweetness) can be significantly enhanced using congruent aroma sensations

© Woodhead Publishing Limited, 2011

2.3   Role of fat in the texture of foods

Fat has a complex function in foods, i.e. it can play multiple roles in the texture. The dominant role is dependent on the properties of the matrix and the interactions with other ingredients. Especially in liquid products, we consider the most important roles of fat as being a texturizer, a lubricant or an aroma carrier. These roles will be discussed separately in further detail in the following three subsections.

2.3.1   Fat as texturizer

The contribution of fat to texture is highly product specific, perhaps more so than any other aspect of fat functionality. In fact, it is easy to think of examples of two very similar products in which the contribution of fat to texture is, in broad terms, the opposite. Consider yoghurt and cheese. In both, texture is built by a network of (primarily) casein proteins, aggregated due to the decrease in solvent quality at low pH. Their fat compositions do not differ – both are nearly always produced with the dairy fat naturally occurring in milk. And yet, in yoghurt fat is structure building, while in cheese fat induces structure breaking. Understanding why and how this difference occurs demonstrates additional factors of importance for fat functionality. In short, the contribution of fat to texture building in water-continuous foods must be interpreted through the lens of the fat–water interface.

Fat in water-continuous systems is essentially unstable; given the opportunity, the system will phase separate. In many but not all water-continuous foods, phase separation is avoided by creating a stable fat–water interface in the form of emulsion droplets. This requires the presence of surface-active compounds, often proteins or small molecule surfactants. In the extreme view, a very well-emulsified fat droplet can behave as an inert colloid with surface properties of the surfactant. The stability of the surface coating and its interaction with the food matrix then determine the contribution of the fat to the food texture (McClements, 2004).

As examples, we will consider two food products in which the stability of the surface of emulsion droplets is crucial in building texture – mayonnaise and ice cream. Full-fat mayonnaise is an emulsion of about 70% oil in water. Egg proteins act as the surfactant. In a traditional recipe, no other texturizing agents are present – the fat droplets fully determine the texture. In part, mayonnaise texture is built by the close packing of the emulsion droplets. However, at low pH, when the water solvent quality becomes less for the proteins on the surface of the droplets, interactions between surfaces lead to the build-up of a continuous network. Thus the pH stability of the surface material is essential to texture. Another type of surface instability is induced in ice cream production. In this case, small molecule surfactants are used to displace part of a protein surface layer and thus ensure an uneven surface coating. Because some of the fat surface is exposed, and in combination with crystalline fat in the interior of the droplets, partial coalescence between droplets occurs. Partial coalescence of fat around air bubbles leads to stabilization of the air in the final product. Partial coalescence in the bulk provides

© Woodhead Publishing Limited, 2011

a semi-continuous fat network which contributes to a creamy mouthfeel. Since the solid fat content is an essential factor here, reducing the fraction of saturated fats will have a direct effect on the air stabilization in ice cream, and thus on its texture.

Not only is the surface itself important for determining the role of fat in texture, but also the interactions of the surface with the food matrix. In yoghurt, for example, fat is well emulsified and covered by a layer of dairy protein. The emulsion droplets participate actively in building the protein network. In the other extreme, in the absence of surface-active material, fat can be kinetically or physically trapped in a water-continuous matrix. In cheese, for example, the fat is essentially free and phase separation is prevented by the gel strength of the surrounding casein network. This free fat is inactive in the matrix and thus acts as a breaking point which softens the overall texture. Work by Sala *et al.* (2008) characterized the contributions of active and inactive emulsion droplets in protein matrices in relation to creaminess perception in semi-solids.

2.3.2   Fat as lubricant

Upon eating, the structure of a food product changes. The product is exposed to severe mechanical forces as a result of the oral movements. In addition, saliva is mixed with the product and the temperature will change towards body temperature. In fat-continuous systems, like margarine or chocolate, a phase inversion will take place in the mouth. In water-continuous systems, the fat- or oil-containing emulsion droplets might become unstable. The droplets can coalesce into larger droplets, they can agglomerate, or they can disrupt and release the oil/fat (van Aken *et al.*, 2007). Emulsion droplets and free fat are known to play a role in lubrication of the oral surfaces (Giasson *et al.*, 1997; Luengo *et al.*, 1997; Malone *et al.*, 2003a; de Wijk and Prinz, 2006).

In liquid dairy products, it has generally been found that the presence of emulsion droplets results in a decrease in friction between tongue and palate mimics. Simultaneously, the creamy perception is increased (Dresselhuis *et al.*, 2008a). This can be explained by the fact that released oil is adhered to the oral surfaces, which will lower the friction between these surfaces (Dresselhuis *et al.*, 2008b). In addition, the protein content influences the friction, since proteins also adhere to the oral surfaces, thereby changing the adhesion between the two surfaces (Dresselhuis *et al.*, 2007). Tribology measurements give sometimes contradictory results concerning the dependence of the friction on sample composition, which mostly can be traced back to the experimental conditions (Dresselhuis *et al.*, 2007). The properties of the surfaces used in the friction measurements are crucial for the results. The most important properties should mimic the oral surfaces as closely as possible, including the hydrophobicity, roughness and elasticity. Figure 2.1 shows results for some commercial dairy products measured with a tribometer. For these products, the friction force measured was reduced upon increase of the fat content for each type of product.

In gelled emulsion samples, the lubrication properties depend on the type and concentration of the gelling ingredient. Interactions between emulsifier and matrix

© Woodhead Publishing Limited, 2011

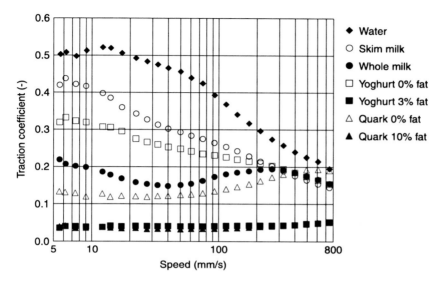

Fig. 2.1   Friction coefficient as a function of speed for commercial dairy products varying in fat content. An increase in fat content corresponds to a decrease in friction.

determine the friction behaviour. If there is an interaction between them, an increase in oil content results in a decrease of friction force measured. In the case where there is no interaction between emulsifier and matrix, there is also a decrease in friction when some fat is present, but further increase of fat content does not affect the friction force. This implies that the dependence of the friction on the oil content is not straightforward, but is influenced by the composition and the presence of other ingredients (Chojnicka *et al.*, 2009).

In oral processing of solid products, the first step is the breakdown of the structure into smaller pieces, followed by hydration of the product to form a bolus that is appropriate for swallowing (Chen, 2009). The fat content will have an effect on the breakdown behaviour of the product in the mouth. At later stages of bolus formation, the same principles as for liquids and gels are valid for the influence of the fat content on the lubrication properties.

2.3.3   Fat as aroma carrier

Aroma, i.e. the odour of a product, is considered the earliest sensory cue for the (caloric) quality of a food. There are many examples illustrating the importance of aromas in the sensory perception of other modalities such as taste and texture. A typical example is that furaneol, a compound having a strong caramel aroma, enhances the perceived sweetness in the same way as ethyl esters enhance the sweet perception in apple juice (Knoop *et al.*, 2008), while sotolon with a soup seasoning flavour top note increases the savoury character, enhancing salt perception (Lawrence *et al.*, 2009). Volatile compounds derived in lipid oxidation

© Woodhead Publishing Limited, 2011

and short-chain fatty acids derived from hydrolysis provide odour cues for assessing the fat content of a product, or are interpreted as rancid off-notes if too strong. The latter induces a strong warning sensory signal to provoke aversive reactions, as highly oxidized lipid materials are prone to generate radical induced cell damage. Recently, the metal-like perception of metal foil has been shown to be the result of the generation of volatile compounds derived from oxidation of the oily materials covering the metal when producing the foil or just from the residues of skin lipids deposited by human touch (Glindemann *et al.*, 2006). Similarly, the same set of compounds can induce a metallic off-note in high-fat products (such as margarines) without any trace of metals in the product. These examples exemplify that aroma compounds are being used as an early diagnosis assessing the nutritive and safety content of a food. As aroma perception is largely subconscious, one can easily expect the aroma of a food to affect the overall emotional state of a consumer as well as specific consumer appreciation attributes such as liking, wanting or indulgence. As a result, low-fat products may not only 'suffer' from low metabolic calorie indicators (Laugerette *et al.*, 2005), but their modified aroma patterns may also be recognized by consumers to reflect that of low-fat (or low-caloric) products.

Fat affects the aroma in two ways: an aroma developed for a high-fat product requires reformulation for similar sensory quality (perceived aroma intensity and aroma quality) when applied in low-fat products, while fat also changes the timely release of the aroma from the food. Both factors are to be taken into consideration in developing low-fat equivalents of high-fat products.

Fat as an aroma solvent
Every aroma (or taste) compound distributes itself amongst the oil- and water-phases of an emulsion in accordance to its so-called partition coefficient, which all differ for different aroma compounds (Hansch *et al.*, 1995). In order to maintain the same head space concentration under equilibrium conditions above high- and low-fat products, the concentrations of all aroma compounds in both the oil and water phases need to be retained. However, as in a low-fat product the volume fraction of fat is lower, the amount to be added to the product of a flavour compound that preferentially partitions in the oil phase needs to be decreased. Hence the overall concentration in the emulsions needs decreasing. Likewise, when reducing the amount of fat, concentrations of hydrophilic compounds need to be enhanced in the overall product concentrations. This phenomenon results in the fact that the concentration ratios of compounds need to be adapted when converting an aroma for application in high-fat foods to an aroma recipe for low-fat food systems. One can imagine that in foods in which the aroma is generated during the production of the food (such as cheese), the manufacturing process of the food needs to be adapted.

Aromas which are not adapted accordingly are judged to be poor in quality, out of balance or too strong or weak. Hence the products prepared with them are considered low quality.

Similarly to the behaviour of aromas, the intensity of taste compounds is also affected by the volume fraction of fat in a product. As most of the taste compounds preferentially partition in the aqueous phase, resulting in very low (if not negligible) concentrations in the fat phase, one would expect that the overall product concentrations of the taste compounds need correction in line with the increase of the volume fraction of the aqueous phase. Indeed, Malone *et al.* (2003b) showed that taste compound product concentrations also need correction for the phase volume of oil in a product.

Fat affecting aroma release
As mentioned earlier, fat has a strong impact on the texture, the (dynamic) viscosity and breakdown of a product. This translates into dynamic differences in diffusivity of aromas through the product into the head space of the nose. Moreover, fat destabilization results in building an oral coating that can produce a stagnant reservoir for lipophilic compounds in the mouth, resulting in many cases in a much more timed release of lingering aroma sensation.

In order to measure the release of aromas from reduced-fat matrices during consumption, atmospheric pressure chemical ionisation-mass spectrometry (APcI-MS) technology (Weel *et al.*, 2003; de Kok *et al.*, 2006) can be employed. In Fig. 2.2 this is illustrated for yoghurt. Figure 2.2 (left) shows the effect of fat reduction on a lipophilic aroma compound's head space concentration of the yoghurt. Reduction of fat results in a strong increase of the headspace concentration in accordance with what one would expect of a compound which partitions in the fat phase. In Fig. 2.2 (right), this increased intensity is corrected to yield maximum intensity, simulating the aroma concentration correction accordingly. Figure 2.2 (right) clearly shows that the time intensity profile of the high-fat variant is much

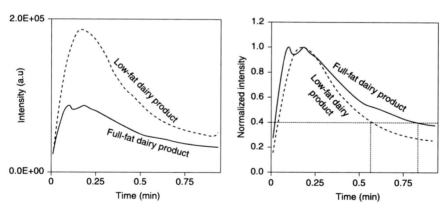

Fig. 2.2   Example of average *in vivo* flavour release curves of an aroma compound of two yoghurts with different amounts of fat as measured with APcI-MS. Left figure shows that removing fat induces a pronounced enhancement of the head space concentration due to the partitioning behaviour of the compound. In the right figure this effect has been cancelled out by equalling the maximum intensity simulating in-product concentration correction. At 40% intensity of the maximum intensity (dotted line), the effect of delayed aroma release from 0.55 to 0.81 minutes is 47%.

© Woodhead Publishing Limited, 2011

more prolonged compared to the aroma release observed in the low-fat system. At 40% of the maximum intensity (see horizontal dotted line in the graph), this effect of delayed aroma release from 0.55 to 0.81 minutes is 47%. It is generally accepted that in products in which the aroma levels have been corrected to produce similar levels of maximum intensity, low-fat products produce short aroma release profiles for hydrophobic compounds, whereas high-fat products sustain prolonged release (Bayarri *et al.*, 2006 and references cited therein). Possible effects of timely aroma release on appetite regulation and consumer reward are illustrated below.

During the consumption of a meal, aroma molecules reach the olfactory epithelium retro-nasally (perceived as arising from the mouth transported via the pharynx). As one would probably expect, there are large interpersonal differences for retro-nasal aroma release efficiency. The latter depends on factors that are likely to be uncontrolled by a person, e.g. saliva production, nasal anatomy and oral processing habits (Buettner *et al.*, 2002). Within a subject, the rates of release are highly reproducible (Ruijschop *et al.*, 2009a). For each individual, irrespective of being an efficient releaser or a poor one, the brain response, i.e. neural brain activation to a retro-nasally sensed food odour, signals the perception of food (Small *et al.*, 2005). Although there are differences in release profile per individual, this will not necessarily lead to differences in sensory perception rating as each individual is calibrated to his/her own sensory system. The hypothesis is that, for each individual, the extent of sensory stimulation induces sensory satiation and thereby provokes meal termination (Ruijschop *et al.*, 2009a). Obviously, the level of sensory stimulation depends on the timed release of the aromas and hence differs for different food structures and compositions. After all, the physical structure of a food that is consumed is important for the extent of retro-nasal aroma release during consumption, i.e. solid foods generate a longer, more pronounced retro-nasal aroma release than liquid foods (Fig. 2.3; Lethuaut *et al.*, 2004). Relatively prolonged aroma release, as observed for solid foods as well as for high-fat products, is believed to be a major factor in generating an enhanced level of satiation compared to the level resulting from consuming an equally calorie-rich beverage (Mattes, 2005b; Ruijschop and de Kok, 2009). With respect to high-fat products, the prolonged aroma release is expected to cue for a high-fat content in a product, which is interpreted as a more pronounced sensory level of satiation.

2.4   Engineering fat to tailor appetite

The ultimate aim is to develop a good-tasting, indulging and rewarding low-fat product that also induces an increased level of satiation, which will prevent consumers from overeating not by rationally restraining a person's diet but merely by early induction of the desired level of reward. In contrast to dietary energy intake restrictions, the latter strategy is expected to satisfy the consumer, preventing the frustration of having to discontinue eating a meal before being satisfied and satiated.

© Woodhead Publishing Limited, 2011

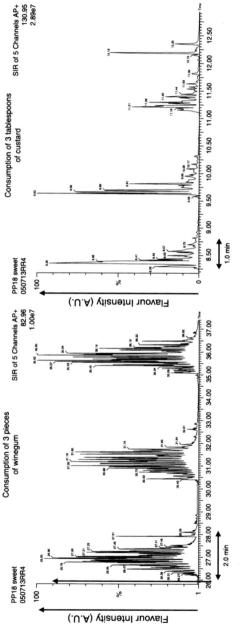

Fig. 2.3 Example of one subject, taken from Ruijschop *et al.* (2009a), illustrating the differences in the extent of retro-nasal aroma stimulation between (left) the consumption of three times one mouthful (on average 5 g per mouthful) of winegum candy ((soft) solid food) and (right) three times one mouthful (on average 19 g per tablespoon) of custard (liquid food), measured by in vivo APcI-MS technology (Weel *et al.*, 2003; Lethaut *et al.*, 2004). As appears from the triplicate measurements, people are reproducible in the morphology and intensity of their aroma release profile.

© Woodhead Publishing Limited, 2011

In order to test the induced level of satiation resulting from either short versus prolonged aroma release profiles, tailored virtual aroma release profiles superimposed on a single product would need to be generated. Using a computer-controlled stimulator based on air dilution olfactometry, aroma stimuli can be administered separately from other stimuli, such as different ingredients, textures and tastes. Hence the relative importance of aroma stimuli apart from other stimuli on satiation mechanisms can be investigated. As described by Visschers *et al.* (2006), delivering food-related aroma stimuli to subjects via an olfactometer involves fine tuning of many parameters, and delivery of aroma stimuli in a manner that reflects aroma release during food intake is a complex undertaking. The generally used approach is based on data from *in vivo* studies with real-time measurement of aroma release, using APcI-MS (Weel *et al.*, 2003; de Kok *et al.*, 2006). It has indeed been demonstrated that the aroma profile that is generated with an APcI-MS-calibrated olfactometer closely resembles the concentration of volatiles in the oro-nasal cavity measured in individuals during ingestion of a specific food product (de Kok *et al.*, 2006). This enables the design of complete aroma release profiles that mimic those obtained by *in vivo* measurement during food consumption (Visschers *et al.*, 2006).

Using this technology it was investigated whether a beverage becomes more satiating when the retro-nasal aroma release profile coincides with the profile of a (soft) solid food (Ruijschop *et al.*, 2008). In a double-blind placebo-controlled randomized cross-over full factorial design, 27 healthy subjects were administered aroma profiles by a computer-controlled stimulator based on air dilution olfactometry (Burghart OM4). Profile A consisted of a profile that is obtained during consumption of normal beverages. Profile B was normally observed during consumption of (soft) solids. The two profiles were produced with strawberry aroma and administered in a retro-nasal fashion, while the subjects in both cases consumed a single sweetened pink-coloured non-aromatized milk drink. Before, during and after the sensory stimulation, satiation measurements were performed. A significant increase was demonstrated in perceived satiation after an olfactometer delivery of a soft solid aroma profile compared to the perceived satiation after an olfactometer delivery of a classical beverage aroma profile. As depicted in Fig. 2.4, subjects felt significantly more satiated if they were subjected to a longer aroma stimulation ($F = 4.24$; $p = 0.04$).

Summarizing, this study showed that satiation can be influenced by making use of differences in retro-nasal aroma release profiles. It has been demonstrated that perceived satiation can be increased by altering the extent of aroma release during food consumption. Aroma-induced satiation (accelerating meal termination) is expected to be related to the degree of indulgence consumers experience. Indulgence is strongly linked to consumer food appreciation and food quality perception. By adopting the timely aroma delivery profile of low-fat products, the level of the hedonic quality experience can be improved in order to match the sensory experience of high-fat products.

Besides aroma, taste and mouthfeel, other sensory modalities contribute to flavour perception, and these may interact, leading to cross-modal effects. The

© Woodhead Publishing Limited, 2011

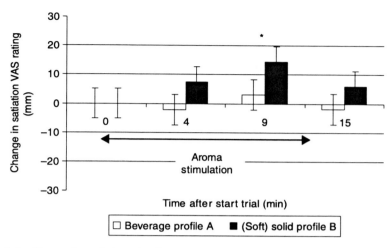

Fig. 2.4 Change in satiation visual analogue scale rating after stimulation with aroma profile A vs. aroma profile B. Data are means with their standard errors represented by vertical bars. * denotes effect of *type* of aroma stimulation (profile A or B) on change in satiation VAS rating with $p < 0.05$ (adapted from Ruijschop *et al.*, 2008).

perceptual match of aroma with taste and mouthfeel is referred to as aroma–taste and aroma–texture congruency. Assuming that the total amount of exposure to a food's sensory properties determines the degree of indulgence consumers experience, it is expected that an enhancement of sensory properties by, for example, a congruent aroma will further enhance the sensory experience, and boost indulgence (*cf.* Harthoorn *et al.*, 2008).

2.5   Consequences for strategies to reduce fat

Strategies to reduce fat must follow from fat functionality, including texture effects, oral breakdown, lubrication, and aroma/taste release and delivery. Texture is typically restored by use of polysaccharides or proteins. Products in which fat acts as a structure breaker are generally more difficult to optimize for low-fat versions. Particulate structure breakers present one possible solution. Alternative strategies may include optimization of fat droplet size and matrix interaction to most efficiently design matrix breaking points.

It has been shown that more effective lubrication from fat can yield equal sensory creaminess from emulsions reduced in fat (Dresselhuis *et al.*, 2008a). Lubrication from other macronutrients is more difficult to achieve. Work has been done on the lubricating properties of proteins and fibres (Chojnicka *et al.*, 2008), but the way the tongue surface coating is perceived is still not fully understood.

In terms of flavour release, a rebalancing of the flavour compounds can restore flavour intensity, but re-engineering time release of flavours remains a challenge.

© Woodhead Publishing Limited, 2011

Flavour release can be altered by adapting texture breakdown or the emulsion properties, but this places restrictions on the texture. Encapsulation of flavours to deliver timed aroma release provides intriguing possibilities, but effective capsules to retain flavour compounds in high-water environments have not yet been developed. During product shelf-life hermetically sealed encapsulates are still a utopia, although controlled leakage can provide an elegant option to induce timed delivery. In these concepts, the partitioning model can help, keeping the bulk phase of aromas specifically designed for this purpose inside the capsule awaiting the moment of consumption.

Fats that are solid at storage temperature, but melt in the mouth during oral processing, have a special effect on the perception. The melting is appreciated in the case of milk fat and cocoa fat. Besides the special aromas of these fats, the melting has an effect on the mouthfeel perception. Saturated fats in general are mostly solid at room temperature. Reducing or replacing these fats in foods will have an effect on the breakdown behaviour in the mouth and therefore affect the perception. Fat-reducing strategies should compensate for these properties.

Digestibility differences between fats will also affect satiety. Generally, the absorption of fats is less for saturated triglycerides (Livesey, 2000). Reducing the saturated fat content will therefore have an effect on satiety sensations through metabolic mechanisms, and should be compensated for.

2.6   Future trends

The perception of fat is complicated. It comprises olfaction, gustation and texture perception, but also gut signalling, metabolic effects and emotional links (Chalé-Rush et al., 2007a). The focus has been on elucidating the mechanisms of fat perception on the various parameters separately. However, the interplay between the various factors should be considered in more detail when developing products with a reduced content of saturated fats.

Nowadays, a lot of attention is paid to mouthfeel and the optimization of fat-reduced products within that perspective. Mechanoreceptors in the mouth contribute to a large extent to the mouthfeel of food products. Gaining more insight into the morphology and mechanisms involved would help to improve the mouthfeel of low-fat products.

The application of aroma to enhance the rewarding value of reduced-fat foods seems promising and appealing. By being able to administer well-defined aroma and taste sensations with designed timely delivery and compositions, the hedonic food experience of reduced-fat foods can be virtually optimized before actual products are being developed, prepared and tested. With the optimized aroma and taste profiles established, product development can be focused using exact defined criteria. This targeted approach provides great opportunities in the development of low-fat products that deliver good consumer food appreciation and food quality perception. For example, foods could be designed with an increase in aftertaste by lingering aroma, or with a long-chewable structure leading to substantially more oral processing and increased oral transit time and higher retro-nasal aroma release efficiency. These applications could evoke a higher quality or quantity of sensory stimulation, leading to enhanced feelings of satiation and, ultimately, decreased food intake. The decreased food intake, in this particular case, would not be the result of rationally limiting consumption (the latter resulting in an increased stress level and discomfort) but merely by early induction of a state of reward. As such, enhancing the sensory stimulation from food influences consumers' motivational state.

2.7   Sources of further information and advice

The review article by Le Révérend *et al.* (2010) on 'Colloidal aspects of eating' gives an overview of the advances in the microstructural approach to reducing unhealthy ingredients. *Designing functional foods*, published by Woodhead Publishing in 2009 (McClements, 2009) provides a comprehensive overview of the current understanding of measuring and controlling food structure breakdown and nutrient absorption.

Food Emulsions: Principles, Practice and Techniques edited by McClements (2004) concentrates on an explanation of the basic concepts of emulsion science, applicable to all types of food emulsion. Details of the properties of particular types of food emulsions are described in *Food Emulsion*, edited by Friberg, Larsson and Sjöblom (2004). *Food Colloids; Self-Assembly and Material Science* edited by Dickinson and Leser (2007) illustrates the basic concepts of food texture. The relation between aroma release and appetite and satiation has been described in more detail by Ruijschop *et al.* (2009b, 2009c).

2.8   Acknowledgements

The authors thank Veronica Galindo Cuspinera for her valuable contribution to the manuscript.

2.9   References

van Aken G A, Vingerhoeds M H and de Hoog E H A (2005), 'Colloidal behaviour of food emulsions under oral conditions', in Dickinson E, *Food colloids*, Cambridge, The Royal Society of Chemistry, 356–66.

van Aken G A, Vingerhoeds M H and de Hoog E H A (2007), 'Food colloids under oral conditions', *Current Opinion in Colloid & Interface Science*, **12**, 251–62.

Bayarri S, Taylor A J and Hort J (2006), 'The role of fat in flavor perception: effect of partition and viscosity in model emulsions', *J Agric Food Chem*, **54**, 8862–8.

Brown R L (1958), 'Wrapper influence on the perception of freshness in bread', *J. Applied Psychology*, **42**, 257–60.

Buettner A, Beer A, Hanning C, Settles M and Schieberle P (2002), 'Physiological and analytical studies on flavor perception dynamics as induced by eating and swallowing process', *Food Qual Pref*, **13**, 497–504.

© Woodhead Publishing Limited, 2011

Chalé-Rush A, Burgess J R and Mattes R D (2007a), 'Multiple routes of chemosensitivity to free fatty acids in humans', *Am J Physiol Gastrointest Liver Physiol*, **292**, G1206–12.
Chalé-Rush A, Burgess J R and Mattes R D. (2007b), 'Evidence for human orosensory (taste?) sensitivity to free fatty acids', *Chem Senses*, **32**, 423–31.
Chen J (2009), 'Food oral processing – A review', *Food Hydrocolloids*, **23**, 1–25.
Chojnicka A, de Jong S, de Kruif C G and Visschers R W (2008), 'Lubrication properties of protein aggregate dispersions in a soft contact', *Journal of agricultural and food chemistry*, **56**, 1274–82.
Chojnicka A, Sala G, de Kruif C G and van de Velde F (2009), 'The interactions between oil droplets and gel matrix affect the lubrication properties of sheared emulsion-filled gels', *Food Hydrocolloids*, **23**, 1038–46.
DeNigris S J, Hamosh M, Kasbekar D K, Lee T C and Hamosh P (1988), 'Lingual and gastric lipsases: species differences in the origin of prepancreatic digestive lipases and in the localization of gastric lipase', *Biochimica et Biophysica Acta*, **959**, 38–45.
Dresselhuis D M, Klok H J, Cohen Stuart M A, de Vries R J, van Aken G A and de Hoog E H A (2007), 'Tribology of o/w emulsions under mouth-like conditions: determinants of friction', *Food Biophysics*, **2**, 158–71.
Dresselhuis D M, de Hoog E H A, Cohen Stuart M A, Vingerhoeds M H and van Aken G A (2008a), 'The occurence of in-mouth coalescence of emulsion droplets in relation to perception of fat', *Food Hydrocolloids*, **22**, 1170–83.
Dresselhuis D M, Cohen Stuart M A, van Aken G A, Schipper R G and de Hoog E H A (2008b), 'Fat retention at the tongue and the role of saliva: adhesion and spreading of protein-poor versus protein-rich emulsions', *Journal of Colloid and Interface Science*, **321**, 21–9.
Dickinson E and Leser M (2007) *Food Colloids; Self-assembly and material science*, Cambridge, RSC Publishing.
Engelen L (2004), *A rough guide to texture: oral physiology and texture perception of semi-solids*, thesis, Wageningen.
Friberg S, Larsson K and Sjöblom J (2004), *Food emulsion*, New York, Marcel Dekker Inc.
Fukuwatari T, Kawada T, Tsuruta M, Hiraoka T, Iwanaga T, Sugimoto E and Fushiki T (1997), 'Expression of the putative membrane fatty acid transporter (FAT) in taste buds of the circumvallate papillae in rats', *FEBS Letters*, **414**, 461–4.
Fukuwatari T, Shibata K, Iguchi K, Saeki T, Iwata A, Tani K, Sugimoto E and Fushiki T (2003), 'Role of gustation in the recognition of oleate and triolein in anosmic rats', *Physiology & Behaviour*, **78**, 579–83.
Giasson S, Israelachvili J and Yoshizawa H (1997), 'Thin film morphology and tribology study of mayonnaise', *Journal of food science*, **62**, 640.
Glindemann D, Dietrich A, Staerk H J and Kuschk P (2006), 'The two odors of iron when touched or pickled: (skin) carbonyl compounds and organophosphines', *Angew. Chem. Int. Ed.* 2006, **45**, 7006–9.
Hansch C, Leo A J and Hoekman D (1995), *Exploring QSAR. Hydrophobic, Electronic, and Steric Constants*, ACS Professional Reference Book, Washington, American Chemical Society.
Harthoorn L F, Ruijschop R M A J, Weinbreck F, Burgering M J M, de Wijk R A, Ponne C T and Bult J H F (2008), 'Effects of aroma–texture congruency within dairy custard on satiation and food intake', *Food Qual Pref*, **19**, 644–50.
Kamphuis M M J W, Saris W H M and Westerterp-Plantenga M S (2003), 'The effect of addition of linoleic acid on food intake regulation in linoleic acid tasters and linoleic acid non-tasters', *British Journal of Nutrition*, **90**, 199–206.
Kawai T and Fushiki T (2003), 'Importance of lipolysis in oral cavity for orosensory detection of fat', *The American Journal of Physiology*, **285**, R447–54.
Knoop J E, Bult J H F and Smit G (2008), 'Masking Undesirable Effects of Ethylhexanoate on Apple Flavour' at the XVIIIth Congress of European Chemoreception Research Organization, ECRO–2008, Portorož, Slovenia.

© Woodhead Publishing Limited, 2011

de Kok P M T, Boelrijk A E M, de Jong C, Burgering M J M and Jacobs M A (2006), 'MS-nose flavour release profile mimic using an olfactometer', in Bredie W and Petersen M A, *Developments in Food Science; Flavour Science, Recent Advances and Trends*, London, Elsevier, 585–99.

Laugerette F, Passilly-Degrace P, Patris B, Niot I, Febbraio M, Montmayeur J-P and Besnard P (2005), 'CD36 involvement in orosensory detection of dietary lipids, spontaneous fat preference, and digestive secretions', *The Journal of Clinical Investigation*, **115**, 3177–84.

Laugerette F, Gaillard D, Passilly-Degrace P, Niot I and Besnard P (2007), 'Do we taste fat?', *Biochimie*, **89**, 265–9.

Lawrence G, Salles C, Septier C, Busch J and Thomas-Danguin T (2009), 'Odour–taste interactions: A way to enhance saltiness in low salt content solutions' *Food Quality and Preference*, **20**, 241–8.

Lethuaut L, Weel K G, Boelrijk A E M and Brossard C D (2004), 'Flavor perception and aroma release from model dairy desserts', *J Agric Food Chem*, **52**, 3478–85.

Livesey G (2000), 'The absorption of stearic acid from triacylglycerols: an inquiry and analysis', *Nutr. Res. Rev.*, **13**, 185–214.

Luengo G, Tsuchiya M, Heuberger M and Israelachvili J (1997), 'Thin film rheology and tribology of chocolate', *Journal of food science*, **62**, 767.

Malone M E, Appelqvist I A M and Norton I T (2003a), 'Oral behaviour of food hydrocolloids and emulsions. Part 1. Lubrication and deposition considerations' *Food Hydrocolloids*, **17**, 763–73.

Malone M E, Appelqvist I A M and Norton I T (2003b), 'Oral behaviour of food hydrocolloids and emulsions. Part 2. Taste and aroma release', *Food Hydrocolloids* **17**, 775–84.

Mattes R D (2005a), 'Fat taste and lipid metabolism in humans', *Physiology & Behaviour*, **86**, 691–7.

Mattes R (2005b), 'Soup and satiety', *Physiol Behav*, **83**, 739–47.

McClements D J (2004), *Food emulsions: Principles, Practice and Techniques*, Boca Raton, CRC Press.

McClements D J (2009), *Designing functional foods*, Cambridge, Woodhead Publishing.

Le Révérend B J D, Norton I T, Cox P W and Spyropoulos F (2010), 'Colloidal aspects of eating', *Current Opinion in Colloid & Interface Science*, **15**, 84–9.

Ruijschop R M A J, Boelrijk A E M, de Ru J A, de Graaf C and Westerterp-Plantenga M S (2008), 'Effects of retro-nasal aroma release on satiation', *Br J Nutr*, **99**, 1140–8.

Ruijschop R M A J, Burgering M J M, Jacobs M A and Boelrijk A E M (2009a), 'Retro-nasal aroma release depends on both subject and product differences: A link to food intake regulation?', *Chem Senses*, **34**, 395–403.

Ruijschop R M A J, Burseg K M M, Lambers T T and Overduin J. (2009b), 'Designing foods to induce satiation – a flavour perspective' in McClements D J and Decker E D, *Designing functional foods: Measuring and controlling food structure breakdown and nutrient absorption*, Cambridge, Woodhead Publishing Ltd & CRC Press, 623–46.

Ruijschop R M A J, Boelrijk A E M, de Graaf C and Westerterp-Plantenga M S (2009c), 'Retro-nasal aroma release and satiation: a review', *J. Agric. Food Chem.*, **57**, 9888–94.

Ruijschop R M A J and de Kok P M T (2009), 'Induction of satiation via aroma in foods', *Food Sci Technol*, **23**, 25–7.

Sala G, de Wijk R A, van de Velde F and van Aken G A (2008), 'Matrix properties affect the sensory perception of emulsion-filled gels', *Food Hydrocolloids*, **22**, 353–63.

Sanz T, Primo-Martin C and van Vliet T (2007), 'Characterization of crispness of French fries by fracture and acoustic measurements, effect of pre-frying and final frying times', *Food research international*, **40**, 63–70.

Schiffman S S, Graham B G, Sattely-Miller E A and Warwick Z S (1998), 'Orosensory perception of dietary fat', *Current Directions in Psychological Science*, **7**, 137–43.

© Woodhead Publishing Limited, 2011

Small D M, Gerber J C, Mak Y E and Hummel T (2005), 'Differential neural responses evoked by orthonasal versus retro-nasal odorant perception in humans', *Neuron*, **47**, 593–605.

Toepel U, Knebel J F, Hudry J, le Coutre J, Murray M M (2009), 'The brain tracks the energetic value in food images', *NeuroImage*, **44**, 967–74.

Trulsson M and Essick G K (1997), 'Low-treshold mechanoreceptive afferents in the human lingual nerve', *J Neurophys*, **77**, 737–48.

Visschers R W, Jacobs M A, Frasnelli J, Hummel T, Burgering M and Boelrijk A E M (2006), 'Cross-modality of texture and aroma perception is independent of orthonasal or retro-nasal stimulation', *J Agric Food Chem*, **54**, 5509–15.

Weel K G C, Boelrijk A E M, Burger J J, Gruppen H, Voragen A G J and Smit, G (2003), 'A protocol for measurement of in vivo aroma release from beverages', *J Food Sci*, **68**, 1123–28.

Weel K G C (2004), *Release and perception of aroma compounds during consumption*, thesis, Wageningen.

de Wijk R A and Prinz J F (2006), 'Mechanisms underlying the role of friction in oral texture', *Journal of Texture Studies*, **37**, 413–27.

Zampini M and Spence C (2004), 'The role of auditory cues in modulating the perceived crispness and staleness of potato chips', *J. Sensory Studies* **19**, 347–63.

3

Sources of saturated and other dietary fats

G. Talbot, The Fat Consultant, UK

Abstract: Saturated fat in the diet comes from a number of vegetable and animal sources. The main vegetable oil sources are palm oil, palm kernel oil, coconut oil, cocoa butter and the fats generally used in cocoa butter equivalents. The most common animal sources are either in the form of milk fats or from the carcass of an animal. Cow's milk fat is by far the most commonly consumed milk fat, not only in its basic form in milk but in other dairy products such as butter and cheese. Animal carcass fats are consumed both as part of the meat of the animal (with beef, lamb or mutton, pork and venison being the most important of these) or as a component of other food products. A further source of saturates is from hydrogenated vegetable oils.

Key words: palm oil, palm kernel oil, coconut oil, cocoa butter, milk fats, animal carcass fats, lard, beef tallow, hydrogenation, *trans* fatty acids.

3.1 Introduction

All edible oils, be they vegetable, animal or marine based, contain saturated fatty acids to some extent. The problems as far as nutrition and the effects of dietary saturated fats are concerned lie with those oils that contain significant levels of saturated fat. It is mainly those oils that will be considered in this chapter (and in this book as a whole). To put these into the total context of commonly consumed oils, Table 3.1 lists the typical saturated, monounsaturated and polyunsaturated fatty acids of a range of these oils.

Because all of these oils contain saturates to some extent, where do we draw the line between an 'acceptable' level of saturates and one which is considered high enough to warrant further investigation and possible replacement? This is a difficult question to answer (a) because such a distinction is likely to be an arbitrary one and (b) because it is not always possible for both legal and functional reasons to replace high saturates fats with lower ones or even significantly reduce

© Woodhead Publishing Limited, 2011

Table 3.1   Typical fatty acid contents (%) of a range of common fats and oils

	Saturates	Monounsaturates	Polyunsaturates
Palm oil	51.1	37.8	10.8
Soyabean oil	15.0	23.5	60.5
Rapeseed oil	6.0	62.2	31.8
Sunflower oil	11.7	19.7	68.6
High-oleic sunflower oil	10.5	81.0	8.5
Groundnut oil	19.0	39.6	41.4
Cottonseed oil	30.4	19.1	50.5
Shea butter	48.9	45.6	5.5
Cocoa butter	61.7	35.1	3.2
Coconut oil	94.1	4.5	1.4
Palm kernel oil	81.9	15.3	2.4
Dairy butterfat	62.3	31.3	4.4
Lard	40.1	48.4	11.4
Beef tallow	36.9	61.3	2.8

their level. In the context of this chapter, a level of 40% saturates has been used to divide 'low'-saturates vegetable oils from 'high'-saturates vegetable oils.

This means that as far as saturated fat in our diet is concerned we can divide its sources into four main categories:

- vegetable oils rich (>40%) in saturates
- mammalian milk fats
- animal carcass fats
- hydrogenated fats.

3.2   Vegetable oils rich in saturated fats

3.2.1   Palm oil
The oil palm is arguably the most useful of all oil-bearing plants. Not only does it produce the highly functional palm oil but it is also the source of palm kernel oil. Although there are many different kinds of palm, only two varieties produce palm oil and palm kernel oil. These are the African oil palm (*Elaeis guineensis*) and the American oil palm (*Elaeis olifera*). In both kinds of tree a soft fleshy fruit with a hard kernel is produced.

Palm oil is found in the soft fleshy outer mesocarp while palm kernel oil is found in the hard kernel. The two oils differ considerably in terms of their fatty acid and triglyceride compositions. Palm kernel oil will be discussed in more detail in section 3.2.2 (along with coconut oil, with which it shares many common attributes). Palm oil contains three distinctly different groups of triglyceride, each with different melting profiles and functionalities. The versatility that palm oil offers to the food technologist is one of the reasons why its usage has increased over the past 10 or 20 years to now make it the leading vegetable oil in terms of tonnage.

© Woodhead Publishing Limited, 2011

In 2008, the global market for oils and fats was about 160 million metric tonnes (REA Holdings, 2010). Of this, 48 million metric tonnes were palm oil and palm kernel oil together. By far the largest volumes of palm oil are produced in Indonesia and Malaysia. Together these two countries account for 85–90% of the total global volume. In 2006, Indonesia produced 15.9 million metric tonnes of palm oil (44% of the global volume) while Malaysia produced 15.88 million metric tonnes of palm oil (43% of the global volume) (Malaysian Palm Oil Council, 2008). In contrast, the next largest individual countries were Thailand, Nigeria and Colombia, each producing about 2% of the global volume. By 2008 the production of palm oil in Indonesia had grown to about 18.3 million metric tonnes and in Malaysia to about 17.7 million metric tonnes (Global Oils & Fats Business Magazine, 2009).

Typical fatty acid compositions of palm oil from different origins are shown in Table 3.2. These can translate into the triglyceride compositions shown in Table 3.3. Palm oil is unusual among vegetable oils in being an oil with more than 33% unsaturation but which also has a significant proportion of saturated fatty acid in the 2-position of the triglyceride. Normally vegetable oils follow a 1,3-random-2-random distribution in which the 2-position is firstly filled with a random distribution of unsaturated fatty acids and then the 1- and 3-positions are filled randomly with whatever is left. Palm oil does not follow this. The result is a significant level of SSS (trisaturated triglycerides) and a significant level of SSU (asymmetrical monounsaturated triglycerides).

As well as triglycerides, palm oil also contains a number of nutritionally beneficial components. The palm fruit and the crude oil produced from it are deep red in colour because of the 500–700 ppm of carotenoids present in the oil (Sundram, 2009). These include beta-carotene, alpha-carotene and lycopene and are the same components that give the red and orange colours to tomatoes and carrots. Crude palm oil is one of the richest sources of these provitamin A carotenoids, containing 15 times as much as in carrots and 300 times more than in tomatoes and is used to treat vitamin A deficiency (Fife, 2010). When the oil is refined, however, much of the colour – and therefore much of the carotenoids – is removed.

Table 3.2   Fatty acid compositions of palm oils from different origins

	Malaysia	Sumatra	Ivory Coast
C12:0	0.1–0.3	0.1–0.2	0.1–0.2
C14:0	0.7–1.3	1.1–1.3	0.8–1.0
C16:0	42.6–45.4	44.2–47.0	43.4–45.2
C18:0	4.0–4.8	4.1–4.6	4.9–5.5
C18:1	37.7–38.8	36.6–38.4	37.1–39.9
C18:2	10.0	9.6–11.5	9.6–10.9
C20:0	0.1–0.4	0.2–0.4	0.2–0.4

Source: Rossell *et al.*, 1983, 1985

© Woodhead Publishing Limited, 2011

Table 3.3 Triglyceride compositions of African and Asian palm oils

	Congo palm oil	Sumatran palm oil
Total SSS (trisaturated triglycerides)	**6.6**	**8.5**
SOS (symmetrical monounsaturated triglycerides)	**33.8**	**30.3**
– MOP	1.2	1.3
– POP	24.1	25.9
– POSt	7.0	3.1
– StOSt	0.5	
SSO (asymmetrical monounsaturated triglycerides)	**5.3**	**7.3**
– PPO	3.6	6.0
– Others	1.7	1.3
Diunsaturated triglycerides	**35.0**	**35.0**
– POO	18.9	18.9
– StOO	2.8	2.6
– OPO	1.0	1.2
– PLiP	7.8	6.8
– StLiP	2.3	1.9
– Others	2.2	3.6
Triunsaturated triglycerides	**19.8**	**18.4**
– OOO	2.7	3.2
– POLi	4.0	2.6
– PLiO	4.5	4.3
– Others	8.6	8.3
Triglycerides with more than three double bonds	**0.5**	**0.2**

Source: Jurriens, 1968

M = myristic acid; P = palmitic acid; St = stearic acid; O = oleic acid; Li = linoleic acid

Palm oil also contains up to 600–1000 ppm of tocopherols and tocotrienols (Han *et al.*, 2006). These are natural antioxidants that help to give a good oxidative stability to the oil and also have vitamin E activity. These do carry through the oil refining process and continue to act as antioxidants in the refined oil.

Historically, palm oil has been processed by all three of the main oil modification processes – hydrogenation, fractionation and interesterification. In recent years hydrogenation has largely been phased out as an oil modification process because of the levels of *trans* fatty acids that are produced. Hydrogenation is considered in more detail in section 3.5. It is worth mentioning, however, that complete hydrogenation of palm oil produces a very high-melting fat that is effectively 100% saturated and virtually free of *trans* fatty acids. It is composed mainly of palmitic and stearic acid and is used at very low levels (usually less than 2–3%) to give structure and stability to systems that are rich in liquid oil, e.g. soft confectionery fillings, nut spreads, etc. The fat still needs to be labelled as 'hydrogenated' and so, to a large extent, it has been replaced even in these applications by a hard palm stearine (see below).

© Woodhead Publishing Limited, 2011

It has already been mentioned that palm oil contains three distinctly different groups of triglycerides. Reference to Table 3.3 will show that these can be split into a group of high melting trisaturated triglycerides, a second group which contains one double bond (with the remaining saturated fatty acids being configured both symmetrically in the 1- and 3-positions and asymmetrically in the 1- and 2-positions), and a third group containing more unsaturated fatty acids. Depending on the origin of the oil about 6–8% of the oil falls into the first group, about 37–38% of the oil into the second group and about 53–55% of the oil into the third group. These groups can be separated by a process of fractional crystallization (fractionation).

This is a process which separates the major triglycerides in palm oil into two or three parts (fractions). It is a process of partial crystallization and filtration and can be carried out in either the presence or absence of an organic solvent. The process without solvent is called 'dry' fractionation. The oil is cooled to such a temperature that crystallization of the higher melting triglycerides (SSS and SOS) takes place. These crystals are separated by filtration and are what is then known as palm stearine. The liquid phase is known as palm oleine. In some instances the stearine fraction is fractionated again by holding at a higher temperature such that mainly SSS triglycerides crystallize out. The crystalline fraction is again separated by filtration and is known as either palm top-fraction or hard palm stearine. The liquid fraction is called palm mid-fraction.

The process using solvent is called 'wet' fractionation. In this, the oil is dissolved in a solvent such as acetone or hexane and the solution is cooled to a low temperature to induce crystallization. Usually, the SOS and SSS triglycerides form the major part of the crystals. These are then separated by filtration. Solvent is removed from the filtrate to give palm oleine. The crystalline fraction can, as with dry fractionation, be refractionated at a higher temperature to give palm top-fraction (or hard palm stearine) and palm mid-fraction. Solvent fractionation is a more expensive process than dry fractionation and is mainly used to produce high-value components such as those needed for cocoa butter equivalents. It gives very sharp solid fractions with very little entrainment of the oleine. Dry fractionation, on the other hand, gives more liquid oleine fractions. The improvements that have been made in dry fractionation in recent years are such that, for palm oil, this is by far the more predominant of the two processes.

In terms of the fractions that can be produced, the most useful situation is when the oil is separated into three fractions: the top (stearine), middle (mid) and bottom (oleine) fractions. Each of these fractions differs in terms of fatty acid composition, melting profile and usage. Typical fatty acid compositions of the three fractions are shown in Table 3.4; their melting profiles can be seen in Fig. 3.1. Palm stearine is very high melting and more saturated than palm oil. It has a wide variety of uses in foods, albeit at a relatively low level of use (because its melting point is above body temperature). It is often used to 'structure' foods such as nut butters, margarines and spreads. It helps to maintain an aerated structure in yeast-raised bread doughs by crystallizing around the bubbles in the bread (Brooker, 1996). It is used to provide part or all of the fat in powdered soups and sauces (Talbot and Slager, 2010). The mid-fraction has a very specific use in confectionery. Because

© Woodhead Publishing Limited, 2011

Table 3.4 Typical fatty acid compositions (%) of palm fractions

	Palm stearine (top-fraction)[a]	Palm mid-fraction[b]	Palm oleine[a]
C12:0	0.1	0.1	0.1
C14:0	1.5	0.6	1.0
C16:0	62.0	56.5	37.0
C16:1		0.1	
C18:0	5.5	4.1	4.0
C18:1	24.0	34.4	45.0
C18:2	6.0	3.7	12.5
C18:3			0.2
C20:0	0.4	0.3	0.7
Total saturates	69.5	61.6	42.8

[a] Gunstone (1987)
[b] Wong Soon (1991)

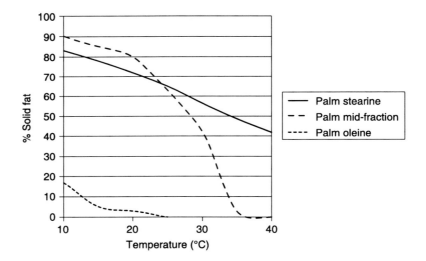

Fig. 3.1 Melting profiles of palm fractions.

its triglyceride composition is similar to that of cocoa butter it finds extensive use as a component of cocoa butter equivalents (Talbot, 2009). The oleine is extensively used as an oxidatively stable frying oil (Talbot and 't Zand, 2006).

Whereas hydrogenation generally increases the level of saturates in an oil and fractionation separates the oil on the basis of saturation, such that some fractions are more saturated and others less saturated than the original oil, interesterification has no effect at all on the fatty acid composition as a whole. The interesterification process changes the positions on the triglyceride molecules of all the fatty acids in the oil. It can be carried out in two ways. In the first type of interesterification, traditionally catalysed by sodium or sodium alkoxide, the distribution of the fatty acids on the

© Woodhead Publishing Limited, 2011

glycerol backbone of the triglyceride molecule is randomized. The second type of interesterification uses an enzyme catalyst. Some types of enzyme catalyst are 1,3-specific. This means that only the fatty acids in the 1- and 3-positions of the triglyceride molecule are randomly redistributed while the fatty acids in the 2-position are left alone. Other types of enzyme act in the same way as the traditional chemical catalysts and fully randomize the distribution. Since, however, interesterification does not in itself alter fatty acid composition it does not therefore reduce saturates. It is, though, useful, in some circumstances, in allowing very unsaturated oils such as palm oleine to be blended with low levels of highly saturated oils such as palm stearine. Normal blending of such oils will often result in a waxy meltdown because of the high-melting triglycerides that are present. Interesterification completely changes the melting profile, allowing a much more palatable product to be made. More detailed information about the nutritional characteristics of palm oil, both in terms of its fatty acid composition and its minor components, is given in Chapter 6.

3.2.2   Palm kernel and coconut oils

Despite the fact that palm kernel oil and palm oil are from the same plant source, palm kernel oil is often discussed together with coconut oil rather than with palm oil. The reason for this is the similarity between palm kernel oil and coconut oil. Both are rich in lauric acid (C12:0) and for this reason are known as 'lauric fats'. They are the most common of the lauric fats, with babassu oil being the only other one that has any real commercial availability.

In terms of their origins, palm kernel oil is obviously grown in the same parts of the world as palm oil and so predominantly comes from Indonesia and Malaysia. Global production of palm kernel oil in 2005 was about 2.5 million metric tonnes, compared with a total of 37 million metric tonnes of palm oil produced in the same year (Dekeloil, 2010). Coconut oil is obtained from copra, the dried endosperm layer of the coconut. This grows within a band 20 degrees north and south of the equator with the Philippines being a major source of coconut oil. Typical annual exports of coconut oil from the Philippines are in the region of more than 800 000 metric tonnes (Commodity Online, 2010).

The fatty acid compositions of palm kernel oil and coconut oil are shown in Table 3.5. Their triglyceride compositions in terms of carbon number[1] are shown in Table 3.6. Coconut oil is very high (>94%) in saturates and such a high level of saturates would be expected to give a very high melting product. However, because the average fatty acid chain length of the saturates in coconut oil is quite low in comparison to most other vegetable fats the solid fat content at ambient temperatures is also quite low (Fig. 3.2). In comparison, palm kernel oil is more unsaturated but the average chain length of its saturated fatty acids is higher, giving it a higher level of solid fat (Fig. 3.2).

---

[1] Carbon number is the sum of the number of carbon atoms in each of the three fatty acids in a triglyceride molecule. In other words, it is the number of carbon atoms in a triglyceride molecule excluding the three that are from the glycerol backbone.

© Woodhead Publishing Limited, 2011

Table 3.5   Typical fatty acid compositions (%) of palm kernel oil and coconut oil

	Palm kernel oil[a]	Coconut oil[b]
C6:0	0.3	1.3
C8:0	3.3	12.2
C10:0	3.5	8.0
C12:0	47.5	48.8
C14:0	16.4	14.8
C16:0	8.5	6.9
C18:0	2.4	2.0
C18:1	15.3	4.5
C18:2	2.4	1.4
Others	0.1	0.1
Total saturates	82.3	94.1

[a] Rossell et al. (1985)
[b] Gunstone et al. (1994)

Table 3.6   Typical carbon number triglyceride compositions of palm kernel oil and coconut oil

	Palm kernel oil[a]	Coconut oil[b,c]
C28	0.4	0.9
C30	1.3	4.2
C32	6.4	15.8
C34	8.4	19.0
C36	21.5	20.3
C38	16.2	17.2
C40	9.7	9.6
C42	9.3	6.4
C44	6.9	3.2
C46	5.6	1.5
C48	6.3	1.0
C50	2.7	0.5
C52	2.8	0.2
C54	2.6	

[a] Rossell et al. (1985)
[b] Bezard (1971)
[c] Bezard et al. (1971)

In the same way as palm oil has been modified by hydrogenation, fractionation and interesterification, so both palm kernel oil and coconut oil have been processed in similar ways. However, their higher level of saturates gives some fundamental differences in comparison to palm oil. Firstly, the higher level of saturates means that when the oils are hydrogenated less *trans* fatty acids are generated. Indeed, the very high level of saturates in coconut oil is such that it is very rare to partially hydrogenate coconut oil. It is more usual to hydrogenate to complete saturation. This gives a fat with a melting point of about 32°C. Coconut oil is the only

© Woodhead Publishing Limited, 2011

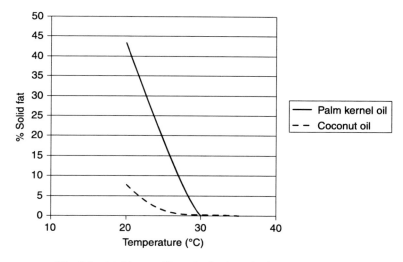

Fig. 3.2 Melting profiles of palm kernel oil and coconut oil.

common vegetable oil that can be fully hydrogenated and still melt below mouth temperature. Palm kernel oil has also been hydrogenated, both partially (to melting points of 32–38°C, often also described by their melting points in degrees Fahrenheit as HPKO90 and HPKO95) and fully hydrogenated to a melting point of 41–42°C. Although fully hydrogenated coconut oil and palm kernel oil contain virtually no *trans* fatty acids, their use has been limited in recent years simply because of the need to still label them as 'hydrogenated'.

Both coconut oil and palm kernel oil are also fractionated, usually by the dry fractionation process. Fractionation of palm kernel oil is more common than that of coconut oil and yields a stearine (PKS) and an oleine fraction. Both of these can then be used directly in these forms or can then also be hydrogenated. The stearine is usually fully hydrogenated to give HPKS. Unlike the fully hydrogenated oil, HPKS melts at mouth temperature. This is because much of the oleic acid in the oil fractionates into the oleine and is therefore not available in the stearine to be converted on hydrogenation into the much higher-melting stearic acid. The melting profiles of fully hydrogenated coconut oil (CN32), palm kernel stearine (PKS) and fully hydrogenated palm kernel stearine (HPKS) are shown in Figure 3.3.

The oils can also be interesterified, and interesterified blends of palm kernel oil and palm oil have been used in various applications but, as with palm oil, this does not change the overall fatty acid composition, just the positional distribution of the fatty acids.

Both palm kernel oil and coconut oil are widely used in confectionery (Talbot, 2009). In their basic state they are used in soft confectionery centres. Coconut oil and, to a certain extent, fully hydrogenated coconut oil have very cool-melting characteristics that make them highly suitable for use in imparting such sensory

© Woodhead Publishing Limited, 2011

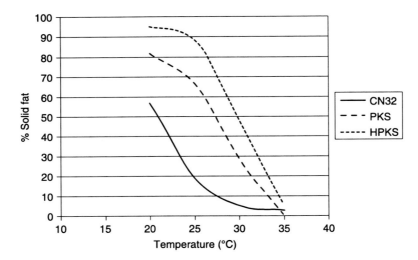

Fig. 3.3   Melting profiles of hydrogenated and fractionated palm kernel oil and coconut oil.

characteristics to confectionery fillings. These 'fillings' are often deposited directly into foil cups and so consumed without any chocolate coating around them and are known as 'ice cups'.

Because of their high level of solid fat at ambient temperatures and sharp melting profile thereafter, PKS and HPKS are used as cocoa butter substitutes. In this context they are blended with a low-fat cocoa powder, sugar and milk powder to make a coating that can substitute for chocolate. Hydrogenated palm kernel oil and, to a lesser extent, hydrogenated palm kernel oleine were, at one time, the preferred industry standard as a toffee fat. In recent years, they have been replaced firstly by hydrogenated palm oil and, more recently, by non-hydrogenated oils. These fats have also been used as analogues of butterfat in non-dairy equivalents to dairy products such as dairy creamers, toppings and coffee creamers.

One of the main uses of palm kernel oil and coconut oil in food is in ice cream, where they form the basis of many non-dairy ice creams. Because they were used in this way in the ice cream they were often also used as the fat base of a chocolate-like coating. Although they are still used in this way in cheaper 'choc ices', many coated ice cream products nowadays use real chocolate coatings – but the ice cream itself may still be based on palm kernel oil.

Coconut oil also has non-food uses in, for example, the soap-making and detergent industries and is also the basis of medium chain triglycerides (MCT). These are triglycerides based mainly on C8 and C10 saturated fatty acids. Fatty acids of such short chain lengths are metabolized differently by the body compared with longer chain-length fats and are able to release their energy more quickly. This makes them particularly suitable for sports nutrition and post-operative nutrition.

© Woodhead Publishing Limited, 2011

3.2.3   Cocoa butter and cocoa butter equivalent fats

Cocoa (*Theobroma cacao*) grows in three main equatorial parts of the world – West Africa (about 70%), South America (about 13%) and Asia/Oceania (about 17%). The largest producing country is Côte d'Ivoire, which accounts for about 35–37% of the total world production of cocoa. Production volumes of cocoa beans for the years 2006 to 2009 are shown in Table 3.7. The cocoa bean is processed by fermentation and roasting before being broken up into nibs and ground into cocoa mass (or cocoa liquor). This process is described in more detail by Beckett (2009). Cocoa mass contains about 55% fat and is either used directly in chocolate, usually supplemented by further quantities of cocoa butter (as well as sugar and, in milk chocolate, milk fat and milk powders) or is separated into a fat phase (cocoa butter) and a non-fat phase (cocoa powder). Although cocoa powder has been described here as being a non-fat phase, in reality it does still contain some fat, the two main types that are commercially available containing 10–12% fat or 20–22% fat.

The fatty acid composition of cocoa butter varies from origin to origin, with Asian cocoa butters generally containing higher levels of stearic acid relative to palmitic acid and South American cocoa butters being more unsaturated (Table 3.8). These differences translate through to the triglyceride compositions of the fats, with South American cocoa butter containing more SOO and Asian cocoa butters containing more POSt and StOSt (Table 3.9). The result of these differences in functional terms is that, in general, cocoa butters from South

Table 3.7   World production of cocoa beans, 2006–2009, thousands of tonnes

	2006/07	2007/08	2008/09
Africa	2361	2688	2424
– Côte d'Ivoire	1229	1382	1222
– Ghana	614	729	662
Americas	423	452	456
– Brazil	126	171	157
Asia and Oceania	650	591	575
– Indonesia	545	485	475
World Total	3439	3731	3515

Source: ICCO, 2009

Table 3.8   Fatty acid compositions of cocoa butters from different origins (%)

	C16:0	C18:0	C18:1	C18:2	C18:3	C20:0	C22:0	Total saturated
Brazil	25.1	33.3	36.5	3.5	0.2	1.2	0.2	59.8
Ivory Coast (Côte d'Ivoire)	25.8	36.9	32.9	2.8	0.2	1.2	0.2	64.1
Malaysia	24.9	37.4	33.5	2.6	0.2	1.2	0.2	63.7

Source: Lipp and Anklam, 1998

© Woodhead Publishing Limited, 2011

Table 3.9   Triglyceride compositions of cocoa butter of different origins

	POP	POSt	StOSt	StOA	SLiS	SOO
South America	19.0	38.0	26.0	0.5	7.4	9.1
Africa	18.4	39.1	28.2	0.6	6.7	6.9
Asia	18.6	40.0	30.8	0.8	5.9	4.1

Source: Chaiseri and Dimick, 1989

America are softer than those from West Africa while those from Asia are harder (Fig. 3.4).

The process of obtaining cocoa butter from cocoa nibs or cocoa mass simply involves pressing the oil out of the mass. This is the reason why there is usually some oil remaining in the cocoa powder – it is impossible to take out all the fat simply by pressing. In some cases, though, further oil can be solvent extracted from the pressed mass. Cocoa butter that has been simply pressed from the cocoa mass (often known as 'prime pressed cocoa butter') is usually used directly in chocolate without any further processing. This makes it unusual among fats in that most fats are refined before use to remove unwanted minor components such as free fatty acids, pigments, oxidation products and off-flavours. The free fatty acid levels in cocoa butter are usually very low (typically less than 1.4%); it has a creamy yellow colour but, since it is usually being used in a product with a distinctive brown colour, it is not necessary to remove these pigments before use; it is a very oxidatively stable fat. When all of these factors are taken into account along with the pleasant cocoa flavours and odours that are naturally present in the fat, it makes no sense to remove them by refining. Usually the only times that

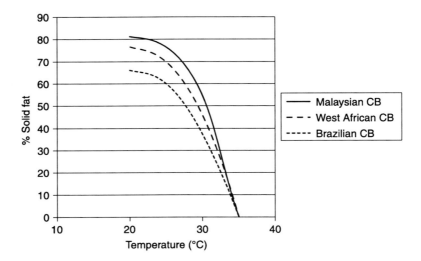

Fig. 3.4   Melting profiles of cocoa butters from different origins.

© Woodhead Publishing Limited, 2011

cocoa butter will be deodorized is if it has been solvent extracted, or it contains some objectionable off-flavours or needs to be 'standardized' in some way.

Fractionation has been mentioned previously in the context of both palm oil and palm kernel oil. Fractionation of cocoa butter was developed (Weyland, 1992) as a means of producing an even harder fraction of cocoa butter (stearine) that is more heat resistant and bloom resistant, and a softer fraction (oleine) that would be suitable for use in more crack-resistant chocolate ice cream coatings. The cost of cocoa butter coupled with the cost of fractionation and the need to be able to use both fractions makes this a process of limited application economically.

The main food use of cocoa butter is in confectionery products, notably, of course, in chocolate. In this context it is also used where chocolate becomes a component of other foods (bakery products, desserts, etc). Outside food, it has more limited applications in cosmetics and in medical applications such as the base for suppositories.

Mention has already been made of the high cost of cocoa butter. To alleviate this somewhat, cocoa butter equivalents (CBEs) were developed by Unilever (Best *et al.*, 1956). These are fats that contain the same basic triglycerides as cocoa butter (i.e. POP, POSt, StOSt) and can therefore be used to replace cocoa butter in chocolate. At least, they can replace cocoa butter in chocolate from a functional point of view. Whether they are able to be used in practice depends on local chocolate regulations. In the European Union, for example, they are permitted to be used at a maximum level of 5% (European Union, 2000) whereas in the United States they are not allowed in chocolate. Functionally, they can be used at levels higher than 5% but, in most countries, the product designation used can no longer be 'chocolate'.

Although any fat that is rich in SOS-type triglycerides can be used in cocoa butter equivalents, in practice the fats used in commercial CBEs are limited to seven types, one of which is produced by enzymically catalysed interesterification. The European Union Chocolate Directive (European Union, 2000) specified six sources of oils that can be used in the vegetable fat part of chocolate and specifically excludes any fat produced by enzymically catalysed interesterification. Although fats from other sources are permitted to be used in other countries that allow the use of vegetable fats in chocolate, it is these six sources that are the most commonly used worldwide. They are:

- palm oil: *Elaeis guineensis* and *Elaeis olifera*
- illipe: *Shorea stenoptera*
- sal: *Shorea robusta*
- shea: *Butyrospermum parkii*
- kokum gurgi: *Garcinia indica*
- mango kernel: *Mangifera indica.*

Each of these oils contains a significant level of either POP, POSt or StOSt, the main triglycerides found in cocoa butter. None of the oils, however, is identical to cocoa butter in terms of the compositional balance of these triglycerides and so CBEs are almost always blends of two or more of these fats. There is an additional complication in that most of these oils also contain significant levels of triglycerides

© Woodhead Publishing Limited, 2011

that are not of the POP, POSt, StOSt type and these need to be removed or, at least, reduced in level before the fat is suitable for use in a CBE. This is usually carried out by fractionation.

Palm oil and its composition has been considered in detail in section 3.2.1. The fatty acid composition of the remaining five oils is shown in Table 3.10. Their triglyceride composition is shown in Table 3.11. Two things are clear from these compositions. Firstly, none of the oils match cocoa butter in terms of their composition and, secondly, some of the oils (notable shea and mango kernel) have levels of total SOS that are much lower than found in cocoa butter. Indeed, the closest match overall to cocoa butter, both in terms of total SOS and the balance of the individual triglycerides, is illipe. The low levels of total SOS in some oils means that, like palm oil, they need to be fractionated to concentrate these triglycerides to a higher, more useful, level. Thus, rather than use all of these oils in their basic form in CBEs the components that are actually used are: palm mid-fraction (see section 3.2.1), illipe, sal (usually as a stearine, although a good quality sal oil can be used as it is), shea stearine, kokum gurgi (usually used unfractionated but fractionation can give a very high-quality component) and mango kernel stearine.

Table 3.10   Typical fatty acid compositions of the base oils (other than palm oil) used in cocoa butter equivalents

	Illipe[a]	Sal[b]	Shea[c]	Kokum gurgi[a]	Mango kernel[d]
C14:0				1	
C16:0	19.3	6.3	3.3	4	10
C18:0	43.5	44.6	44.3	53	40
C18:1	35.3	41.6	45.6	40	44
C18:2	1.0	1.7	5.5	2	5
C20:0	1.3	5.7	1.3		1

[a] Bracco et al. (1970)
[b] Bhattacharyya and Bhattacharyya (1991)
[c] Sawadogo and Bezard (1982)
[d] Sridhar and Lakshminarayana (1991)

Table 3.11   Typical SOS triglyceride compositions of the base oils (other than palm oil) used in cocoa butter equivalents

	Cocoa butter[a]	Illipe[b]	Sal[c]	Shea[a]	Kokum gurgi[a]	Mango kernel[a]
POP	16	7	5	<1	<1	6
POSt	37	34	16	6	6	13
StOSt	26	45	36	30	72	18
Total SOS	79	80	67*	36	78	37

* Includes 9% StOA and 1% AOA
[a] Talbot (2006)
[b] Jurriens (1968)
[c] Sridhar and Lakshminarayana (1991)
P = palmitic acid; St = stearic acid; O = oleic acid; S = total saturates (palmitic, stearic and arachidic acids)

© Woodhead Publishing Limited, 2011

Table 3.12   Typical triglyceride compositions of CBE components

	Cocoa butter	Palm mid-fraction	Shea stearine	Illipe butter	Sal stearine	Kokum gurgi	Mango kernel stearine
POP	16	66	1	7	<1	<1	1
POSt	37	12	7	34	10	6	16
StOSt	26	3	74	45	60	72	59
Total SOS	79	81	82	86	81*	78	76

* includes 11% StOA
P = palmitic acid; St = stearic acid; A = arachidic acid; S = total satuarated acids; O = oleic acid
Source: Talbot, 2006

Typical triglyceride compositions of the components actually used in CBEs are shown in Table 3.12. Usually, two or three of these components are blended together to produce a CBE. More information about the composition and use of CBEs is given by Talbot (2006, 2009). The main thing to point out in the context of saturated fats, though, is that generally the saturated fat content of CBEs is very similar to that of cocoa butter (because they are intended to match cocoa butter both chemically and physically) and is therefore in the region of 60–65%. In theory, lower saturated vegetable fats could be used, e.g. palm oleine would fall within the scope of the EU Chocolate Directive, but these would soften chocolate significantly. Such proposals are considered in more detail in Chapter 16.

One potential component of CBEs that has been mentioned but has not been discussed above is the type produced by enzymic interesterification. Such fats are prohibited by the EU Chocolate Directive (European Union, 2000) but can be used in other countries that allow the use of vegetable fats in chocolate. As a process, this has been referred to in section 3.2.1. In terms of producing SOS triglycerides it is necessary to have a source of triglycerides rich in 2-position oleic acid together with stearic (and palmitic) acids. Suitable sources of triglycerides rich in 2-position oleic acid are palm oleine and high-oleic sunflower oil. When interesterified with stearic acid in the presence of a suitable lipase catalyst the fatty acids on the 1- and 3-positions of the oil (high-oleic sunflower oil, for example) interchange with stearic acid. The result is a mix of triglycerides including unreacted sunflower oil (mainly OOO), triglycerides in which one of the fatty acids on the 1- or 3-position has interchanged with stearic acid to give StOO and triglycerides in which both acids have interchanged with stearic acid to give StOSt. This mix is then firstly deacidified to remove free fatty acids and is then fractionated to concentrate the StOSt for use in CBEs. Yet again, though, the total level of saturates in the end product is similar to that found in cocoa butter.

3.3   Mammalian milk fats

All mammals produce milk for their young but, in terms of human consumption, the most common one used in food is that derived from cow's milk, followed by

© Woodhead Publishing Limited, 2011

sheep's milk and goat's milk. However, in terms of total human consumption then, clearly, human breast milk plays an important role in infant nutrition. Although the focus in this section will be mainly on cow's milk fat and dairy products that include this, mention will also be made of the compositions of the other three types of milk fat referred to above.

Milk is an oil in water emulsion with the fat being present in a globular form. Over 90% of cow's milk is water with the fat content being about 4%. This fat content can vary from species to species with buffalo milk and ewe's milk containing over 7% fat while (horse) mare's milk contains less than 2% fat. Human breast milk typically contains about 3.5% fat (Chambon, 1996).

The fatty acid compositions of mammalian milk fats are much more complicated than those of vegetable oils. Whereas vegetable oils are mainly composed of fatty acids with even numbers of carbon atoms and a straight carbon chain, milk fats contain a wide range of different fatty acids including odd chain lengths and branched chains. Typical fatty acid compositions of cow's, sheep's, goat's and human milk fats are shown in Table 3.13. It is clear from this that human milk fat is significantly less saturated than any of the other three 'animal' milk fats.

Table 3.13 Typical fatty acid compositions[a] of some common milk fats

	Cow[b]	Cow[e]	Sheep[c]	Goat[c]	Human[d]
C4:0	8.8	3–4	4.4	5.1	
C6:0	5.0	2–3	3.6	4.4	
C8:0	2.5	1–2	2.4	2.6	
C10:0	5.3	2–4	5.5	7.8	0.5
C12:0	5.2	3–4	3.5	3.8	3.0
C14:0	13.8	9–12	9.8	3.6	5.8
C14:1[a]	1.7	1–2	0.6	0.2	0.7
C15:0	1.0	1–2	2.8	2.0	0.7
C15:1[a]	0.2	<0.4			
C16:0	28.0	23–32	21.2	26.0	26.6
C16:1[a]	2.3	2–3	1.7	1.8	5.3
C17:0	0.6	1–2	1.0	0.8	0.8
C17:1[a]	0.2	<1			
C18:0	8.3	13	14.0	9.9	6.7
C18:1	14.1	29	21.8	20.6	36.4
C18:2	1.1	2	4.4	2.7	11.1
C18:3[a]	0.9	<1	2.6		0.9
Others	1.0		0.7	2.7	1.5
Total saturates	78.5	57–76	68.2	66.0	44.1

[a] The C14:1, C15:1, C16:1 and C17:1 acids include C15:0br, C16:0br, C17:0br and C18:0br acids respectively; C18:3 includes C18:2c,t conjugated
[b] from Parodi (1982)
[c] from Marai et al. (1969)
[d] from Breckenbridge et al. (1969)
[e] from Chambon (1996)

© Woodhead Publishing Limited, 2011

The fatty acid composition of milk fat also varies depending on what the animal is being fed and the season of the year. Cow's milk fat shows considerable seasonal variations and the composition shown in Table 3.13 may be considered to be extreme, particularly in terms of the total saturates level. More recent studies generally find lower levels of the shorter chain acids than those shown in Table 3.13. For example, Chambon (1996) gives ranges of the main fatty acids in milk fat suggesting that saturates can range from 57% to 76%. Typically we would expect to find between 60% and 65% saturates in cow's milk. Not shown in the compositions shown for cow's milk fat in Table 3.13 is the level of *trans* fatty acids in cow's milk. This is produced by biohydrogenation of lipids in the rumen of the animal and levels of between 2% and 11% have been measured with a range of 4–8% being more common (Deman and Deman, 1983). Unlike the *trans* fatty acids found in partially hydrogenated vegetable oils, which show a range of positional distribution along the fatty acid chain (but mainly centred on a double bond at n-9, elaidic acid) the main *trans* fatty acid in cow's milk is vaccenic acid with the double bond at position n-7.

This variation in fatty acid composition of cow's milk fat then can carry through to differences in the physical properties of the milk fat. Summer milk fat is generally higher melting and higher in solid fat than is spring milk fat (Fig. 3.5, from Timms and Parekh, 1980). The effect of animal feed and, particularly, the fatty acid composition of the feed can be of importance in altering the fatty acid composition of milk fat. Any changes made to the milk fat in this way will, of course, carry through to any dairy product made from that milk (butter, cheese, etc). So, changes to animal feed may well be one of the major strategies that the food and agricultural industries can use to reduce saturates in dairy products and this will be considered in more detail in later chapters.

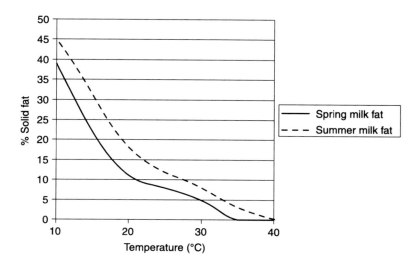

Fig. 3.5   Melting profiles of spring and summer milk fats.

© Woodhead Publishing Limited, 2011

The main fat-containing material that is produced from milk and then goes on to be used as an ingredient in food manufacture is butter. Butter is made by churning cream, converting it from an oil-in-water emulsion into a water-in-oil emulsion. The total fat content of butter is about 80–82% with most of the remainder being water. This can be used directly in food products such as cakes, biscuits, pastries and caramels. Alternatively it can be used in an anhydrous form in which effectively all the water is removed. The production of anhydrous milk fat is described in detail by Illingworth and Bissell (1994). Anhydrous milk fat is known by a variety of names (anhydrous milk fat [AMF], anhydrous butter oil, butter oil), each of which has slightly different specifications defined by the International Dairy Federation but all of which contain greater than 99% fat. Also, under the heading of anhydrous milk fat, we can consider ghee. Ghee is a clarified butter produced and used in the cuisine of the Indian subcontinent and Middle East. It is produced from cream that has been allowed to ripen overnight. The cream is skimmed off and is then boiled to remove the water. This process also results in some caramelization of the non-fat solids in the milk.

Milk fat can also be fractionated to give different physical characteristics to the fat. The melting profiles of milk fat stearine and milk fat oleine are shown in Fig. 3.6 (from Timms and Parekh, 1980). The softer oleine fractions can be used to produce a more spreadable butter while the harder stearine fractions have beneficial properties when used in pastries, for example. The stearine is also a better inhibitor of fat bloom in chocolate than is whole milk fat. Whether it can actually be used in this way within the scope of many countries' chocolate regulations, though, is debatable since many countries specify that milk components in chocolate need to be present in the ratios found in whole milk.

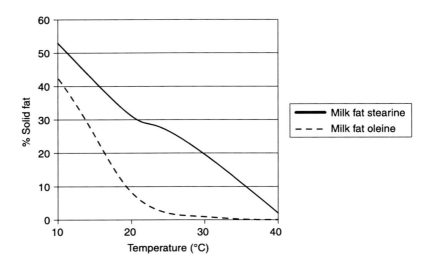

Fig. 3.6   Melting profiles of milk fat stearine and milk fat oleine.

© Woodhead Publishing Limited, 2011

3.4   Animal carcass fats

In this section the focus will be on the fats obtained from four-legged land animals. Arguably fats from fish and fats from poultry could be classed as animal fats; however, but fish oils are excluded because they are very low in saturates but, from a nutritional point of view, very rich in long-chain polyunsaturates. Poultry fats are also low in saturates compared with the animals which will be considered here. Chicken fat, for example, contains about 28–29% saturates (mainly palmitic acid); duck fat contains about 32–33% saturates (again, mainly palmitic acid) and turkey fat contains about 28% saturates (also mainly palmitic acid)

In terms of the fats that will be considered in more detail in this section, two are used for cooking and frying as well as being consumed in combination with the muscle meats from those animals, while the fats from the other two are mainly consumed as part of the meat. The fats that are used for cooking and frying are lard (from pigs) and tallow (from cattle). These two fats are also consumed when either pork or beef is eaten. The remaining two fats that will be mentioned are from sheep and deer – these are mainly consumed along with lamb or mutton meat or venison rather than used as cooking fats.

3.4.1   Lard, beef tallow, sheep and deer fats

As with milk fats, it is difficult to quote specific fatty acid compositions as being representative of the fat in a specific animal because the carcass fats also depend upon what the animal is fed on. Reducing the saturates in cattle feed, for example, not only reduces saturates in the milk but also in the meat. This, too, will be considered in more detail in later chapters. The situation in animal carcass fats is complicated further by fat from different parts of the animal having different fatty acid compositions. For example, the total level of saturates in the fat found in different parts of the pig and beef carcasses is shown in Table 3.14. However, typical fatty acid compositions of the four animal fats being considered here are given by Gunstone *et al.* (1994) and are summarized in Table 3.15.

Table 3.14   Saturated fat content of fats from various parts of pig and beef carcasses

	Pig	Beef
Back fat layer rump – bottom	46.4	54.0
Back fat layer rump – top	49.5	48.4
Back fat layer shoulder – upper 1 cm	38.0	
Back fat layer shoulder – lower 1 cm	42.8	
Perinephric	43.6	60.8
Flank	43.2	
Visceral pericardial		63.2
Ribs		52.6

Source: Chacko and Perkins, 1965

© Woodhead Publishing Limited, 2011

Table 3.15 Typical fatty acid compositions of common animal carcass fats

	Lard	Beef	Mutton	Red deer[a]
C12:0	tr	tr	0.6	0.3
C14:0	2.0	2.5	5.6	5.7
C14:1	tr	3.0		0.4
C16:0	27.1	27.0	27.0	30.9
C16:1	4.0	10.8	1.6	2.0
C18:0	11.0	7.4	31.7	35.7
C18:1	44.4	47.5	31.7	15.4
C18:2	11.4	1.7	1.6	1.1
C18:3	tr	1.1	0.2	
C20:0	tr	tr	tr	

[a] Also contain significant levels of C15:0 and C17:0 fatty acids not included here
Source: Gunstone *et al.*, 1994

Both lard and beef tallow are extracted from the animal tissue by a process of rendering. Essentially, rendering involves heating chopped-up fatty tissues from pigs or cattle to a temperature below 100°C (although in some rendering processes steam can be used). Pure rendered lards, for example, are obtained by melting the fat from pig adipose tissue at a temperature below 80°C. The fat is separated from the remaining tissue by centrifugation. If steam or hot water has been used to help render the fat from the tissue this will, in the first extraction, be centrifuged off with the liquid fat. The water is then separated from liquid fat by a second centrifugation. Because these fats contain very little natural antioxidant they are often supplemented after refining by the addition of natural tocopherols to protect them against oxidation. Beef tallow is often also known as beef dripping or premier jus.

Both lard and beef tallow will fractionate into a liquid portion and solid crystals if left to stand. The lard crystals are very fine and difficult to separate by filtration. Beef tallow, on the other hand, produces crystals that are very easy to separate and so beef tallow can be split into the liquid oleo oil or oleomargarine and the solid oleostearine. Oleomargarine formed the fatty base for the first margarine to be developed by Mège-Mouriés in France in 1869.

Lard is an excellent pastry fat because it crystallizes in a form that makes it ideal for promoting the flakiness of pastry. Beef tallow is mainly used in the form of beef suet in suet pastries (both savoury, as in steak and kidney puddings, and sweet, as in fruit or jam-filled suet rolls). Beef tallow does give a slightly meaty flavour to products either using it or cooked in it. For many years it was the fat of choice for frying potatoes in fish and chip shops in the United Kingdom (particularly in the north of England) but, for reasons of both nutrition and ethical and religious concerns, it has largely been replaced by vegetable oils. It also used to be used in some kinds of biscuit and again gave a distinctive flavour to the biscuit.

© Woodhead Publishing Limited, 2011

3.5   Hydrogenated fats

Hydrogenation is a modification process that was widely used in the oils and fats industry until a few years ago. It is essentially the reaction of hydrogen with the unsaturated carbon–carbon double bonds in the fatty acid chains of a triglyceride. In vegetable oils almost all of the carbon–carbon double bonds are in the *cis* configuration (see Fig. 3.7). When these are reacted with hydrogen in the presence of a catalyst two competing reactions can take place.

In the first reaction hydrogen is 'added' to the double bond, converting it into a saturated single bond and hence producing a saturated fat from what was an unsaturated fat. In the second reaction the *cis* double bond can partially break and while it is in this state can rotate and re-form. Some will re-form back in the original *cis* configuration while others will re-form in a *trans* configuration (Fig. 3.7). Both the saturated fatty acids formed during the first reaction and the *trans* fatty acids formed during the second reaction have higher melting points than the original *cis* fatty acids, and so higher melting, more solid fats can be produced from a basic liquid vegetable oil. Indeed, one of the alternative names for hydrogenation is 'hardening'.

The reaction to convert *cis* unsaturates to saturates is a one-way reaction – once the saturates have been formed they do not then lose hydrogen to become unsaturated again. The reaction between *cis* and *trans* formation is, though, an equilibrium reaction, and a balance between the two forms results. There is also an equilibrium between the two competing reactions of saturation and isomerization. The position of these equilibria is determined by both the reaction conditions and the choice of catalyst. Finely divided nickel is the most common catalyst for hydrogenation. If this has been 'poisoned' by a reaction with sulphur then there will be a greater tendency for *trans* fatty acids to result rather than saturates. Similarly if the pressure (i.e. amount) of hydrogen that is used is low then *trans* formation will predominate over saturates formation.

Many reasons have been given as to why hydrogenated fats were developed but, undoubtedly, the driving force behind their development was initially the

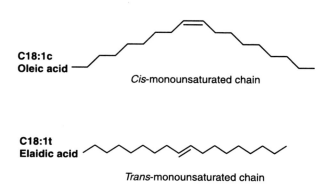

C18:1c
Oleic acid

Cis-monounsaturated chain

C18:1t
Elaidic acid

Trans-monounsaturated chain

Fig. 3.7   Structures of *cis* and *trans* fatty acids.

© Woodhead Publishing Limited, 2011

ability to produce solid fats from liquid oils and this has probably been the main reason for their continued use – until recently, that is. However, as hydrogenated fats began to be used in more applications other beneficial attributes came to the fore. The *trans* fatty acids that are produced during hydrogenation have a greater oxidative stability than do their corresponding *cis* fatty acids. This meant that foods with a greater stability and longer shelf-life could be manufactured using partially hydrogenated vegetable fats. It also meant that partially hydrogenated fats became the oils of choice for industrial frying, again to enhance oxidative stability of both the oils themselves and of materials fried in them. As far as bakery and confectionery are concerned, partially hydrogenated oils were used in both malleable cake coatings that could be cut easily without shattering and in aerated confectionery centres. The problem, though, was the level of *trans* fatty acids that was produced during hydrogenation. In some instances over 50% of a hydrogenated fat consisted of fatty acids in the *trans* configuration.

Clinical nutritional studies over the past two to three decades have shown that *trans* fatty acids have a considerable adverse effect on blood cholesterol and that this, in turn, can be related to an elevated risk of coronary heart disease (Mensink *et al.*, 2003). In essence, *trans* fatty acids increase the levels of 'bad' low-density lipoprotein (LDL) cholesterol and lower the levels of 'good' high-density lipoprotein (HDL) cholesterol. In contrast, *cis* unsaturated fatty acids have the opposite effect, lowering LDL cholesterol and raising HDL cholesterol. Saturated fatty acids, taken as a whole, raise the levels of both types of cholesterol (Mensink *et al.*, 2003). However, individual saturated fatty acids have different effects on these two types of cholesterol. This is an aspect that will be dealt with in more detail in later chapters.

A distinction needs to be made, though, between partial and full hydrogenation. Only partial hydrogenation results in the formation of *trans* fatty acids. When a fat is *fully* hydrogenated, all the unsaturated fatty acids, whether they are in the *cis* or the *trans* configuration, are converted into saturates. A fully hydrogenated fat is, therefore, effectively 100% saturated. Since most unsaturated fatty acids occurring naturally in common vegetable oils contain 18 carbon atoms (i.e. oleic, linoleic and linolenic acids) when they are fully hydrogenated, the result is the formation of stearic acid. Stearic acid and fully hydrogenated fats that contain predominantly stearic acid are, however, very high melting (the typical melting point of a fully hydrogenated liquid oil such as rapeseed oil or soyabean oil is about 70°C, well above mouth temperature). While such fats can be and are used at very low levels in a variety of foods for very specific functions, any usage at high levels would result in an unpalatable, waxy product. Even simple blending with the corresponding unhydrogenated oil would also result in a high-melting 'tail'. Interesterifying such a blend, though, completely rearranges the positions of the fatty acids in the triglycerides and can result in an end product that is solid at room temperature yet melts readily in the mouth (Nor Aini and Miskandar, 2007). Indeed, the only common vegetable oil that melts below mouth temperature even when fully hydrogenated is coconut oil, with a melting point in its fully hydrogenated form of about 32°C.

Different countries have responded to the issue of hydrogenation and *trans* formation in different ways. Denmark, for example, has limited the levels of *trans*

© Woodhead Publishing Limited, 2011

fats produced 'industrially' to a maximum of 2% of the fats used in any food product (Danish Veterinary and Food Administration, 2003). *Trans* fats found in the milk and meat of ruminant animals are, however, excluded from these constraints. The United States responded differently and, rather than putting limits on the amount of *trans* fats that can be present in fats for use in food, they imposed labelling legislation in which the *trans* fatty acid contents of foods needs to be declared as part of their nutritional composition (Food and Drug Administration, 2003). However, since that legislation came into force, some individual states and cities (notable California and New York City) have introduced legislation banning the use of *trans* fats in foods served in restaurants, etc. 'Zero' *trans* is, however, defined as less than 0.5 g per serving, which means that if the serving is small enough (for example, an individual portion of margarine or spread served with bread in a restaurant) there could still be a significant percentage of *trans* fatty acids in the product. The United Kingdom, along with many other countries, has taken a voluntary approach in which food manufacturers have been encouraged to replace hydrogenated fats with unhydrogenated alternatives. Although initially media-led, this approach was quickly adopted by the major retailers in the UK, who all declared that hydrogenated fats were being removed from their own-label brands. Branded producers followed suit to the extent that the consumption of *trans* fatty acids in the UK has fallen considerably and is now mainly from ruminant animal sources.

3.6   The *trans* effect

The different approaches taken by each of the three countries mentioned above – Denmark, the USA and the UK – has resulted in different approaches to the replacement of hydrogenated fats and *trans* fatty acids in foods. This is particularly apparent if the United States and the United Kingdom are compared. During the years leading up to the past decade in which *trans* fatty acids have been removed, the main sources of 'solid' fats in the United States were partially hydrogenated domestic oils such as soyabean and cottonseed oils. Very little palm oil, for example, was used because in the 1980s there was a campaign against so-called 'tropical' oils such as palm oil, palm kernel oil and coconut oil, claiming that these oils were leading to high numbers of deaths from diseases such as coronary heart disease in the United States. The United Kingdom, along with many other European countries, however, was not subjected to this campaign and so palm oil was a readily accepted source of the 'solid' fat needed for applications such as bakery products. These differences have meant that there have been substantially different approaches to replacing *trans* fats in these countries.

In the United States the emphasis has largely been on replacing *trans* fatty acids and not necessarily on replacing hydrogenation. When this is coupled with the greater use of domestic oils such as soyabean and cottonseed oils and still a reluctance (although this is diminishing) to use tropical oils such as palm oil, the result has been to replace some partially hydrogenated oils with interesterified blends of fully hydrogenated and unhydrogenated oils. In the United Kingdom,

© Woodhead Publishing Limited, 2011

however, this approach would have been less successful because such oils still need to be labelled as 'hydrogenated'. The campaign against hydrogenation as a total process (irrespective of whether it resulted in *trans* fatty acids or saturates) has been such that it would be more difficult to convince the consumer that fully hydrogenated fats are acceptable from the point of view of containing no *trans* fatty acids. The result immediately after removing hydrogenated oils from products was an increased use of palm oil in their place. This led, in some instances, to an increase in saturates in products such as biscuits and pastry. The effect that this has had on the total fat and saturated fat content of different UK biscuits is shown in Table 3.16.

Table 3.16   Changes in total and saturated fat contents of selected UK biscuits

(a) Total fat as a percentage of the biscuit

Biscuit type	1998[a]	2006[b]	2008[c]	2008[d]
Cream Cracker	13.3	12.7	13.5[1]	13.5[1]
Semi-sweet biscuit (e.g. Rich Tea)	13.3	15.5	15.5[2]	15.5[2]
Digestive	20.3	21.5	21.5[3]	21.3[3]
Short sweet biscuit	21.8	n/a	24.8[4]	24.8[4]

(b) Saturated fat as a percentage of the biscuit

Biscuit type	1998[a]	2006[b]	2008[c]	2008[d]
Cream Cracker	5.42	6.5	6.2[1]	6.2[1]
Semi-sweet biscuit (e.g. Rich Tea)	6.25	7.3	7.3[2]	3.5[2]
Digestive	9.0	10.1	10.0[3]	4.8[3]
Short sweet biscuit	11.05	n/a	11.6[4]	11.6[4]

(c) Saturated fat as a percentage of total fat

Biscuit type	1998[a]	1998[a] *trans*	2006[b]	2008[c]	2008[d]
Cream Cracker	40.8	9.3	51.2	45.9[1]	45.9[1]
Semi-sweet biscuit (e.g. Rich Tea)	47.0	4.4	47.1	47.1[2]	22.6[2]
Digestive	44.3	4.7	47.0	46.5[3]	22.5[3]
Short sweet biscuit	50.7	4.1	n/a	46.8[4]	46.8[4]

[a] McCance and Widdowson (MAFF, 1998)
[b] Labelling (2006)
[c] Labelling (pre-November 2008)
[d] Labelling (post-November 2008*)
[1] Jacob's Cream Crackers
[2] McVitie's Rich Tea biscuits
[3] McVitie's Digestive biscuits
[4] Tesco Shortcake biscuits
* On 27 October 2008, United Biscuits announced that McVitie's Digestive, HobNobs and Rich Tea biscuits would contain 50% less saturated fat

© Woodhead Publishing Limited, 2011

Table 3.16(a) shows the total fat contents of four types of biscuit, a savoury biscuit (Cream Crackers) and three sweet biscuits of different total fat levels (Rich Tea, Digestive, Shortcake). Table 3.16(b) shows the saturated fat contents of these biscuits (as a percentage of the total biscuit). Table 3.16(c) shows the saturated fat (and, for 1998, the *trans*) content as a percentage of the fat phase of the biscuit. These latter figures reflect the type of dough fat that was being used. For 1998 information data was taken from McCance and Widdowson (MAFF, 1998) and is based on data collected in 1992. The data for 2006 and 2008 reflected information taken from on-pack nutritional declarations. Two sets of data are given for 2008 because, partway through that year, McVitie's, the UK market leader in biscuits, cut the amount of saturated fat in three of its plain biscuit products by 50% and has since made a further 50% reduction. Two of these products were Digestive and Rich Tea as shown in this table. The data in Table 3.16(c) is particularly relevant in terms of changes made to dough fats. The data from McCance and Widdowson (MAFF, 1998) shows the presence of 50–55% saturates plus *trans* and reflects the fact that the typical dough fat used at that time was mainly palm oil with a small amount (10–15%) of a partially hydrogenated oil. In 2006, by which time hydrogenated oils had been removed from these products, the *trans* had disappeared but, in some cases, saturates had increased, reflecting a greater use of palm oil itself as the dough fat. This effect can also be seen if we try to estimate the average fatty acid consumption over a period of time.

Gunstone (2005) took oil consumption on a global basis, subtracted from this estimates of industrial as opposed to food uses and then calculated the intake of individual fatty acids based on typical fatty acid compositions of each oil. Oil World Annual (1996–2009) publishes information on opening stocks, imports, exports and ending stocks of the major global oils and fats. From this can be calculated the 'domestic disappearance', i.e. the amount of each oil that has been used in a specific country. For the United Kingdom, information is published each year for soyabean oil, cottonseed oil, groundnut oil, sunflower oil, rapeseed oil, corn oil, olive oil, palm oil, palm kernel oil, coconut oil, butteroil, lard, fish oil, linseed oil, castor oil and 'tallow and grease'. Not all of these oils are used in food and, of course, there are other oils which are used in food which are not on the list. Nevertheless, this does allow us to calculate useful information on fatty acids intake.

Gunstone (2005) in his calculations assumes no food use for castor oil, linseed oil or fish oil and that only 50% of tallow, 85% of soyabean oil, 80% of palm oil, 80% of canola oil and 90% of sunflower oil is used in food. Doing this gives the proportion of total production which is used in food to be 79.7–80.9% – this is close to the generally recognized level of 80%. The changes in intakes of palmitic acid, oleic acid, linoleic acid and total saturates for the years 1992 to 2008 are shown in Fig. 3.8. After spending a number of years of about 20% of total fatty acid intake, between 2001 and 2005 the level of palmitic acid increased steadily until in 2005 it comprised about 23% of total fatty acids. Much of this increase was due to the replacement of partially hydrogenated oils by palm oil. Since 2005, however, there has been a reduction in the proportion of palmitic acid in total fat intake back down to about 20%. To a large extent the changes in total saturates

© Woodhead Publishing Limited, 2011

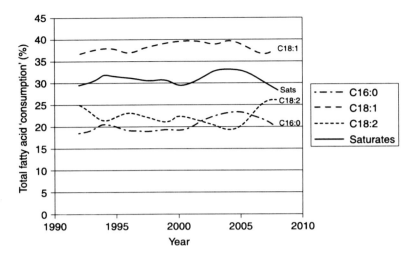

Fig. 3.8   Changes in UK fatty acid 'consumption' (1992–2008).

mirror the changes in palmitic acid levels, also showing a reduction between 2005 and 2008 as manufacturers respond to the UK Government's call for a reduction in saturated fatty acid consumption.

In the United States the trends are not so clear cut and this is because this data only considers the usages of the basic oils themselves. In the United States (Fig. 3.9) it would appear that (a) very few changes have been made between the years 1992 and 2008, and (b) consumption of saturates is much lower than in the

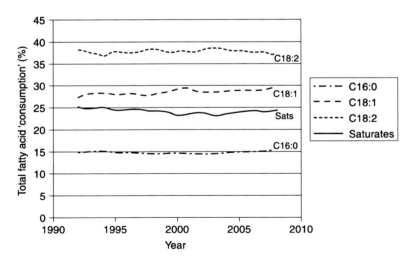

Fig. 3.9   Changes in US fatty acid 'consumption' (1992–2008).

© Woodhead Publishing Limited, 2011

UK and consumption of polyunsaturates such as linoleic acid is much higher. The data, however, takes no account of saturates or *trans* produced by hydrogenation. As has already been mentioned, a proportion of the partially hydrogenated oils originally used in the United States has been replaced by interesterified blends of fully hydrogenated and unhydrogenated oils. This data, as presented in Fig. 3.9, does not make a distinction between the two. As well as not considering saturates or *trans* fatty acids resulting from hydrogenation, the data shown in Fig. 3.8 and 3.9 also omits saturates and other fatty acids from sources other than the oils mentioned above. In other words, saturates from, for example, cocoa butter and from non-oilseed sources such as meat and dairy products (apart from butteroil, lard and tallow themselves) are not included. Despite these drawbacks the data does show, particularly for the UK, the general trends that have taken place in fatty acid consumption over this period of time.

3.7   Future trends

The major sources of saturated fat in our food and diet are likely to stay largely the same, although clearly, from the topic of this book, the amounts consumed may well decrease as consumers are encouraged to reduce their intake of saturated fat. The saturated fatty acid that is likely to show the largest increase in terms of availability may well be stearic acid. For example, cottonseed oil with high levels of stearic acid has been produced using post-transcriptional gene silencing (Liu *et al.*, 2002). Other liquid vegetable oils are also being produced in high-stearic variants using genetic modification, for example, high-stearic soyabean oil (List *et al.*, 2001) and high-stearic sunflower oil (Fernandez-Moya *et al.*, 2002). Many of these developments are taking place in North America where (a) these oils are 'domestic' oils, (b) they have been traditionally partially hydrogenated, and (c) genetic modification is an accepted process. Their introduction into Europe will be more difficult and longer term because of the reluctance in Europe to accept genetic modification as a means of producing new plant varieties.

Similarly, the use of fully hydrogenated liquid oils such as soyabean and cottonseed oils to produce stearic-rich triglycerides is also now an accepted process in the United States and, when combined with blending with unhydrogenated oils and subsequent interesterification, is seen as a potential way of replacing partial hydrogenation. While such a process may not have acceptance problems across Europe in total, it may be difficult to introduce it into those countries, such as the United Kingdom, where hydrogenation as a process (whether this be partial or total) is considered unacceptable.

In addition to these plant and process changes, clinical nutrition may also show that stearic acid is the most acceptable of saturated fatty acids from a health point of view. There are indications of this in a number of papers suggesting that stearic acid has a fairly neutral effect on blood cholesterol levels (German and Dillard, 2004; Sanders and Berry, 2005).

© Woodhead Publishing Limited, 2011

3.8   Sources of further information and advice

Reference has been made in this chapter to *The Lipid Handbook* (Gunstone *et al.*, 1994). A new edition of this definitive text is now available (Gunstone *et al.*, 2007) and contains a wealth of analytical and compositional information on both vegetable and animal fats. *Modifying lipids for use in food* (Gunstone, 2006) contains very useful sections on the main processes used to modify oils and fats – hydrogenation, fractionation and interesterification. More detailed information on fats that are used in confectionery (which tend to be largely solid, more saturated fats such as cocoa butter, palm oil and the lauric fats) can be found in *Science and technology of enrobed and filled chocolate, confectionery and bakery products* (Talbot, 2009).

In addition to these textual sources of information, the main global producers of oils and fats (for example, ADM, Cargill, AAK, Loders Croklaan, Fuji Oils) are all excellent sources of information on oils, products and processes.

3.9   References

Beckett ST (2009). 'Chocolate manufacture' in *Science and technology of enrobed and filled chocolate, confectionery and bakery products* ed. Talbot G. Woodhead Publishing, Cambridge, pp 12–14.

Best RL, Crossley A, Paul S, Pardun H, Soeters CJ (1956). 'Improvements in or relating to cocoa butter substitutes'. *GB Patent 827.172.*

Bézard JA (1971). 'The component triglycerides of palm kernel oil' *Lipids* 6, 630–4.

Bézard JA, Bugaut M, Clement G (1971). 'Triglyceride composition of coconut oil'. *J. Am. Oil Chem. Soc.* **48**, 134–9.

Bhattacharyya AS, Bhattacharyya DK (1991). 'Enzymatic acidolysis of sal fat and its fractions'. *Oléagineux* **46**, 509–13.

Bracco U, Rostagno W, Egli EH (1970). 'A study of cocoa butter–illipe butter mixtures'. *International Chocolate Review* **25**, 41–8.

Breckenbridge WC, Marai L, Kuksis A (1969). 'Triglyceride structure of human milk fat'. *Canadian J. Biochem.* **47**.

Brooker BE (1996). 'The Role of Fat in the Stabilisation of Gas Cells in Bread Dough'. *Journal of Cereal Science* **24**(3), 187–98.

Chacko GK, Perkins EG (1965). 'Anatomical variation in fatty acid composition and triglyceride distribution in animal depot fats'. *J. Am. Oil Chem. Soc.* **42**, 1121–4.

Chaiseri S, Dimick PS (1989). 'Lipid and hardness characteristics of cocoa butter from different geographical areas'. *J. Am. Oil Chem. Soc.* **66**, 1771–6.

Chambon M (1996). 'Milk Fat' in *Oils and Fats Manual* Volume 1, 277–86, ed Karleskind A. Intercept Ltd., Andover, United Kingdom.

Commodity Online (2010). 'Philippines remains world's top coconut oil exporter'. http://www.commodityonline.com/news/Philippines-remains-worlds-top-coconut-oil-exporter-25294-3-1.html. Accessed 3 February, 2010.

Danish Veterinary and Food Administration (2003). Executive Order No. 160 of 11 March 2003 on the Content of Trans Fatty Acids in Oils and Fats.

Dekeloil (2010). 'Palm Oil Global Market'. http://www.dekeloil.com/nrg_pl_global%20market.html. Accessed 3 February, 2010.

Deman L, Deman JM (1983). 'Trans fatty acids in milk fat' *J. Am. Oil Chem. Soc.* **60**, 1095–8.

© Woodhead Publishing Limited, 2011

European Union (2000) 'Directive 2000/36/EC on Cocoa Products and Chocolate' Published 23 June 2000.

Fernandez-Moya V, Martinez-Force E, Garces R (2002). 'Temperature effect on a high stearic acid sunflower mutant'. *Phytochemistry*, **59**(1), 33–7.

Fife B (2010). 'Red palm oil: A daily dose of vitamins from a cooking oil'. http://www.americanpalmoil.com/publications/Red%20Palm%20Oil.pdf. Accessed 5 August 2010.

Food and Drug Administration, 2003. 'Food Labeling; Trans Fatty Acids in Nutrition Labeling; Consumer Research to Consider Nutrient Content and Health Claims and Possible Footnote or Disclosure Statements; Final Rule and Proposed Rule.' *Federal Register – 68 FR 41433 July 11, 2003.*

German JB and Dillard CJ (2004). 'Saturated fats: what dietary intake?' *Am. J. Clin. Nutr.,* **80**(3), 550–9.

Global Oils & Fats Business Magazine (2009) 'Malaysian Palm Oil Industry Performance 2008' vol. 6, issue 1 (Jan–March).

Gunstone FD (1987). *Palm Oil Critical Reports on Applied Chemistry*. Vol. 15. Published for the Society of Chemical Industry by John Wiley and Sons.

Gunstone FD, Harwood JL, Padley FB (1994) *The Lipid Handbook 2nd Edition,* Chapman and Hall, London.

Gunstone FD (2005). 'Fatty acid production for human consumption'. *Inform,* **16**, 736–7.

Gunstone FD (2006). *Modifying lipids for use in foods.* Woodhead Publishing, Cambridge.

Gunstone FD, Harwood JL, Dijkstra AJ (2007). *The Lipid Handbook, 3rd Edition,* CRC Press, Boca Raton, USA.

Han NM, Top AGM, May CY, Hgan MA (2006). 'Palm tocols (tocopherols and tocotrienols) as standard reference materials'. *Malaysian Palm Oil Board Information Series,* June 2006, ISSH 1511–7871.

ICCO (2009). *Quarterly Bulletin of Cocoa Statistics* Vol. XXXV, no. 4, Cocoa year 2008/09. Published 3 December 2009.

Illingworth D, Bissell TG (1994). 'Anhydrous milkfat products and applications in recombination' in *Fats in Food Products*, chapter 4, ed. Moran DPJ and Rajah KK. Blackie Academic and Professional. Glasgow.

Jurriens G (1968). 'Analysis of Triglycerides' in *Analysis and Characterisation of Oils and Fats for Fat Products'*, Vol. 2 ed. Boekenoogen HA. Intersciences Publishers, London, New York, Sydney.

Lipp M, Anklam E (1998). 'Review of cocoa butter and alternative fats for use in chocolate – Part A. Compositional data.' *Food Chemistry*. **62**, 73–97.

List GR, Pelloso T, Orthoefer F, Warner K, Neff WE (2001). 'Soft margarines from high stearic acid soybean oils'. *J. Am. Oil Chem. Soc.* **78**(1), 103–4.

Liu Q, Singh S, Green A (2002). 'High-Oleic and High-Stearic Cottonseed Oils: Nutritionally Improved Cooking Oils Developed Using Gene Silencing'. *Journal of the American College of Nutrition,* **21**(3), 205S–211S.

Marai L, Breckenbridge WC, Kuksis A (1969). 'Specific distribution of fatty acids in the milk fat triglycerides of goat and sheep'. *Lipids,* **4**, 562–70.

MAFF (1998). 'Fatty Acids, Supplement to McCance and Widdowson's The Composition of Foods', Ministry of Agriculture Fisheries and Food, London.

Malaysian Palm Oil Council (2008). 'Malaysian Palm Oil Industry Performance, 2007'. *Global Oils and Fats Business Magazine* **5**(1), 1–8.

Mensink RP, Zock PL, Kester AD, Katan MB (2003). 'Effects of dietary fatty acids and carbohydrates on the ratio of total to HDL cholesterol and on serum lipids and apolipoproteins: a meta-analysis of 60 controlled trials'. *Am. J. Clin. Nutr.* **77**, 1146–55.

Nor Aini I, Miskandar MS (2007). 'Utilization of palm oil and palm products in shortenings and margarines'. *Eur. J. Lipid Sci. Technol.* **109**(4) 422–32.

Oil World (1996–2009). *Consumption of Oils and Fats.* ISTA Mielke GmbH, Hamburg.

Parodi PW (1982). 'Positional distribution of fatty acids in triglycerides from milk of several species of mammals'. *Lipids* **17**, 437–43.

© Woodhead Publishing Limited, 2011

REA Holdings (2010). 'Oils and Fats Market'. http://www.rea.co.uk/market/. Accessed 15 March 2010.

Rossell JB, King B, Downes MJ (1983). 'Detection of Adulteration'. *J. Am. Oil Chem. Soc.* **60**, 333–9.

Rossell JB, King B, Downes MF (1985). 'Composition of oil'. *J. Am. Oil Chem. Soc.* **60**, 221–30.

Sanders TAB, Berry SEE (2005). 'Influence of stearic acid on postprandial lipemia and hemostatic function'. *Lipids*, **40**(12), 1221–7.

Sawadogo K, Bézard J (1982). 'Étude de la structure glyceridique du beurre de karité'. *Oléagineux*, **37**, 69–74.

Sridhar R, Lakshminarayana G (1991). 'Triacylglycerol compositions of some vegetable fats with potential for preparation of cocoa butter equivalents by high performance liquid chromatography'. *J. Oil Tech. Asssoc. Of India*, **23**, 42–3.

Sundram K (2009). 'Combating Vitamin A deficiency through red palm oil'. *International Workshop on Micronutrients and Child Health*. 20–23 October 2009, New Delhi, India.

Talbot G (2006). *Application of Fats in Confectionery*. Kennedy's Publications, London.

Talbot G (2009). 'Compound coatings' in *Science and technology of enrobed and filled chocolate, confectionery and bakery products'* ed. Talbot G. Woodhead Publishing, Cambridge, Chapter 5.

Talbot G, Slager H (2010). 'Fats to Revel In'. *World of Food Ingredients*, April 2010.

Talbot G, 't Zand I (2006). 'Increased industrial use of palm oleine'. *Food Engineering and Ingredients* **31**(3), 34–5.

Timms RE, Parekh JV (1980). 'The possibilities for using hydrogenated, fractionated or interesterified milk fat in chocolate'. *Lebensm. Wiss. Technol.*, **13**, 177–81.

Weyland M (1992). 'Cocoa butter fractions: a novel way of optimizing chocolate performance'. Lecture given at the *Pennsylvania Manufacturing Confectioners' Asssociation 46th Annual Production Conference*, Hershey, PA, 28 April.

Wong Soon (1991). *Speciality Fats versus Cocoa Butter*. Malaysia.

© Woodhead Publishing Limited, 2011

4

Health aspects of saturated fatty acids

J. I. Pedersen, University of Oslo, Norway and B. Kirkhus, Nofima – Food, Fisheries and Aquacultural Research, Norway

Abstract: This chapter presents an overview of the arguments linking intake of saturated fatty acids (SFA) to plasma cholesterol and development of atherosclerosis, the basis of cardiovascular diseases (CVD) like coronary heart disease (CHD) and stroke. A short description of atherosclerosis and the role of low-density lipoprotein (LDL) cholesterol as well as effects of dietary fatty acids on the concentration of total and LDL cholesterol are given with emphasis on the dominating role of palmitic acid in this regard. Effects of fatty acids on haemostasis and inflammation, important elements in atherosclerosis, are also discussed. An overview of the evidence linking LDL cholesterol to CHD is given based on animal, clinical, epidemiological and intervention studies. Possible involvement of SFA in the development of obesity, the metabolic syndrome, type 2 diabetes and cancer is discussed. Finally, the background for the current recommendations of SFA intake is given. These all conclude that limitation in SFA intake is necessary if we are to combat the CVD epidemic.

Key words: saturated fatty acids, cholesterol, lipoproteins, atherosclerosis, cardiovascular disease.

4.1 Introduction

For more than half a century saturated fat has been at the centre of interest in discussions on nutrition and dietary recommendations. All over the developed world people have been advised to reduce total – and in particular saturated – fat in the diet. The food industry has followed this up by marketing low-fat products and designing foods with altered fat composition. The reason behind this trend is the supposed links between saturated fat intake, plasma cholesterol and atherosclerosis, the pathologic basis for cardiovascular diseases (CVD). This is in its simplest form the so-called 'lipid hypothesis' of CVD. We now know that this pathological process is far more complicated. Although most prevalent in rich countries, CVD, like coronary heart disease (CHD), also termed ischemic heart

© Woodhead Publishing Limited, 2011

disease (IHD), and stroke, is a global epidemic and responsible for about one-third of all deaths worldwide (WHO, 2005). Altering dietary fat intake, both quantitatively and qualitatively, is seen as one of the most important aspects of prevention of these diseases and the rationale for this will be discussed in the following sections.

4.2   Atherosclerosis as the basis for cardiovascular diseases (CVD)

4.2.1   The lipid hypothesis in atherogenesis

This hypothesis was generated more than 100 years ago when it was found that feeding high-fat diets and cholesterol to animals resulted in atherosclerosis (for an historical overview see Stamler, 1992). The relationship between blood cholesterol and CHD was strengthened by observations that people with genetically high blood cholesterol (familial hypercholesterolemia) died from CHD at young age. Subsequently it was found that intake of fat and cholesterol influenced the level of plasma cholesterol. In particular, the systematic studies by Keys (1984), Hegsted (1986) and others during the 1950s established the basis for our current understanding of how different fatty acids influence plasma cholesterol. At the population level mean plasma cholesterol is mainly determined by the amount and the quality of fat in the diet. There is a strong positive association between intake of saturated fat and mean cholesterol level between populations (Fig. 4.1; Keys, 1970, Kromhout *et al.*, 1995). Within populations, however, such association has not been possible to demonstrate. The reason is that the biological and analytical variability in plasma cholesterol is larger than variability in fat intake within the population (Keys, 1988). In addition, methods for determining dietary intake have large measuring errors leading to considerable misclassification (Bingham *et al.*, 2003, Prentice, 2003).

4.2.2   Lipoproteins and their role in atherogenesis

The uptake, transport and utilization of dietary lipids require them to be transformed into water-soluble forms. The processes involved are highly complicated (Williams, 2008). Lipids circulate in plasma in the form of lipoprotein particles, among which cholesterol is distributed. These lipoproteins have different functional and pathological significance. They are characterized according to size and density (Table 4.1). They are composed of different proteins, apolipoproteins, facing towards the aqueous face together with other hydrophilic groups (OH, phosphate etc) and containing hydrophobic elements like triacylglycerol (triglyceride (TG)) and cholesterol ester (CE) in the core part. Chylomicrons (CM) that contain about 85% triglycerides and only 2% protein are the largest and have the lowest density. Low-density lipoproteins (LDL) are the most cholesterol-rich lipoproteins. They are derived from circulating very low-density lipoproteins (VLDL) as these lose their TG content. LDL transports cholesterol from the liver

© Woodhead Publishing Limited, 2011

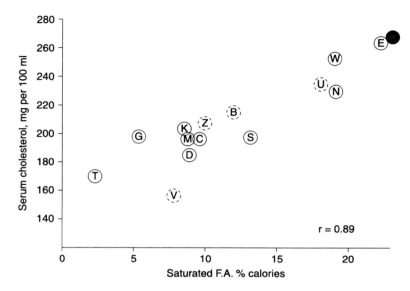

Fig. 4.1 Average percentage of total energy from saturated fatty acids in the diets plotted against median serum cholesterol values of the cohorts (represented by different letters) of the Seven Countries Study (Keys, 1970). The filled circle represents the results from a group of 20 men, 40–49 years selected at random in 1973 before recruitment to the Oslo diet and smoking study. The fatty acids in the diet were chemically analysed by the so called double portion method (G. Riis, Master thesis, University of Oslo 1978).

Table 4.1 Characteristics of the most important lipoproteins

	Chylomicrons	VLDL	LDL	HDL
Density (g/mL)	0.95	0.95–1.006	1.019–1.063	1.063–1.210
Diameter (nm)	>70	30–80	18–22	5–12
Triglyceride (%)	85	50	10	8
Cholesterol (free and esterified) (%)	4	22	48	20
Phospholipid (%)	7	20	22	22
Protein (%)	2	10	20	50
Apolipoproteins	B48, CII, E	B100, CII, E	B100	A1, A2, CI, CIII, E

to peripheral cells. High-density lipoprotein (HDL) contains over 50% protein and has the highest density. This particle is supposed to transport cholesterol from peripheral cells and tissues to the liver for excretion, the so-called reverse cholesterol transport (Cuchel and Rader, 2006). In addition to lipoproteins, a small amount of non-esterified fatty acids circulate in the plasma bound to albumin.

© Woodhead Publishing Limited, 2011

4.2.3   Low density lipoprotein (LDL) as the pathogenetic factor

The LDL particle is generally considered the pathogenetic factor in atherogenesis and small dense LDL particles appear to be particularly pathogenic (Berneis and Krauss, 2002). The particles are susceptible to structural modifications by oxidation, particularly the small dense LDL particles. Increased circulating oxLDL concentrations have been related to cardiovascular disease in some studies (Holvoet et al., 2003, Verhove et al., 2009), but the role of circulating oxLDL needs further investigation. At high concentrations LDL particles have the ability to pass through the endothelial cell layer lining the inner vessel wall, possibly after some form of injury to the endothelial cells (Ross 1999, Libby et al., 2009), where they are modified by oxidation or other chemical reactions and taken up in white blood cells or macrophages. These enlarge and become so-called foam cells that may eventually burst and leave their cholesterol-containing content in the vessel wall with atheroma formation and aggravation of the inflammatory process. As lipid accumulation and inflammation progress, different cell types, such as white blood cells, smooth muscle cells and fibroblasts, are recruited and there is formation of fibrous material and calcification in order to delimit the process. This encapsulation process may be more or less stable. It may rupture, empty its content into the vessel and precipitate a clot or thrombus formation, thus inhibiting blood flow. If this happens in a coronary artery the result may be a myocardial infarction; if it happens in an artery to the brain the result may be a stroke.

There is a strong correlation between LDL cholesterol and total cholesterol. Determination of either is thus a marker of total amount of LDL particle mass. A high concentration of total or LDL cholesterol is associated with high risk of CHD (Castelli, 1984, Martin et al., 1986). It is of interest, however, that even if the relative risk may be the same in different populations, the absolute risk at the same cholesterol level may vary considerably between populations even if corrections are made for smoking and blood pressure (Kromhout, 1999). This illustrates that there must be several other factors in addition to LDL cholesterol that influence risk.

4.2.4   The protective role of high density lipoprotein (HDL)

The HDL particle is associated with decreased risk of CHD (Castelli, 1984). A low concentration is associated with metabolic disturbances characterized by increased concentration of triglycerides, impaired glucose tolerance and insulin sensitivity, obesity and often high blood pressure – a cluster of risk factors now defined as the metabolic syndrome (see section 4.6.2 below). Lack of physical activity and smoking is also associated with low HDL cholesterol. A low concentration of HDL cholesterol is thus both a risk indicator and a metabolic marker. However, it has not been documented that altering HDL cholesterol by drugs or diet influences the risk of CHD (Briel et al., 2009). It now appears that the association between HDL cholesterol and risk is more complicated than has been anticipated (van der Steeg et al., 2008, Genest, 2008). The primary target for risk reduction by dietary fat should therefore still be LDL or total cholesterol (Briel et al., 2009).

© Woodhead Publishing Limited, 2011

4.2.5   The roles of other lipoproteins

VLDL and CM are the largest lipoproteins and rich in triglycerides (TG). It has long been debated whether TG is a risk factor for CHD. A high concentration of TG is part of the metabolic risk cluster (see section 4.6.2 below) and when HDL is adjusted for in prospective studies, TG no longer appears as an independent risk factor (Di Angelantonio *et al.*, 2009). Lipoprotein (a) is an LDL-like particle that is independently associated with risk of CHD. It is strongly genetically determined and only to a minor degree influenced by diet.

4.3   Effects of individual fatty acids on plasma total cholesterol, LDL cholesterol, HDL cholesterol and triglycerides (VLDL)

4.3.1   Effects of saturated fatty acids (SFA), monounsaturated (MUFA), polyunsaturated (PUFA) and *trans* fatty acids (TFA)

A large number of metabolic studies have been performed during the last 50 years to establish the effects of fat and fatty acids on the concentration of cholesterol in plasma.[1] It should be mentioned that if a group of individuals are given the same diet over a certain time (plasma cholesterol will stabilize after two to three weeks) the cholesterol values will be almost normally distributed. The cholesterol level is dependent on our genes and the variability among individuals is substantial (Keys, 1988). Also the response to change in diet will differ: some will react more strongly than others and some may not react at all. When we are talking about the effects of fatty acids on plasma cholesterol we are accordingly talking about change in a group of individuals. This being said we now have a fairly precise picture of the effects of different fatty acids on plasma cholesterol. Both Keys (1984) and Hegsted (1986) showed that SFA (lauric, C12:0, myristic, C14:0, and palmitic acid, C16:0) increased serum cholesterol when replacing carbohydrates in the diet. They further showed that PUFA (linoleic acid, C18:2, and α-linolenic acid, C18:3) decreased serum cholesterol, but the decreasing effect was only about half the increasing effect of saturated fat. MUFA (oleic acid, C18:1) was neutral and dietary cholesterol had only a small effect. By regression analysis, predictive equations have been developed and that of Keys (1984) is the most well known:

$$\Delta \text{ cholesterol} = 1.35(2\Delta S - \Delta P) + \sqrt{Z} \qquad [4.1]$$

Δ cholesterol is the change in plasma cholesterol in mg/100 mL. ΔS and ΔP are the changes in SFA (C12:0 – C16:0) and PUFA (C18:2 and C18:3) expressed as % of energy intake, Z is the change in dietary cholesterol expressed as mg/1000 kcal. In those early experiments the effects of TFA were not explored systematically.

---

[1] The concentration of cholesterol in plasma is generally performed on serum. Since the difference between plasma and serum cholesterol is insignificant both expressions are used.

© Woodhead Publishing Limited, 2011

Much later the important paper by Mensink and Katan (1990) documented that elaidic acid (*trans* C18:1) also increases LDL cholesterol.

From intervention studies, reviews and large meta-analyses we now have solid knowledge on the effects of individual dietary fatty acids on blood cholesterol (Clarke *et al.*, 1997, Mensink *et al.*, 2003, Yu *et al.*, 1995, Müller *et al.*, 2001, Sanders, 2009). The different saturated fatty acids have very different effects. The short and medium chain fatty acids (in particular C8:0 and C10:0) are generally considered to have no or insignificant effect on serum cholesterol (St-Onge *et al.*, 2008) although there are studies reporting the contrary (Tholstrup *et al.*, 2004). Also stearic acid (C18:0) has no effect on cholesterol. In most studies lauric acid (C12:0) has been found to only moderately increase cholesterol, but most of this increase may be due to an increase in HDL cholesterol (Mensink *et al.*, 2003). Myristic acid (C14:0) is the most potent cholesterol-increasing fatty acid and increases both LDL cholesterol and HDL cholesterol. Palmitic acid (C16:0) also increases LDL cholesterol and to a minor extent HDL cholesterol, whereas the *trans* C18:1 increases total and LDL cholesterol to about the same extent as palmitic acid (Fig. 4.2). *Trans* fatty acids also decrease HDL cholesterol (Mensink and Katan 1990, Almendingen *et al.*, 1995). This decreasing effect on HDL is unusual since the saturated fatty acids C12:0 to C16:0 all increase HDL (Mensink *et al.*, 2003). It is common to judge health effects of fatty acids according to their

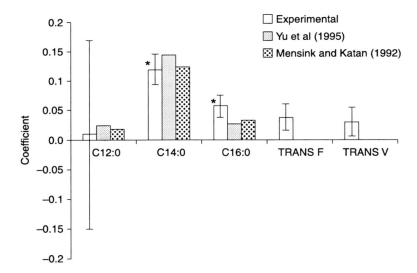

Fig. 4.2 Coefficients of individual cholesterol-increasing fatty acids obtained by constrained linear regression and expressed as mmol total cholesterol/L per energy % change in fatty acid intake (Müller *et al.*, 2001). The standard deviations are calculated by jack-knifing (*regression coefficients are significantly different from zero, p < 0.05). TRANS F = *trans* fatty acids from partially hydrogenated fish oils, TRANS V = *trans* fatty acids from partially hydrogenated vegetable oils. Regression coefficients for individual saturated fatty acids published by Yu *et al.* (1995) and Mensink and Katan (1992) are shown for comparison.

© Woodhead Publishing Limited, 2011

effects on the ratio of total cholesterol to HDL cholesterol (Mensink *et al.*, 2003). Even if the ratio of total to HDL cholesterol in plasma strongly predicts the risk of CHD (Di Angelantonio *et al.*, 2009), identifying health effects of fatty acids according to their effects on the ratio of total to HDL cholesterol may be premature, however, and possibly not relevant (see section 4.2.4). Replacing carbohydrates by SFA will to some extent reduce fasting levels of TG (Mensink *et al.*, 2003). The significance of a high carbohydrate/low fat diet is further discussed in section 4.8.

4.3.2   Effects of palmitic acid

The dietary SFA comprises the whole series of chain lengths, short- and medium-chain fatty acids C4:0 to C10:0, long-chain fatty acids C12:0 to C18:0, and a very small amount of very long-chain fatty acids C20:0–C24.0 (Table 4.2). Most SFA in the Western diet is derived from animal food, meat and dairy products. A smaller part is derived from vegetable sources, e.g. medium-chain fatty acids from coconut and palm kernel oil, long-chain fatty acids from palm oil and stearic acid from cocoa butter, shea fat and fully hydrogenated oils. Palm oil has become an important source of saturated fat in recent years due to its replacement of *trans* fatty acids in the food industry.

In the Western diet myristic acid (C14:0) makes up about 10% of the SFA (Table 4.3) while palmitic acid (C16:0) makes up more than 50%. Even if myristic acid is more cholesterol increasing than the others, the much higher amount in the diet makes palmitic acid the most important cholesterol-increasing fatty acid in the Western diet. This was mentioned by Keys *et al.* (1965) as early as the 1960s. Animal fat, in particular dairy fat, counts for the major part of palmitic acid in the diet but replacement of partially hydrogenated fat (*trans* fat) by palm oil has made margarine and other industrially processed foods an important source. Palmitic acid from palm oil may contribute to serum cholesterol in the population to about the same degree as palmitic acid from meat (Fig. 4.3). From a nutritional point of view the use of palm oil as a replacement for partially hydrogenated fat should be reduced.

Table 4.2   Common SFA in food fats and oils

Common name	Systematic name	Abbreviation	Typical sources
Butyric	Butanoic	C4:0	Dairy fat
Caproic	Hexanoic	C6:0	Dairy fat
Caprylic	Octanoic	C8:0	Dairy fat, coconut oil, palm kernel oil
Capric	Decanoic	C10:0	Dairy fat, coconut oil, palm kernel oil
Lauric	Dodecanoic	C12:0	Dairy fat, coconut oil, palm kernel oil
Myristic	Tetradecanoic	C14:0	Dairy fat, coconut oil, palm kernel oil
Palmitic	Hexadecanoic	C16:0	Most animal fats and vegetable oils
Stearic	Octadecanoic	C18:0	Most animal fats and vegetable oils
Arachidic	Eicosanoic	C20:0	Peanut oil
Behenic	Docosanoic	C22:0	Trace amounts in certain seed fats
Lignoceric	Tetracosanoic	C24:0	Trace amounts in certain seed fats

© Woodhead Publishing Limited, 2011

Table 4.3   Distribution of saturated fatty acids in the US diet

Fatty acid	% of total fat	% of total SFA
	Mean	Mean
C4:0–C10:0	2.1	6.0
C12:0	1.0	2.8
C14:0	3.2	9.1
C16:0	19.3	54.8
C18:0	9.0	25.6
Total SFA	35.2	

Source: Allison *et al.*, 1999

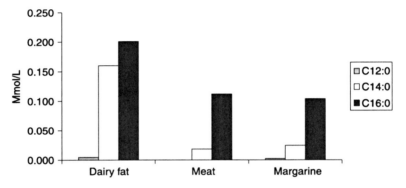

Fig. 4.3   Estimated contribution of lauric, myristic and palmitic acid in the Norwegian diet to serum total cholesterol. The results are expressed as change in serum cholesterol (mmol/L) when carbohydrate corresponding to 20% of energy is replaced by fatty acids. Based on food disappearance data for 2002 and margarine composition in 2008. Estimations according to Müller *et al.*, 2001 and Pedersen and Kirkhus, unpublished.

Fully hydrogenated and interesterified vegetable oils to increase the content of stearic acid at the expense of palmitic acid might be a better alternative (Pedersen and Kirkhus, 2008). Predictive equations based on how individual fatty acids affect serum cholesterol (see section 4.3.1 above) would be a valuable tool in product development, making it possible to optimize the fatty acid composition of margarines as well as other fat-containing products (Müller *et al.*, 2001, Pedersen *et al.*, 2003).

4.4   Effects of fatty acids on other biomarkers related to coronary heart disease (CHD)

It is now recognized that the original 'lipid hypothesis in atherosclerosis' is too simplistic and that many pathological processes in addition to atheroma formation may be involved in CHD such as thrombotic processes, inflammation, formation of oxygen reactive species (ROS), factors affecting blood pressure, arrhythmia,

© Woodhead Publishing Limited, 2011

etc. Particular interest has focused on the effects of fatty acids on haemostasis and inflammation.

4.4.1   Haemostatic factors

Thrombus formation or blood clotting that stops the blood flow in a coronary artery is a common complication of atherosclerosis leading to myocardial infarction. In the body there is a complex balance between factors promoting clot formation and clot dissolution or fibrinolysis. There is evidence that some of these factors, such as Factor VII, fibrinogen and plasminogen activator inhibitor-1 (PAI-1), are associated with increased risk of CVD. The effects of fatty acid intake on these factors have been difficult to study and the data are too conflicting to draw definitive conclusions (for a review see Lefevre *et al.*, 2004). Differences in *ex vivo* platelet aggregation in small population groups have been found to be associated with SFA intake and in particular with stearic acid (Renaud *et al.*, 1986). It should be noted, however, that the intake of SFA was very high in these groups and the variation in stearic acid very small (less than 2% of energy). Also, dietary studies have not confirmed increased tendencies of platelet aggregation with diets high in stearic acid (Lefevre *et al.*, 2004). High SFA intake may moderately increase Factor VII coagulant activity and thus contribute to risk of CVD. Intake of dietary fat is followed by an increase in large triglyceride-rich particles. This postprandial lipemia is reported to have an effect on the haemostatic status and in particular on the activation of Factor VII (Duttaroy, 2005). The importance of the dietary fatty acid composition for this postprandial effect is still unclear, however (Lefevre *et al.*, 2004, Duttaroy, 2005).

4.4.2   Markers of inflammation

Inflammation appears to be an integral part of the atherosclerotic process (Ross, 1999, Libby *et al.*, 2009). The effects of saturated fatty acids on inflammatory markers have so far only been studied *in vitro*. Thus palmitate (esters of palmitic acid) has been shown to induce expression of interleukin-6 (IL-6) in human myotubes (Weigert *et al.*, 2004), endothelial cells (Staiger *et al.*, 2004) and adipocytes (Ajuwon and Spurlock, 2005). Furthermore, both palmitate and stearate induce the proinflammatory cytokines TNF-α, IL-1ß and IL-8 in human macrophages (Håversen *et al.*, 2009). The relevance of these findings for the *in vivo* situation must await further studies, however.

4.5   Evidence linking LDL cholesterol to the development of atherosclerosis and CHD

4.5.1   Animal experiments

Since the initial animal studies by Anitschkow 100 years ago, hypercholesterolemia and atherosclerosis have been induced by cholesterol and fat feeding in virtually every species of laboratory animals (Stamler, 1992). Of special interest are

© Woodhead Publishing Limited, 2011

experiments in primates, where it has been possible to induce serious atheroclerosis and myocardial infarction after a relatively short time feeding with an ordinary high-fat western diet (Taylor *et al.*, 1962).

4.5.2   Clinical observations

The most well-known example is that of familial hypercholesterolemia, a genetic disorder affecting the LDL receptor (Yuan *et al.*, 2006), the discovery of which was awarded the Nobel price in 1985. The reduced uptake of cholesterol in the liver results in high serum cholesterol and development of CHD leading to myocardial infarction at young age. Those that are homozygote for the defect may die from myocardial infarction in early childhood.

4.5.3   Epidemiological studies

Identification of risk factors: plasma cholesterol, one of several risk factors
A large number of prospective cohort studies in different parts of the world have identified modifiable risk factors such as smoking, high blood pressure and serum cholesterol. Although the relative risk associated with serum cholesterol, after correcting for smoking and blood pressure, is the same between different populations, the absolute risk may be very different. The risk of dying from a myocardial infarction is thus five times higher in northern Europe than in the Mediterranean region or in Japan at the same cholesterol level (Kromhout *et al.*, 1995, Kromhout, 1999). This shows that there must be other factors that modify the risk of cholesterol. Such factors may be physical activity, intake of fruits and vegetables, fish, *trans* fatty acids, etc.

Associations between dietary fatty acids and CHD
Considering the strong effect of saturated fatty acids on serum cholesterol one would assume that there would be a strong association between intake of saturated fat and risk of CHD. In the Seven Countries Study (Keys, 1970, Kromhout, 1999) as well as in international comparisons (Artaud-Wild *et al.*, 1993) (so-called ecological studies) this correlation has been very high (Fig. 4.4). However, such comparisons may be distorted by other factors than those under study, so-called confounders, and may thus not disclose a true picture. Prospective cohort studies are generally considered to be more reliable. Some recent meta-analyses of such studies have failed to find consistent associations between intake of saturated fat and risk of CHD (Skeaff and Miller, 2009, Siri-Tarino *et al.*, 2010). This does not mean, however, that no such association exists. One problem with these studies is the adjustment for confounders, as seriously criticized in an editorial to the most recent of these meta-analyses (Stamler, 2010). A major error in that analysis is adjustment for serum cholesterol in six of the 16 studies that included CHD as endpoint. SFA strongly affect serum cholesterol, which means that adjustment for serum cholesterol will bias the results of the meta-analyses towards finding no association

© Woodhead Publishing Limited, 2011

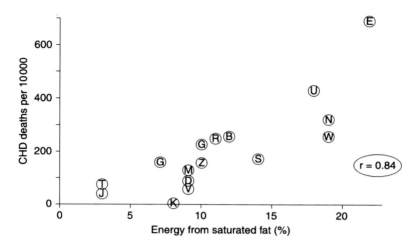

Fig. 4.4   Correlation between mean saturated fat intake and number of CHD deaths in the cohorts of the Seven Countries Study after ten years' follow-up. Each circle represents the mean of a cohort (adapted from Keys, 1980).

between dietary saturated fat intake and CHD. Another major problem with studies on the effects of diet on health outcomes is the difficulty of obtaining reliable data for food intake. The misclassification is considerable (Bingham *et al.*, 2003, Prentice, 2003). Any misclassification or random errors in the measurements will most likely result in reduced association compared to any truly existing association. This means that the finding of even a small association may be of importance. Finally, as mentioned above (section 4.2.1), the small variation in fat intake within a population compared to the large biological variation in serum cholesterol contributes to the lack of finding an association between SFA and CHD.

Changing one nutrient will inevitably result in change in another and when investigating the effect of exchanging saturated fat with other nutrients it has been convincingly shown that replacing SFA by PUFA is associated with a reduction in CHD risk (Jacobsen *et al.*, 2009). Replacing SFA by carbohydrates increases the risk slightly, while replacing by monounsaturated fat (oleic acid) has no effect (Jacobsen *et al.*, 2009).

4.5.4   Intervention studies

Dietary interventions
In the 1960s and 1970s both secondary and primary prevention studies were performed. The dietary modification was based on reducing SFA and increasing PUFA in order to reduce total cholesterol. The Oslo secondary prevention study (Leren, 1970) and the Los Angeles Veterans Administration study with elderly men (Dayton *et al.*, 1969) both resulted in reduction of serum cholesterol (13% and 14% compared to the controls, respectively) and a significant reduction in atherosclerotic events, although no significant reduction in mortality. The Finnish mental hospital

© Woodhead Publishing Limited, 2011

study, which was a cross-over study that lasted for 12 years, also showed that during the periods on low SFA and high PUFA the event rate and CHD mortality were significantly reduced (Miettinen *et al.*, 1972). The most successful of all dietary intervention studies was the so-called Oslo Diet and Smoking Study (Hjermann *et al.*, 1981). Intervention with a diet low in total and saturated fat and attempts to reduce smoking resulted after five years in a 13% reduction in serum cholesterol and 47% reduction in CHD events. By following the individuals for another 3.5 years reduction in mortality also became significant (Hjermann *et al.*, 1986). It was estimated that 59% of the effect could be accounted for by reduction in serum cholesterol and 24% by reduced smoking while 17% remained unexplained (Holme *et al.*, 1985).

Interventions at national level
In most Western countries the populations have been advised to change their lifestyles in order to reduce the burden of chronic diseases, CHD in particular. CHD mortality has declined in these countries during the last 30 to 40 years. The estimated contribution of reduction in serum cholesterol to this decline has in most studies been around 35% (Kuulasmaa *et al.*, 2000, Ford *et al.*, 2007, Aspelund *et al.*, 2009). The most remarkable result of the population strategy has been seen in Finland, where mortality from CHD has shifted from being the highest in the world to now being among the lowest. It has been estimated that reduction in serum cholesterol due to reduced intake of saturated fat, in particular milk fat, and increase in intake of PUFA can explain most of this decline (Puska, 2009). Similarly, in Norway dietary changes with reduction in saturated and *trans* fat (dairy and margarine) and increase in PUFA and the resulting cholesterol reduction can explain a major part of the decline in CHD mortality (Pedersen *et al.*, 2004).

Interventions with cholesterol-reducing drugs
Statins are a group of drugs that inhibit the synthesis of cholesterol, thereby reducing serum total and LDL cholesterol. An impressive reduction in CHD mortality has been observed in long-term clinical intervention studies both in individuals with previous CHD (secondary prevention studies) (Scandinavian Simvastatin Survival Study, 1994) and in individuals free of disease at entry (primary prevention studies) (Shepherd *et al.*, 1995). A large number of similar studies with different statins show similar results. This has led to an almost unanimous acceptance of LDL cholesterol as a causative factor in atherosclerotic disease (Thompson, 2009).

4.6   Effects of saturated fatty acids (SFA) on disease states related to CVD

4.6.1   Obesity
It is a general belief that high-fat diets promote overweight and obesity. In fact, obesity is prevalent in populations with high-fat (and high-sugar) diets while it is less prevalent in poor populations with low-fat/high-carbohydrate diets. High-fat diets have a high caloric density and it is conceivable that high calorie content per

© Woodhead Publishing Limited, 2011

mouthful may disturb energy balance. A large number of intervention studies have been performed to study the importance of dietary fat content in relation to energy balance. The results are conflicting. A previous meta-analysis of 16 studies demonstrated that low-fat diets, high in protein and complex carbohydrates, had beneficial effects on blood lipids and maintained weight in subjects with normal body mass index (BMI) whereas overweight subjects reduced their weight (Astrup et al., 2000). A more recent review concluded, however, that there is insufficient evidence for an association between total fat intake and body weight and probable evidence that increased intake of SFA results in increased weight (Melanson et al., 2009). In a recent intervention study it was found that a non-restricted-calorie, relatively low-carbohydrate (41% of energy) high-fat (39% of energy) diet resulted in an appreciable weight loss of 4.7 kg over a two-year period (Shai et al., 2008). From the available literature one must conclude that in order to maintain or lose weight, calorie adjustment and physical activity appear to be more important than the proportion of fat in the diet. It should be noted, however, that with Western diets an increase in total fat will invariably increase the intake of saturated fat and thus increase serum cholesterol and contribute to the CVD risk of obesity.

4.6.2   Metabolic syndrome

The metabolic syndrome is defined as a cluster of risk factors that predisposes for type 2 diabetes and CVD. To characterize the metabolic syndrome at least three of the criteria listed in Table 4.4 should be satisfied (Alberti et al., 2009). It has been convincingly shown that increased physical activity and a hypocaloric moderately low-fat diet will favourably influence traits of the metabolic syndrome and prevent development of diabetes type 2 (Tuomilehto et al., 2001, Knowler et al., 2002). No conclusion about the effects of specific fatty acids can be made from these studies, however. In a large recent review on the relationship between dietary fat and the metabolic syndrome it was concluded that there is insufficient evidence at this time to determine the association between diabetes risk and intake of total fat

Table 4.4   Criteria for diagnosis of the metabolic syndrome

Measure	Cut points
Waist circumference*	≥94 cm (men) ≥80 cm (women)
Serum triglycerides	1.7 mmol/L (150 mg/dL)
Serum HDL-cholesterol	<1.0 mmol/L (40 mg/dL) in men <1.3 mmol/L (50 mg/dL) in women
Blood pressure	Systolic ≥130 and/or diastolic ≥85 mm Hg
Fasting glucose	≥5.6 mmol/L (100 mg/dL)

* Limits as proposed by the International Diabetes Federation and WHO
Source: modified from Alberti et al., 2009

© Woodhead Publishing Limited, 2011

or of any particular type of fat. However, there is a sufficient number of studies suggesting that total fat and saturated fat intakes increase the risk of having components of the metabolic syndrome, and that higher intakes of MUFA and PUFA may reduce this risk (Melanson *et al.*, 2009).

4.6.3   Insulin sensitivity and type 2 diabetes

Both dietary fat quantity and quality influence insulin resistance and insulin sensitivity (Risérus, 2008). In particular, intervention studies have shown that reducing saturated fatty acids and replacing them by *cis*-unsaturated fatty acids improves insulin sensitivity (Vessby *et al.*, 2001, Risérus, 2008). In a study on the association between fatty acids in adipose tissue and insulin sensitivity a negative correlation was found between palmitic acid (16:0) and insulin sensitivity (Iggman *et al.*, 2010). Some minor fatty acids, C12:0, C14:0, C17:0 and C18:0, as well as polyunsaturated fatty acids were positively correlated with insulin sensitivity. The question has therefore been raised of whether some fatty acids, in particular palmitic acid, may promote insulin resistance more efficiently than others (Vessby *et al.*, 2002). Epidemiological evidence also suggests that replacing SFA by PUFA or MUFA has beneficial effects on insulin sensitivity and is likely to reduce the risk of type 2 diabetes (Risérus *et al.*, 2009).

4.7   Cancer

The high incidence of certain cancers like colorectal cancer, prostate cancer and breast cancer in rich countries suggests a strong influence of lifestyle factors. To what extent dietary factors and fat in particular are involved has been difficult, if not impossible, to clarify in spite of numerous studies. The current status was recently summarized in an extensive review (Gerber, 2009). For colorectal cancer an association has been found with total fat, and thus also with SFA, but the association disappears when adjusted for energy. The World Cancer Research Fund (WCRF) (2007) states that there is limited but suggestive evidence that foods containing animal fat increase colorectal cancer risk. To what extent this is due to SFA is unknown. Data indicate a possible relationship between total fat and endometrial cancer, ovarian cancer and breast cancer. There is also some evidence that SFA moderately increase breast cancer risk but not at an intake level <11% of energy (E%). Progression of prostate cancer has been reported to be more rapid on a high SFA intake. Otherwise, data are not sufficient to conclude on any specific effect of SFA on cancer (Gerber, 2009).

4.8   Dietary recommendations related to SFA

In 1957 the American Heart Association (AHA) prepared a report that summarized the evidence on the relation between diet and atherosclerotic disease. Since that time the Nutrition Committee of the AHA has at regular intervals prepared updated

© Woodhead Publishing Limited, 2011

reports and issued nutrition recommendations and dietary guidelines for primary prevention of CVD. The latest report was published in 2006 (Lichtenstein *et al.*, 2006). As knowledge has accumulated the AHA has updated the recommendations to include both nutrition recommendations (distribution of the energy-yielding nutrients) and dietary guidelines. These reports have been the model for all subsequent national and international reports by expert committees, such as WHO, ESC (the European Society of Cardiology), EFSA (European Food Safety Agency), etc. The initial AHA reports emphasized the importance both of fat quantity and quality. In more recent reports priority is given to fat quality. Quantitative recommendations for fat intake were first issued during the 1960s. Intake of total fat was set at about 30% of energy (E%) with a distribution of one third for SFA, one third for MUFA and one third for PUFA. This initial recommendation to limit SFA to 10 E% was based on the known association between serum cholesterol and atherosclerosis, early epidemiological studies and the effects of fatty acids on serum (total) cholesterol. The goal was to reduce the population's cholesterol level to < 200 mg/dL (<5.2 mmol/L) because at that level CHD was not considered a major public health problem (Blackburn *et al.*, 1979, WHO, 1982). From epidemiological (Keys, 1970) and metabolic studies (Clarke *et al.*, 1997) it was estimated that a mean of 10 E% from SFA corresponds to a mean cholesterol level in the population of about 200 mg/L (5.17 mmol/L). An intake of up to 10 E% from SFA has subsequently been adopted as a recommendation by most expert groups and it is still the generally accepted recommendation. When it became clear that *trans* fatty acids increase serum cholesterol similar to SFA, *trans* fatty acids were included in these 10 E%.

As stated above, there is no lower limit of cholesterol where risk of CHD disappears. In the Seven Countries Study CHD mortality was very low in the Japanese and Greek populations (Keys, 1970). Mean cholesterol was of the order of 140–170 mg/dL and 200 mg/dL, and saturated fat intake below 5 E% and 7–8 E%, respectively. CHD has been shown to be almost non-existent in rural China where mean cholesterol was of the order of 3.5 mmol/L (135 mg/dL), total fat intake about 15 E%, and saturated fat intake extremely low. This has raised the question of whether the goal for total cholesterol in the population should be set lower than 200 mg/dL (5.17 mmol/L). Based on the Chinese studies it has been suggested that in order to reduce CHD mortality to a minimum level the population mean should be reduced to 150 mg/dL (3.88 mmol/L) (Campbell *et al.*, 1998). This would require the amount of SFA to be reduced to a level of around 5 E% (Clarke *et al.*, 1997). In the latest report from the AHA the recommended level of SFA intake is set at 7 E% (Lichtenstein *et al.*, 2006). A similar recommendation has been made for developing countries in Asia with total fat intake set at 21 E%, SFA at 7 E%, MUFA at 7 E% and PUFA at 7 E% (Singh *et al.*, 1996). So far no other expert groups have recommended such low levels of saturated fat intake. But it is not unreasonable to assume that we may see recommendations for SFA below the actual 10 E% in the years to come.

What should replace SFA? In metabolic experiments replacing SFA by carbohydrates reduces total- and LDL cholesterol (Clarke *et al.*, 1997, Mensink

© Woodhead Publishing Limited, 2011

et al., 2003). In individuals with dyslipidemia and the metabolic syndrome, however, carbohydrates may actually result in increased triglycerides (VLDL) and lower HDL cholesterol, which may increase CVD risk. Large prospective studies in Western populations have in fact shown increased risk when replacing SFA by carbohydrate (Jacobsen *et al.*, 2009). This may appear a paradox since in many parts of the world – China in particular as mentioned above – it has been found that CVD risk is very low on low-fat, high-carbohydrate diets (Campbell *et al.*, 1998). The reason for this discrepancy may be that these populations are characterized by consuming high-fibre, complex carbohydrates and having considerably higher energy expenditure and lower BMI compared to affluent populations (Campbell and Chen, 1999).

Replacing saturated fat by PUFA is the most efficient way of reducing serum cholesterol (Clarke *et al.*, 1997, Mensink *et al.*, 2003). Prospective studies also show that replacing saturated fat by PUFA lowers the risk of CHD mortality (Jacobsen *et al.*, 2009). Recommendations for PUFA are generally set at 5 to 10 E%. Replacing SFA by MUFA is less efficient for cholesterol reduction (Clarke *et al.*, 1997, Mensink *et al.*, 2003) and epidemiological studies show that replacing SFA by MUFA does not alter the risk (Jacobsen *et al.*, 2009).

4.9   Trends in consumption of SFA as related to trends in mortality and incidence of CVD

Recent dietary surveys in European countries have shown intake of saturated fat varying between 8.8 and 14.6 E% (after excluding Romania as an outlier with 26.3 E%) (Elmadfa, 2009a). The decline in CHD mortality in the US and most European countries can to a large extent be explained by cholesterol reduction due to altered dietary habits (Ford *et al.*, 2007, Kuulasmaa *et al.*, 2000). The general trend has been a reduction in animal fat and an increase in vegetable oils. Finland is a particularly good example (see section 4.5.4) where saturated fat declined from around 20 E% in 1980 to 12 E% in 2007 mainly due to a reduction in butter intake from 18 kg/capita/yr to 3 kg in 2005 while PUFA were at around 5-6E% (Puska, 2009). In Norway saturated fat declined from around 17 E% in the 1970s to 14 E% and *trans* from 4 E% to <0.5 E% while PUFA have increased to 7 E%, the changes being mainly due to reduction in margarine and to some extent to reduction in dairy fat (Pedersen *et al.*, 2004).

The mean cholesterol levels in the European populations are still high, however. The MONICA study indicated values near 5.8 mmol/L in the early 1990s (Kuulasmaa *et al.*, 2000) while more recent data from a smaller selection of eight countries gave a mean of 5.3 mmol/L (Elmadfa, 2009b). A further reduction is thus desirable which would justify further reductions in SFA intake compared to today's level. One should keep in mind, however, that the main health problem in the affluent world is overfeeding and inactivity and as long as they prevail CVD will probably continue to be a serious health problem irrespective of any change in dietary SFA intake.

© Woodhead Publishing Limited, 2011

4.10   Conclusion

'The lipid hypothesis in atherosclerosis' has been tested in innumerable ways during the last 100 years but it has stood the test of time. The hypothesis has been modified as the complexity of the atherosclerotic process has become evident but it has not been falsified. The model that derives from the hypothesis predicts that an increased intake of saturated fat increases the amount of circulating LDL particles (of which LDL cholesterol is a marker). By penetrating the arterial wall these particles act as a pathogenic agent in the development of atherosclerosis. The consequences of increased LDL cholesterol have been demonstrated in animal, clinical and epidemiological studies. The model further predicts that reduction in SFA intake and reduction in plasma LDL cholesterol should favourably influence CHD risk, which again has been verified in clinical and epidemiological studies. This now forms the basis for preventive measures by diet or drugs. The lack of unanimous acceptance of the lipid hypothesis is generally that more importance is given to single discordant studies than to the totality of the vast array of concordant multidisciplinary research evidence that the hypothesis is based on.

4.11   References

Ajuwon KM, and Spurlock ME (2005), 'Palmitate activates the NF-κB transcription factor and induces IL-6 and TNFα expression in 3T3-L1 adipocytes', *J Nutr*, 135, 1841–6.

Alberti KG, Eckel RH, Grundy S M, Zimmet PZ, Cleeman J I, Donato KA, Fruchart J–C, James WPT, Loria CM and Smith SC (2009), 'Harmonizing the metabolic syndrome: a joint interim statement of the International Diabetes Federation Task Force on Epidemiology and Prevention; National Heart, Lung, and Blood Institute; American Heart Association; World Heart Federation; International Atherosclerosis Society; and International Association for the Study of Obesity', *Circulation*, 120, 1640–5.

Allison DB, Egan SK, Barraj LM, Caughman C, Infante M and Heimbach JT (1999), Estimated intakes of *trans* fatty and other fatty acids in the US population, *J Am Diet Assoc* 99, 166–74.

Almendingen K, Jordal O, Kierulf P, Sandstad B and Pedersen JI (1995), 'Effects of partially hydrogenated fish oil, partially hydrogenated soybean oil, and butter on serum lipoproteins and Lp[a] in men', *J Lipid Res*, 36, 1370–84.

Artaud-Wild SM, Connor SL, Sexton G and Connor WE (1993), 'Differences in coronary mortality can be explained by differences in cholesterol and saturated fat intakes in 40 countries but not in France and Finland. A paradox', *Circulation*, 88, 2771–9.

Aspelund T, V Gudnason, B Magnusdottir, K Andersen, G Sigurdsson, J Critchley, M O'Flaherty and S Capewell (2009), 'Explaining the massive declines in coronary heart disease mortality rates in Iceland 1981–2006', *European Journal of Cardiovascular Prevention and Rehabilitation*, 16, 80–1. [Abstract].

Astrup A, Ryan L, Grunwald GK, Storgaard M, Saris W, Melanson E and Hill JO (2000), 'The role of dietary fat in body fatness: evidence from a preliminary meta–analysis of ad libitum low fat dietary intervention studies', *Br J Nutr*, 83 (suppl 1), 25–32.

Berneis KK and Krauss RM (2002) Metabolic origins and clinical significance of LDL heterogeneity, *J Lipid Res*, 43, 1363–79.

Bingham SA, Luben R, Welch A, Wareham N, Khaw KT and Day N (2003), 'Are imprecise methods obscuring a relation between fat and breast cancer?', *Lancet*, 362, 212–14.

© Woodhead Publishing Limited, 2011

Blackburn, H. Berenson GS, Christakis G et al. (1979), 'Conference on the health effects of blood lipids: Optimal distribution for populations', Prev Med, 8, 612–78.

Briel M, Ferreira-Gonzalez I, You JJ, Karanicolas PJ, Akl EA, Wu P, Blechacz B, Bassler D, Wei X, Sharman A, Whitt I, Alves da Silva S, Khalid Z, Nordmann AJ, Zhou Q, Walter SD, Vale N, Bhatnagar N, O'Regan C, Mills EJ, Bucher HC, Montori VM, Guyatt GH (2009), 'Association between change in high density lipoprotein cholesterol and cardiovascular disease morbidity and mortality: systematic review and meta-regression analysis', BMJ, 338:b92doi:10.1136/bmj.b92.

Campbell TC and Chen J (1999), 'Energy balance: Interpretation of data from rural China', Toxicol Sciences, 52 (suppl), 87–94.

Campbell TC, Parpia B and Chen J (1998), 'Diet, lifestyle, and the etiology of coronary artery disease: the Cornell China study', Am J Cardiol, 26, 82(10B), 18–21.

Castelli WP (1984), 'Epidemiology of coronary heart disease: the Framhingham study', Am J Med, 76, 4–12.

Clarke R, Frost C, Collins R, Appleby P and Peto R (1997), 'Dietary lipids and blood cholesterol: quantitative meta-analysis of metabolic ward studies', BMJ, 314, 112–17.

Cuchel M and Rader DJ (2006), 'Macrophage reverse cholesterol transport: key to the regression of atherosclerosis?' Circulation, 113, 2548–55.

Dayton S, ML Pearce, S Hashimoto, WJ Dixon and U Toniyasu (1969), 'A controlled clinical trial of a diet high in unsaturated fat in preventing complications of atherosclerosis', Circulation, 39 (suppl 2), 1–63.

Di Angelantonio E, Sarwar N, Perry P, Kaptoge S, Ray KK, Thompson A, Wood AM, Lewington S, Sattar N, Packard CJ, Collins R, Thompson SG and Danesh J. (2009), 'Major lipids, apolipoproteins, and risk of vascular disease', JAMA, 302, 1993–2000.

Duttaroy AK (2005), 'Postprandial activation of hemostatic factors: role of dietary fatty acids', Prostaglandins Leukot Essent Fatty Acids, 72, 381–91.

Elmadfa I (2009a), 'Energy and nutrient intake in the European Union based on national data', European nutrition and health report 2009, Basel, Switzerland, Karger, pp 68–156.

Elmadfa I (2009b), 'Health and lifestyle indicators in the European Union', European nutrition and health report 2009, Basel, Switzerland, Karger, pp 157–201.

Ford ES, Ajani UA, Croft JB, et al. (2007), 'Explaining the decrease in U.S. deaths from coronary disease 1980–2000', N Engl J Med, 356, 2388–98.

Genest J (2008), 'The yin and yang of high-density lipoprotein cholesterol', J Amer Coll Cardiol, 51, 643–44.

Gerber M (2009), 'Background review paper on total fat, fatty acid intake and cancers', Ann Nutr Metab, 55,140–61.

Håversen L, Danielsson KN, Fogelstrand L and Wiklund O (2009), 'Induction of proinflammatory cytokines by long-chain saturated fatty acids in human macrophages', Atherosclerosis, 202, 382–93.

Hegsted DM (1986), 'Serum-cholesterol response to dietary cholesterol: A re-evaluation', Am J Clin Nutr 44, 299–305.

Hjermann I, Velve Byre K, Holme I and Leren P (1981), 'Effect of diet and smoking intervention on the incidence of coronary heart disease, Report from the Oslo Study Group of a randomised trial in healthy men', Lancet, 12, 2(8259), 1303–10.

Hjermann I, Holme I and Leren P (1986), 'Oslo Study Diet and Antismoking Trial. Results after 102 months', Am J Med, 80, 7–11.

Holme I, Hjermann I, Helgeland A and Leren P (1985), 'The Oslo Study: diet and antismoking advice, Additional results from a 5-year primary preventive trial in middle-aged men', Prev Med, 14(3), 279–92.

Holvoet P, Harris TB, Tracy RP, Verhamme P, Newman AB, Rubin SM, Simonsick EM, Colbert LH and Kritchevsky SB (2003), 'Association of high coronary heart disease risk status with circulating oxidized LDL in the well-functioning elderly: findings from the

© Woodhead Publishing Limited, 2011

Health, Aging, and Body Composition study', *Arterioscler Thromb Vasc Biol* 1, 23(8), 1444–8.

Iggman D, Arnlöv J, Vessby B, Cederholm T, Sjögren P and Risérus U (2010), 'Adipose tissue fatty acids and insulin sensitivity in elderly men', *Diabetologia* Feb 3. [Epub ahead of print].

Jacobsen MU, O'Reilly EJ, Heitmann BL Pereira MA, Bälter K, Fraser GE, Goldbourt U, Hallmans G, Knekt P, Liu S, Pietinen P, Spiegelman D, Stevens J, Virtamo J, Willett WC and Ascherio A (2009), 'Major types of dietary fat and risk of coronary heart disease: a pooled analysis of 11 cohort studies', *Am J Clin Nutr*, 89, 1425–32.

Keys A (ed.) (1970), 'Coronary heart disease in seven countries', *Circulation*, 41 (Suppl 1), 1–211.

Keys A (1980), 'Diet' Chapter 14, in: Seven Countries. A multivariate analysis of death and coronary heart disease. Harvard University Press, Cambridge, Massachusetts and London, 248–62.

Keys A (1984), 'Serum-cholesterol response to dietary cholesterol', *Am J Clin Nutr*, 40, 351–9.

Keys A (1988), 'Diet and blood cholesterol in population surveys – lessons from analysis of the data from a major survey in Israel', *Am J Clin Nutr*, 48, 1161–5.

Keys A, Anderson JT and Grande F (1965), 'Serum cholesterol response to change in the diet. IV. Particular saturated fatty acids in the diet', *Metabolism*, 14, 776–87.

Knowler WC, Barrett-Connor E, Fowler SE, Hamman RF, Lachin JM, Walker EA and Nathan DM (2002), 'Reduction in the incidence of type 2 diabetes with lifestyle intervention or metformin', Diabetes Prevention Program Research Group, *N Engl J Med*, 346, 393–403.

Kromhout D, Menotti A, Bloemberg B, Aravanis C, Blackburn H, Buzina R, Dontas AS, Fidanza F, Giaipaoli S, Jansen A, Karvonen M, Katan M, Nissinen A, Nedeljkovic S, Pekkanen J, Pekkarinen M, Punsar S, Rasanen L, Simic B and Toshima H (1995), 'Dietary Saturated and *trans* Fatty Acids and Cholesterol and 25-Year Mortality from Coronary Heart Disease: The Seven Countries Study', *Preventive Medicine*, 24, 308–315.

Kromhout D (1999), Serum cholesterol in cross-cultural perspective. The Seven Countries Study, *Acta Cardiol*, 54,155–8.

Kuulasmaa K, Tunstall-Pedoe H, Dobson A, Fortmann S, Sans S, Tolonen H, Evans A, Ferrario M and Tuomilehto J (2000), 'Estimation of contribution of changes in classic risk factors to trends in coronary-event rates across the WHO MONICA Project populations', *Lancet*, 355, 675–87.

Lefevre M, Kris-Etherton PM, Zhao G and Tracy RP (2004), 'Dietary fatty acids, hemostasis, and cardiovascular disease risk', *Am Diet Assoc*, 104, 410–19.

Lichtenstein AH, Appel LJ, Brands M, Carnethon M, Daniels S, Franch HA, Franklin B, Kris-Etherton P, Harris WS, Howard B, Karanja N, Lefevre M, Rudel L, Sacks F, Van Horn L, Winston M and Wylie-Rosett J (2006), 'Diet and lifestyle recommendations revision 2006: a scientific statement from the American Heart Association Nutrition Committee'. *Circulation* 4, 114(1), 82–96.

Leren P (1970), 'The Oslo diet–heart study – eleven-year report', *Circulation*, 42, 935–42.

Libby P, Ridker PM and Hansson GK (2009), 'Inflammation in atherosclerosis: from pathophysiology to practice', *J Am Coll Cardiol*, 54, 2129–38.

Martin MJ, Hulley SB, Browner WS, Killers LH and Wentworth D (1986), 'Serum cholesterol, blood pressure, and mortality: implications from a cohort of 361.662 men', *Lancet*, 2(8513), 933–36.

Melanson EL, Astrup A and Donahoo WT (2009), 'The relationship between dietary fat and fatty acid intake and body weight, diabetes, and the metabolic syndrome', *Ann Nutr Metab*, 55, 229–43.

Mensink RP and Katan MB (1990), 'Effect of dietary *trans* fatty acids on high-density and low-density lipoprotein cholesterol levels in healthy subjects', *N Engl J Med*, 323, 439–45.

© Woodhead Publishing Limited, 2011

Mensink RP and Katan MB (1992), 'Effect of dietary fatty acids on serum lipids and lipoproteins. a meta-analysis of 27 trials', *Arterioscl. Thromb.* 12, 911–19.

Mensink RP, Zock PL, Kester ADM and Katan MB (2003), 'Effects of dietary fatty acids and carbohydrates on the ratio of serum total to HDL cholesterol and on serum lipids and apolipoproteins: a meta-analysis of 60 controlled trials', *Am J Clin Nutr,* 77, 1146–55.

Miettinen M, Turpeinen O, Karvonen MJ, Elosuo R and Paavilainen E (1972), 'Effect of cholesterol lowering diet on mortality from coronary heart-disease and other causes: A 12 year clinical trial in men and women', *Lancet,* 21, 2(7782), 835–8.

Müller H, Kirkhus B, and Pedersen JI (2001), 'Serum cholesterol predictive equations with special emphasis on *trans* and saturated fatty acids, An analysis from designed controlled studies', *Lipids,* 36, 783–91.

Pedersen JI and Kirkhus B (2008), 'Fatty acid composition of post *trans* margarines and their health implications', *Lipid Technology,* 20, 132–5.

Pedersen JI, Kirkhus B and Müller H (2003), 'Serum cholesterol predictive equations in product development', *Eur J Med Res* 8, 325–31.

Pedersen JI, Tverdal A and Kirkhus B (2004), 'Diet changes and the rise and fall of cardiovascular disease mortality in Norway', *Tidsskr Nor Laegeforen* 3, 124(11), 1532–36. (Norwegian, English abstract)

Prentice RL (2003), 'Dietary assessment and the reliability of nutritional epidemiology reports', *Lancet,* 362, 182–3.

Puska P (2009), 'Fat and heart disease: yes we can make a change – the case of North Karelia (Finland)', *Ann Nutr Metab,* 54 Suppl 1, 33–8.

Renaud S, Morazain R, Godsey F, Dumont E, Thevenon C, Martin JL and Mendy F (1986), 'Nutrients, platelet function and composition in nine groups of French and British farmers', *Atherosclerosis,* 60, 37–48.

Risérus U (2008), 'Fatty acids and insulin sensitivity', *Curr Opin clin Nutr metab Care,* 11, 100–5.

Risérus U, Willett WC and Hu FB (2009), 'Dietary fats and prevention of type 2 diabetes', *Prog Lipid Res,* 48, 44–51.

Ross R (1999), 'Atherosclerosis – an inflammatory disease', *N Eng J Med,* 340, 115–26.

St-Onge MP, Bosarge A, L. L. T. Goree LLT, and Darnell B (2008), 'Medium chain triglyceride oil consumption as part of a weight loss diet does not lead to an adverse metabolic profile when compared to olive oil', *J. Am Coll Nutr,* 27, 547–52.

Sanders TAB (2009), 'Fat and fatty acid intake and metabolic effects in human body', *Ann Nutr Metab,* 55, 162–72.

Shai I, Schwarzfuchs D, Henkin Y, Shahar DR, Witkow S, Greenberg I, Golan R, Fraser D, Bolotin A, Vardi H, Tangi-Rozental O, Zuk-Ramot R, Sarusi B, Brickner D, Schwartz Z, Sheiner E, Marko R, Katorza E, Thiery J, Fiedler GM, Blüher M, Stumvoll M and Stampfer MJ (2008), 'Dietary Intervention Randomized Controlled Trial (DIRECT) Group. Weight loss with a low-carbohydrate, Mediterranean, or low-fat diet', *N Engl J Med,* 359, 229–41.

Shepherd J, Cobbe S, Ford I, Isles CG, Lorimer AR, MacFarlane PW *et al.* (1995), 'Prevention of coronary heart disease with pravastatin in men with hypercholesterolemia. West of Scotland Coronary Prevention Study Group', *N Engl J Med,* 333, 1301–7.

Scandinavian Simvastatin Survival Study (1994) [No authors listed]. 'Randomised trial of cholesterol lowering in 4444 patients with coronary heart disease: the Scandinavian Simvastatin Survival Study (4S)', *Lancet,* 344, 1383–9.

Singh RB, Mori H, Chen J, Mendis S, Moshiri M, Zhu S, Kim SH, Sy RG and Faruqui AM (1996), 'Recommendations for the prevention of coronary artery disease in Asians: a scientific statement of the International College of Nutrition', *J Cardiovasc Risk,* 3(6):489–94.

Siri-Tarino PW, Sun Q, Hu FB and Krauss RM (2010), 'Meta-analysis of prospective cohort studies evaluating the association of saturated fat with cardiovascular disease', *Am J Clin Nutr,* 91, 535546.

© Woodhead Publishing Limited, 2011

Skeaff CM and Miller J (2009), 'Dietary fat and coronary heart disease: Summary of evidence from prospective cohort and randomised controlled trials', *Ann Nutr Metab*, 55, 173–201.

Staiger H, Staiger K, Stefan N, Wahl HG, Günther H, Machicao F, Kellerer M and Häring HU (2004), 'Palmitate-induced interleukin-6 expression in human coronary artery endothelial cells', *Diabetes*, 53, 3209–16.

Stamler J (1992), 'Established major coronary risk factors', in: Marmot M, Elliott P, eds. *Coronary heart disease epidemiology: from aetiology to public health*. London, Oxford University Press, 32–70.

Stamler J (2010), 'Diet–heart: a problematic revisit', *Am J Clin Nutr*, 91, 497–9.

Taylor CB, Cox GE, Manalo-Estrella P, Southworth J, Patton DE and Cathcart C (1962), 'Atherosclerosis in rhesus monkeys, II. Arterial lesions associated with hypercholesterolemia induced by dietary fat and cholesterol', *Arch Pathol*, 74, 16–34.

Tholstrup T, Ehnholm C, Jauhiainen M, Petersen M, Hoy CE, Lund P, and Sandstrom B (2004), Effects of medium-chain fatty acids and oleic acid on blood lipids, lipoproteins, glucose, insulin, and lipid transfer protein activities, *Am J Clinl Nutr*, 79, 564–9.

Thompson GR (2009), 'History of the cholesterol controversy in Britain', *QJM*, 102, 81–6.

Tuomilehto J, Lindström J, Eriksson JG, Valle TT, Hämäläinen H, Ilanne-Parikka P, Keinänen-Kiukaanniemi S, Laakso M, Louheranta A, Rastas M, Salminen V and Uusitupa M (2001), 'Prevention of type 2 diabetes mellitus by changes in lifestyle among subjects with impaired glucose tolerance', *N Engl J Med*, 344, 1343–50.

van der Steeg WA, Holme I, Boekholdt SM, Larsen ML, Lindahl C, Stroes ESG, Tikkanen MJ, Wareham NJ, Faergeman O, Olsson AG, Pedersen TR, Khaw K-T and Kastelein JJP (2008), 'High-Density Lipoprotein Cholesterol, High-Density Lipoprotein Particle Size, and Apolipoprotein A-I: Significance for Cardiovascular Risk: The IDEAL and EPIC-Norfolk Studies', *J Am Coll Cardiol*, 51, 634–42.

Verhove E, Langlois MR and Asklepios Investigators (2009), 'Circulating oxidized low-density lipoprotein: a biomarker of atherosclerosis and cardiovascular risk?', *Clin Chem Lab Med*, 47(2), 128–37.

Vessby B, Unsitupa M, Hermansen K, Riccardi G, Rivellese AA, Tapsell LC, Nälsén C, Berglund L, Louheranta A, Rasmussen BM, Calvert GD, Maffetone A, Pedersen E, Gustafsson IB and Storlien LH (2001), 'Substituting dietary saturated for monounsaturated fat impairs insulin sensitivity in healthy men and women', The KANWU Study. *Diabetologia*, 44, 312–19.

Vessby B, Gustafsson IB, Tengblad S, Boberg M and Andersson A (2002), 'Desaturation and elongation of Fatty acids and insulin action', *Ann N Y Acad Sci*, 967, 183–95.

WCFR/AICR (2007), *Food, nutrition, physical activity and the prevention of cancer: A global perspective*. Washington, American Institute for Cancer Research.

Weigert C, Brodbeck K, Staiger H, Kausch C, Machicao F, Häring HU and Schleicher ED (2004), 'Palmitate, but not unsaturated fatty acids, induces the expression of interleukin-6 in human myotubes through proteasome-dependent activation of nuclear factor-kappaB', *J Biol Chem*, 279, 23942–52.

WHO (1982), *Prevention of coronary heart disease. Report of a WHO expert committee*, Technical Report Series 678, Geneva, World Health Organization.

WHO (2005), *Preventing Chronic Diseases. A Vital Investment*, Geneva, World Health Organization.

Williams KJ (2008), 'Molecular processes that handle and mishandle dietary lipids', *J Clin Invest*, 118(10), 3247–59.

Yu S, Derr J, Etherton TD and Kris-Etherton PM (1995), 'Plasma cholesterol-predictive equations demonstrate that stearic acid is neutral and monounsaturated fatty acids are hypocholesterolemic', *Am J Clin Nutr*, 61(5), 1129–39.

Yuan G, Wang J and Hegele RA (2006), 'Heterozygous familial hypercholesterolemia: an underrecognized cause of early cardiovascular disease', *CMAJ*, 174, 1124–29.

© Woodhead Publishing Limited, 2011

5

Chronic disease risk associated with different dietary saturated fatty acids

D. I. Givens and K. E. Kliem, University of Reading, UK

Abstract: This chapter compares the risks of chronic disease, and cardiovascular disease in particular, associated with consumption of different saturated fatty acids. Emphasis is placed on the effects of stearic acid as this has potential to replace *trans* fatty acids in certain manufactured food products. The chapter first reviews the effects of individual saturated fatty acids on blood lipids, including cholesterol, as these are commonly used as markers of disease risk. It then looks directly at evidence in relation to health outcomes. Finally, recent evidence specifically on the effect of stearic acid relative to other fatty acids, including *trans* fatty acids, is summarised.

Key words: individual saturated fatty acids, chronic disease, stearic acid, palmitic acid.

5.1   Introduction

Early ecological studies suggested a positive association between consumption of saturated fats and rates of coronary heart disease (CHD). One of the most widely reported ecological studies of diet and CHD is the Seven Countries Study (Keys, 1970). This examined 16 cohorts of middle-aged men in seven different countries between 1958 and 1964. This showed that death rates from CHD during a 10- and 15-year follow-up period were positively associated with saturated fatty acid (SFA) intake and negatively related to intake of monounsaturated fat (MUFA) (Keys *et al.*, 1986). The Seven Countries Study also showed a strong positive relationship between SFA consumption and serum cholesterol concentrations. Support for these ecological studies has been seen in some prospective cohort studies (e.g. Hu *et al.*, 1997; Oh *et al.*, 2005) and in some long-term dietary intervention studies (e.g. Turpeinen *et al.*, 1979). Some studies have not supported such a relationship, however (e.g. Gordon *et al.*, 1981; Ascherio *et al.*, 1996), and indeed recent meta-analyses of cohort studies (Skeaff and Miller, 2009;

© Woodhead Publishing Limited, 2011

Siri-Tarino *et al.*, 2010) have failed to show a clear association between SFA intake and CHD, although a meta-analysis of intervention studies involving increasing the polyunsaturated:saturated fat ratio in diets did show that this significantly reduced risk of total CHD events (relative risk 0.83, 95% confidence interval (CI) 0.69–1.00, *P* = 0.050; Skeaff and Miller, 2009). There has, however, been less attention paid to the relative effects of the various different SFA typically present in the diet.

5.2   Key dietary saturated fatty acids

Dietary fats are mainly comprised of triglycerides made up of three fatty acids esterified to a glycerol molecule. Saturated fatty acids are those which contain no carbon–carbon double bonds, and in most diets the SFA in greatest abundance are lauric (C12:0), myristic (C14:0), palmitic (C16:0) and stearic (C18:0) acids. Most diets will also contain some short and medium chain SFA (C4:0. C6:0. C8:0, C10:0), mainly of milk origin as milk fat typically contains about 12 g of these SFA per 100 g (Givens and Kliem, 2009). Intake of these is, however, low and their effect on plasma cholesterol is likely to be small (Kris-Etherton and Yu, 1997; Hu *et al.*, 1999). The major biological role of short and medium chain SFA is an energy source, following β-oxidation. SFA are thought to be the preferred energy substrate of the heart (Huber *et al.*, 2007) and during low- and moderate-intensity exercise regimes fatty acid oxidation is an important fuel of skeletal muscles (Romijn *et al.*, 1993). In addition to fuel, some of the short chain SFA have other minor roles within biological systems. Butyric acid (C4:0) has been shown to modulate genetic regulation (Smith *et al.*, 1998), while C6:0, C8:0, C10:0 and C12:0 have antiviral, antibacterial or antitumour activities (German and Dillard, 2004). In mammals, dietary C16:0 and C18:0 are among the fatty acids thought to be involved in transcriptional activation of oxidative enzymes, shifting energy metabolism to fatty acid oxidation from glucose/lactate utilisation which is typical of the foetal heart (Barger and Kelly, 2000). Both C16:0 and C18:0 are also important constituents of cell membranes, with 20 to 40% of tissue phospholipids containing C16:0 and C18:0 (Cunnane and Griffin, 2002). Short and medium chain SFA (C4:0, C6:0, C8:0 and C10:0) are rapidly oxidised in the liver to acetyl CoA and so do not alter the composition of the circulating lipid pool. As such, these SFA are biologically neutral with respect to regulation of serum cholesterol concentrations and will not be considered further in this chapter.

There appear to be few sources of data providing intakes of individual SFA but Table 5.1 shows intakes from the TRANSFAIR study (Hulshof *et al.*, 1999) for men in selected EU member states for total SFA, C12:0+C14:0+C16:0, C18:0 and, by difference, other SFA. Although the intake of total SFA varied markedly between countries in this selection, the proportion of SFA from C12:0+C14:0+C16:0 was fairly consistent (all between 62 and 72%). Intakes of C18:0 were in the range of approximately 6 to 12 g/d for men, equating to about 14 to 25% of total SFA.

© Woodhead Publishing Limited, 2011

Table 5.1   Intakes of saturated fatty acids (SFA) by men in 11 EU member states

Country	Intake (g methyl esters/d) of:				
	Total SFA	C12:0+C14:0+C16:0	C18:0	Others[1]	C12:0+C14:0+C16:0 as % total SFA
Belgium	47.3	29.6	11.6	6.1	62.6
Finland	34.6	23.4	8.0	3.2	67.6
France	36.0	23.7	7.3	5.0	65.8
Germany	51.6	37.0	7.3	7.3	71.7
Greece	23.8	14.7	4.4	4.7	61.8
Italy	32.5	21.9	6.1	4.5	67.4
Netherlands	42.1	27.9	9.4	4.8	66.3
Portugal	29.6	19.9	6.2	3.5	67.2
Spain[2]	35.2	23.0	7.8	4.4	65.3
Sweden	39.7	26.0	8.1	5.6	65.5
UK[2]	28.5	19.4	6.0	3.1	68.1

[1] calculated as total SFA – (C12:0+C14:0+C16:0+C18:0)
[2] includes men and women
Source: adapted from Hulshof et al., 1999.

5.3   Chronic disease risk differences between different saturated fatty acids

5.3.1   Effects on serum lipids and lipoproteins

Traditionally, the effects of SFA on CHD risk have been assessed from their effect on serum total cholesterol. There is general agreement that dietary SFA increase the concentrations of serum low-density lipoprotein (LDL)-cholesterol, an identified risk factor for cardiovascular disease (CVD) in general and particularly for CHD (Zock, 2006). While in general, SFA raise total and LDL-cholesterol, early studies showed that individual fatty acids have markedly different effects. In particular, lauric (C12:0), myristic (C14:0) and palmitic (C16:0) acids have been associated with elevated serum LDL-cholesterol concentrations. Katan et al. (1995) concluded based on a review of several studies that substituting 1% energy as carbohydrates with all three of these SFA is associated with elevated total, LDL and high-density lipoprotein (HDL) cholesterol levels. The cholesterol-raising potential of C16:0 has been confirmed by many well-controlled intervention studies (e.g. Denke and Grundy, 1992). The same authors also concluded that C12:0 had two-thirds of the cholesterol-raising potential of C16:0 (Denke and Grundy, 1992), whereas Temme et al. (1996) demonstrated that dietary C12:0 increased serum total, LDL and HDL cholesterol to a greater extent than dietary C16:0. A summary of the outcome of the study of Temme et al. (1996) is shown in Table 5.2. A total of 30 healthy men and women consumed isoenergetic diets providing either 10.6, 13.2 and 19.0% of energy intake (EI) from lauric (C12:0),

© Woodhead Publishing Limited, 2011

palmitic (C16:0) and oleic (C18:1) acids respectively over six-week periods (separated by two-week washout periods) and Table 5.2 summarises the serum cholesterol concentrations at the end of each period. Essentially, Temme *et al.* (1996) found that the diet high in C12:0 increased serum total cholesterol concentrations significantly more than did the diet high in C16:0. However, this was due to an increase in both LDL- and HDL-cholesterol concentrations and while the total to HDL cholesterol ratio was lower for the lauric acid diet, potentially indicating reduced CHD risk, no statistics are available for these values. Also, as pointed out by the authors, a possible confounding factor may be the higher myristic acid (C14:0) content (4.2% EI) of the C12:0 diet than the other two diets (2.2, 1.9% EI; palmitic, oleic respectively). Other studies suggest that C12:0 and C14:0 acids have more potent effects on serum LDL-cholesterol than C16:0 while others suggest that C14:0 and C16:0 are more potent than C12:0 (see review of Gurr, 1999). Also noteworthy is the study of Nestel *et al.* (1994), which showed in hypercholesterolemic men, at the amounts consumed (4% EI) at least, that palmitoleic acid (C16:1) behaves very much like an SFA and not a MUFA with respect to effects on LDL-cholesterol. Since much of the C12:0, C14:0 and C16:0 in the human diet is derived from milk fat (Gunstone *et al.*, 1994), the consumption of conventional milk and dairy foods would be expected to have adverse effects on serum LDL-cholesterol levels. However, research has demonstrated that the typical fatty acid profile of milk can be altered by targeted changes in the dairy cow diet (Givens and Shingfield, 2006).

An important meta-analysis of the effect of dietary SFA on serum cholesterol pools was reported by Mensink *et al.* (2003). A total of 60 well-controlled intervention trials met the specified criteria and these provided 159 diet data points and involved 1672 volunteers (70% men). For 35 of the studies where individual fatty acids were reported, a meta-analysis confirmed that when dietary carbohydrate is replaced with an isoenergetic amount of C12:0, C14:0 or C16:0, significant increases in serum total and LDL-cholesterol occur (Table 5.3) and the effect is greatest for C12:0 followed in turn by C14:0 and C16:0. This analysis also noted that there was also a tendency for all SFA to increase in HDL-cholesterol with the greatest effect being due to C12:0 ($P < 0.001$). Mensink *et al.* (2003) suggested

Table 5.2   Effect of three different diets on serum cholesterol concentrations (mean of men and women)

Serum cholesterol (mmol/L)	Lauric acid diet	Palmitic acid diet	Oleic acid diet
Total cholesterol	5.90[a,b]	5.69[a]	5.42
LDL-cholesterol	3.84[a]	3.71	3.49
HDL-cholesterol	1.59[a,b]	1.47	1.44
Total:HDL†	3.71	3.87	3.76

[a] significantly different from oleic acid $P < 0.02$.
[b] significantly different from palmitic acid $P < 0.02$.
† calculated from published data hence no statistical analysis.
Source: Temme *et al.*, 1996.

© Woodhead Publishing Limited, 2011

Table 5.3   Effect of replacing 1% dietary energy as carbohydrates with lauric, myristic, palmitic and stearic acids on mean changes in serum lipids and lipoproteins

Lipid or lipoprotein	Replacement of carbohydrate with saturated fatty acid:			
	Lauric	Myristic	Palmitic	Stearic
Total cholesterol (mmol/L)	0.069*	0.059*	0.041*	−0.010
LDL-cholesterol (mmol/L)	0.052*	0.048*	0.039*	−0.004
HDL-cholesterol (mmol/L)	0.027*	0.018	0.010	0.002
Total:HDL-cholesterol	−0.037*	−0.003	0.005	−0.013
Triacylglycerol (mmol/L)	−0.019*	−0.017*	−0.017*	−0.017*
Apo B (mg/L)	5.6	1.9	4.2	−3.8
Apo A1 (mg/L)	13.8*	10.4*	7.5*	−1.6

* $P < 0.01$.
Source: meta-analysis of Mensink *et al.*, 2003.

that the ratio of total to HDL-cholesterol provides the most powerful predictor of the effect of dietary fatty acids on risk of CHD with low values being associated with reduced risk. This interpretation implies that diet-induced increases in HDL-cholesterol reduce the risk of CVD. Mensink *et al.* (2003) admit that no causal role for such an interpretation has been shown though they cite other evidence supporting the use of total to HDL-cholesterol ratio. This interpretation suggests that the effects of C12:0 may be somewhat beneficial as it significantly ($P < 0.001$) reduced the total to HDL-cholesterol ratio when compared with carbohydrates while the effect of C14:0 was neutral. Replacing dietary carbohydrate with C16:0 tended to increase the total to HDL-cholesterol ratio though in the meta-analysis this did not reach significance. These data are summarised in Fig. 5.1, and seem to suggest that replacing small amounts of dietary carbohydrates with these SFA does not have overall adverse affects on lipoprotein profile.

Mensink *et al.* (2003) also demonstrated that there was little effect of C18:0 on total to HDL cholesterol (Table 5.3). Other studies have shown that C18:0 is relatively neutral in its effects on serum cholesterol levels. Compared with a C16:0-rich diet, a diet enriched with C18:0 resulted in lower total and LDL-cholesterol concentrations, with no effect on HDL cholesterol (Bonanome and Grundy, 1988). The neutral effect of C18:0 on plasma lipoproteins is thought to partially reflect rapid desaturation of C18:0 to *cis*-9 C18:1 in the liver (Grundy and Denke, 1990). Also, C18:0 (along with C6:0, C8:0 and C10:0) has been found to have neutral effects on hepatic LDL-receptor activity in hamsters, which controls uptake of LDL from the circulation (Dietschy, 1998). This is in contrast to C12:0, C14:0 and C16:0, which have been found to reduce hepatic LDL-receptor activity (Dietschy, 1998), thus providing evidence of variation in effect of specific SFA in lipoprotein metabolism.

The observed effects of SFA on circulating lipoprotein levels summarised above are based on assessment of clinical trials. However, caution must be

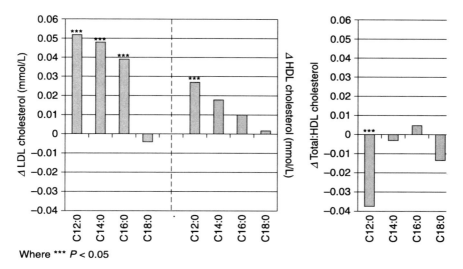

Where *** $P < 0.05$

Fig. 5.1   Predicted changes in the ratio of serum total to HDL cholesterol and in LDL- and HDL-cholesterol concentrations when carbohydrates constituting 1% of energy are replaced isoenergetically with C12:0, C14:0, C16:0 or C18:0 (from Mensink *et al.*, 2003).

employed when directly comparing results of clinical trials as additional factors can influence lipoprotein responses to dietary fat change. For example, women have higher concentrations of circulating HDL-cholesterol than men (Schaefer, 2002) due to hormonal factors, suggesting women have a lower total to HDL cholesterol ratio than men. A meta-analysis comparing the results of seven trials examining the replacement of 9% EI as SFA with MUFA or PUFA demonstrated that the decline in total and LDL-cholesterol is greater in men than in women (Weggemans *et al.*, 1999). These results suggest that men would benefit more from a reduction in SFA intake. However, effects of specific SFA were not reported.

There is also an important effect of genotype. Individuals with the homozygous apoE4 genotype have demonstrated a greater reduction in circulating LDL-cholesterol levels after changing from a high-fat to a low-fat diet than individuals with other genotypes (Dreon *et al.*, 1995). Homozygous apoE4 is present at a frequency of 1–2% in the human population worldwide (Minihane *et al.*, 2007) so it is possible that this may affect the outcome of intervention studies. However, research into the effect of apoE genotype on serum lipoprotein response to changes in dietary fat type has shown inconsistent results (Masson *et al.*, 2003).

Mensink *et al.* (2003) concluded that, overall, the risk of CHD would be most effectively reduced by the replacement of dietary SFA with either *cis*-MUFA or PUFA. The benefits, with respect to cholesterol profile of the two replacement strategies, were broadly similar. They also concluded that effects of dietary fatty acids on biomarkers such as cholesterol can never replace studies which have disease events or death as an outcome.

© Woodhead Publishing Limited, 2011

5.3.2   Effects on disease outcome

Intervention and prospective studies have attempted to overcome the possible weakness of using biomarkers like cholesterol by studying the effect of dietary lipid change on CVD events and all-cause mortality. One prospective cohort study reported that increased intake of C12:0-C18:0 SFA was associated with increased risk of coronary heart disease over 14 years (Hu *et al.*, 1999). A weakness with long-term prospective studies is the error associated with assessment of dietary fatty acid intake from diets. A recent systematic review (Hooper *et al.*, 2009) of all available intervention trials of at least six months' duration, carried out to assess the effect of reducing fat intake or changing dietary fat type on total and CVD mortality and CVD morbidity, found little effect of dietary fat changes in trials lasting less than two years. This suggests that dietary interventions aimed at assessing disease events need to be long term and highly powered, both of which are challenging to achieve and expensive. Warensjö *et al.* (2008) suggested that measurement of serum esterified fatty acids may be a better approach for assessing dietary fat quality citing studies where serum lipids high in C16:0 and C16:1 and low in linoleic acid (C18:2 n-6) were associated with CHD and stroke events (e.g. Öhrvall *et al.*, 1996).

Warensjö *et al.* (2008) reported the results of a population-based prospective study examining the effects of dietary fat quality (SFA in particular) on total and CVD mortality. Warensjö *et al.* (2008) used not only the fatty acid composition of serum cholesteryl esters as predictors of CVD and total mortality but also the fatty acid ratios C16:1/C16:0, C18:3n-6/C18:2n-6 and C20:4n-6/C20:3n-6, which served as indices of Δ^9, Δ^6 and Δ^5-desaturase activities since they argued that serum fatty acid composition is influenced not just by dietary fat but also by endogenous fatty acid metabolism. The study involved a cohort of men (the Uppsala Longitudinal Study of Adult Men) born between 1920 and 1924 and was originally established in 1970, with this study using follow-up data to the end of 2003 (median period 30.7 years). Some of the key findings of this study are summarised in Table 5.4. Of the SFA measured, serum C16:0 was associated with increased mortality and especially CVD mortality. The effect of C14:0 was less and there was no effect of C18:0. Interestingly, of all the serum fatty acids, the greatest mortality risk was associated with palmitoleic acid (*cis*-9, C16:1). Since, as the authors point out, C16:1 in the diet is normally low, most C16:1 in serum is a result of Δ^9-desaturase action on C16:0 and it is notable that the estimate of Δ^9-desaturase activity was also significantly associated with increased CVD and total mortality. Overall, this study tended to agree with the conclusions of cholesterol-based studies that of the dietary SFA, C16:0 poses the greatest risk and that C16:1 of dietary or endogenous origin is probably of greater risk. The study also showed that an individual's inherent Δ^9-desaturase activity may be of equal or greater importance, a factor that will be at least partly under genetic control. In this study it was reported that 78% of men in the highest quartile of Δ^9-desaturase activity (C16:1/C16:0) at age 50 years remained in the top two quartiles at age 70 years. This also raises the question as to what proportion of the negative effect of C16:0 is a direct one and what proportion is exerted through desaturation to C16:1.

© Woodhead Publishing Limited, 2011

Table 5.4 Hazard ratios for selected fatty acids in serum cholesteryl esters and desaturase activities in relation to CVD and total mortality

Fatty acid and estimated desaturase activity	Adjusted[1] hazard ratio[2] for:	
	CVD mortality	Total mortality
Myristic acid (C14:0)	1.12 (1.02–1.23)	1.06 (0.99–1.13)
Palmitic acid (C16:0)	1.15 (1.04–1.26)	1.09 (1.02–1.17)
Palmitoleic (C16:1)	1.18 (1.07–1.30)	1.19 (1.11–1.27)
Stearic acid (C18:0)	1.04 (0.94–1.15)	0.98 (0.91–1.04)
Δ^9 desaturase (C16:1/C16:0)	1.15 (1.04–1.27)	1.18 (1.10–1.26)

[1] Adjusted for total cholesterol, BMI, smoking, physical activity and hypertension.
[2] each with 95% confidence interval.
Source: Warensjö et al., 2008.

Although most attention has been focused on the relationship between SFA and CVD, an interesting case-control study was reported by Nkondjock et al. (2005) examining the association between intake of different fatty acids and pancreatic cancer. The odds ratios for pancreatic cancer in those in the highest versus the lowest quartile of intake were 0.73 (95% CI 0.56–0.96), 0.70 (95% CI 0.51–0.94) and 0.75 (95% CI 0.55–1.02) for C16:0, C18:0 and C18:1 respectively. There were significant interactions with body mass index such that the odds ratios for C18:0, total SFA and total MUFA were 0.36, 0.35 and 0.32 respectively in obese subjects. The authors concluded that substituting PUFA with SFA or MUFA may reduce pancreatic cancer risk, particularly among obese subjects, and this reduction was independent of total EI. It should be noted, however, that evidence from case-control studies is generally regarded as being weaker than from prospective cohort studies.

5.4   The 'stearic acid' effect – chronic disease risk effects of stearic acid

The work cited earlier in relation to the effect of C18:0 on plasma lipids (Bonanome and Grundy, 1988; Mensink et al., 2003, Fig. 5.1) and CVD outcome (Warensjö et al., 2008) suggested its effect was neutral. There has, however, been a resurgence of interest in this SFA since oils high in C18:0 represent a valuable, stable product that can be used to replace *trans* fatty acids in foods such as shortenings and baked products that require solid fats for textural characteristics. Hulshof et al. (1999) reported that intakes of C18:0 by European populations were in the range of approximately 6 to 9 g/d for women and 6 to 13 g/d for men, equating overall to 18 to 23% of total SFA. In the UK intake was 6 g/d (men and women), equivalent to 21.1% of total SFA or about 3.1% of EI. This intake for the UK, which is essentially the same as the European average, though now somewhat

© Woodhead Publishing Limited, 2011

dated, is very similar to the recent estimate of 3.0% EI for the US population (Hunter *et al.*, 2010).

Because of the possibility of replacing *trans* fatty acids with C18:0, the relative effects of C18:0 have recently been the subject of a systematic review by Hunter *et al.* (2010). Table 5.5 summarises the main conclusions from this review. Broadly, the results show that relative to other SFA and *trans* fatty acids, C18:0 provides benefit in relation to most markers of CVD risk, though *cis*-MUFA and PUFA provide greater benefit than C18:0. However, there were only four studies found which directly looked at replacing *trans* fatty acids with C18:0 and in general there were only limited data on effects on lipoproteins and inflammatory markers. Not included in Table 5.5 is the summary of effects on plasma glucose and insulin concentrations of feeding diets high in C18:0. Only four studies were reported and while one (Sundram *et al.*, 2007) showed that feeding C18:0 at 12.5% EI for 28 days gave a 19% increase in plasma glucose and a 22% reduction in plasma insulin, the other three studies reported no significant effects. Hunter *et al.* (2010) did confirm that further research on this aspect is required to clarify whether high intakes of C18:0 may have detrimental effects on glucose homeostasis. Overall, the authors concluded that the review supports the idea that C18:0 is a 'reasonable substitute' for *trans* fatty acids and other more hypercholesterolemic SFA in food products requiring a solid fat for textural and mouthfeel reasons, though clearly more research is required in certain areas. In relation to the UK, it is worth noting the recent review of SACN (2007), which confirmed that intake of *trans* fatty acids has more than halved over the last 20 years and is now about 1.0% EI. This will limit further reductions in *trans* fatty acid intake and thus its replacement with C18:0 may be less relevant.

5.5   Future trends

There are major forces at work which will shape food-related policy for decades to come. These include the rapidly increasing burden of obesity, the increasing age of populations and the challenge of increasing world food production by some 50% by 2030 to meet the increasing demands (House of Commons, 2009). The first two forces in particular will increase the risk of chronic disease substantially and the third may also add to this risk. WHO/FAO (2003) provide data which suggest that by 2020 chronic diseases will account for almost 75% of all deaths worldwide, with the vast majority being related to cardiovascular disease (CVD). At present CVD has been identified by WHO as the top cause of death in Europe (WHO, 2006) and has been estimated to cost the EU in order of €192 billion per year. The associated large increase in the obesity/type 2 diabetes so-called metabolic syndrome is also of particular concern since it is now also beginning to affect younger people. These issues mean that diet, a key moderator of chronic disease risk, will play an increasingly important role and while there will no doubt be continued pressure from government health agencies to further reduce intake of SFA, the need to more clearly understand the relative effects of different SFA will become even greater.

© Woodhead Publishing Limited, 2011

Table 5.5 Summary of cardiovascular disease risk of stearic acid (C18:0) compared with other dietary fatty acids and other factors

Assessment	Assessment of effects of C18:0 based on:				
	Epidemiology	Plasma lipids/lipoproteins[1]	Haemostatic factors and markers of inflammation[2]	Postprandial effects on plasma lipids/lipoproteins	Postprandial effects on haemostatic factors
High vs. low intake of C18:0 on CHD events	Only three studies found that examined intake of individual SFA. No independent effect of C18:0 found but intake strongly associated with that of other SFA				
Effect of C18:0 vs. other SFA[3]		C18:0 had slight lowering or neutral effect on LDL-C and HDL-C and overall directional decrease in TC/HDL-C ratio. Effects on Lp(a) limited, more studies needed		Single meals high in C18:0 reduced TAG compared with other SFA and unsaturates. Overall no responses associated with CVD risk	Single meals giving up to 26%EI as 18:0 showed no evidence of adverse effects
Effect of C18:0 vs. carbohydrate		C18:0 had no effect on LDL-C compared with high carbohydrate diets			
Effect of diets high in C18:0			Diets with at least to 9% EI as C18:0 fed for up to 40d showed no increases thrombogenic risk and no effect on CRP. More work needed on other markers of inflammation		
Replacement of TFA by C18:0		Only four studies but C18:0 decreased or did not change LDL-C and increased or did not change HDL-C. TC/HDL-C ratio directionally reduced	Very limited data		

[1] LDL-C, HDL-C, TC, LDL-cholesterol, HDL-cholesterol, total cholesterol respectively.
[2] CRP, C-reactive protein; [3]SFA, saturated fatty acids.
Source: Hunter et al., 2010.

© Woodhead Publishing Limited, 2011

In relation to CVD, as noted above much of the work on SFA has evaluated risk in terms of effects on cholesterol as an indicator of the atherogenicity of plasma lipids. There is, however, some evidence that fatty acids can directly influence events in the artery that influence atheroma formation. Attention is beginning to focus on the assessment of endothelial function as dysfunction is a key early sign of atheroma formation (West, 2001). Keogh *et al.* (2005) reported that subjects consuming a high (19% EI) SFA diet for three weeks had reduced flow-mediated dilation when compared with PUFA and MUFA enriched diets. Nicholls *et al.* (2006) showed that, relative to PUFA, diets high in SFA significantly reduced arterial endothelial function. Although no information was provided on the relative proportions of individual SFA in the test diet, the source of SFA was coconut oil, which is unusually rich in C12:0. This study therefore cannot confirm that all SFA have an equal effect on endothelial function but this clearly is an area needing attention. The recent review of Hall (2009) concluded that evidence on the effect of types of dietary fat on endothelial function and blood pressure is inconclusive so further research is required.

5.6   Sources of further information and advice

Williams C and Buttriss J (eds) (2006). *Improving the fat content of food*. Woodhead Publishing Ltd, Cambridge, 542 pp.
British Nutrition Foundation: http://www.nutrition.org.uk.

5.7   References

Ascherio A, Rimm EB, Giovannucci EL, Spiegelman D, Stampfer MJ and Willett WC (1996) 'Dietary fat and risk of coronary heart disease in men: cohort follow-up study in the United States', *Br Med J*, 313, 84–90.
Barger PM and Kelly DP (2000), 'PPAR signalling in the control of cardiac energy metabolism', *Trends Cardiovas Med*, 10, 238–245.
Bonanome A and Grundy SM (1988), 'Effect of dietary stearic acid on plasma cholesterol and lipoprotein', *New Eng J Med*, 318, 1244–8.
Cunnane SC and Griffin BA (2002), 'Nutrition and Metabolism of Lipids', in Gibney M, Vorster HH and Kok FJ, *Introduction to Human Nutrition*, Wiley Blackwell, 81–115.
Denke MA and Grundy SM (1992), 'Comparison of the effects of lauric acid and palmitic acid on plasma lipids and lipoproteins', *Am J Clin Nutr*, 56, 895–8.
Dietschy JM (1998) 'Dietary fatty acids and the regulation of plasma low density lipoprotein cholesterol concentrations', *J Nutr*, 128, 444S–448S.
Dreon DM, Fernstrom HA, Miller B and Krauss RM (1995), 'Apolipoprotein E isoform phenotype and LDL subclass response to a reduced-fat diet', *Arterioscler Thromb Vasc Biol*, 15, 105–11.
German JB and Dillard CJ (2004), 'Saturated fats: what dietary intake?', *Am J Clin Nutr*, 80, 550–9.
Givens DI and Kliem KE (2009), 'Improving the nutritional quality of milk', in Paquin P, *Functional and specialty beverage technology*, Woodhead Publishing Ltd, Cambridge.
Givens DI and Shingfield KJ (2006), 'Optimising dairy milk fatty acid composition', in Williams CM and Buttriss J, *Improving the fat content of foods*, Woodhead Publishing Ltd, Cambridge, pp. 252–80.

© Woodhead Publishing Limited, 2011

Gordon T, Kagan A, Garcia-Palmieri M, Kannel WB, Zukel WJ, Tillotson J, Sorlie P and Hjortland M (1981), 'Diet and its relation to coronary heart disease and death in three populations', *Circulation*, 63, 500–15.

Grundy SM and Denke MA (1990) 'Dietary influences on serum lipids and lipoproteins', *J Lipid Res*, 31, 1149–72.

Gunstone FD, Harwood JL and Padley FB (1994), 'Occurrence and characteristics of oils and fats', in Padley FB, Gunstone FD and Harwood JL, *The Lipid Handbook*, Cambridge, Cambridge University Press, 47–224.

Gurr MI (1999), *Lipids in Nutrition and Health: A Reappraisal*, Bridgewater, Somerset, The Oily Press, pp. 1–48.

Hall WL (2009), 'Dietary saturated and unsaturated fats as determinants of blood pressure and vascular function', *Nutr Res Rev*, 22, 18–38.

Hooper L, Summerbell CD, Higgins JPT, Thompson RL, Clements G, Capps N, Davey Smith G, Riemersma R and Ebrahim S (2009), 'Reduced or modified dietary fat for preventing cardiovascular disease (Review)', *The Cochrane Library 2009*, Issue 1. Available at: http://www.thecochranelibrary.com (accessed 2 May 2010).

House of Commons (2009), *Securing Food Supplies up to 2050: The Challenges Faced by the UK*, Environment, Food and Rural Affairs Committee, Fourth Report of Session 2008–09 *Volume I*, London, The Stationery Office Limited.

Hu FB, Stampfer MJ, Manson JE, Rimm E, Colditz GA, Rosner BA, Hennekens CH and Willett WC (1997), 'Dietary fat intake and the risk of coronary heart disease in women', *N Engl J Med*, 337, 1491–9.

Hu FB, Stampfer MJ, Manson JE, Ascherio A, Colditz GA, Speizer FE, Hennekens CH and Willett WC (1999) 'Dietary saturated fats and their food sources in relation to the risk of coronary heart disease in women', *Am J Clin Nutr*, 70, 1001–8.

Huber K, Petzold J, Rehfeldt C, Ender K and Fiedler I (2007), 'Muscle energy metabolism: structural and functional features in different types of porcine striated muscles', *J Muscle Res Cell Motil*, 28, 249–58.

Hunter JE, Zhang J and Kris-Etherton PM (2010), 'Cardiovascular disease risk of stearic acid compared with trans, other saturated and unsaturated fatty acids: a systematic review', *Am J Clin Nutr*, 91, 46–63.

Hulshof K FAM, van Erp-Baart MA, Anttolainen M, Becker W, Church SM, Couet C, Hermann-Kunz E, Kesteloot H, Leth T, Martins I, Moreiras O, Moschandreas J, Pizzoferrato L, Rimestad A H, Thorgeirsdottir H, van Amelsvoort JMM, Aro A, Kafatos AG, Lanzmann-Petithory D and van Poppel G (1999), 'Intake of fatty acids in Western Europe with emphasis on trans fatty acids: The TRANSFAIR study', *Eur J Clin Nutr*, 53, 143–57.

Katan MB, Zock PL and Mensink RP (1995), 'Dietary oils, serum lipoproteins, and coronary heart disease', *Am J Clin Nutr*, 61, 1368S–1373S.

Keogh JB, Grieger JA, Noakes M and Clifton PM (2005), 'Flow-mediated dilation is impaired by a high-saturated fat diet but not by a high carbohydrate diet', *Arterioscler Thromb Vasc Biol*, 25, 1274–9.

Keys A (1970), 'Coronary heart disease in seven countries', *Circulation*, 41, 1–211.

Keys A, Mienotti A, Karvonen MJ, Aravanis C, Blackburn H, Buzina R, Djordjevic BS, Dontas AS, Fidanza F, Keys MH, Kromhout D, Nedeljkovic S, Punsar S, Seccareccia F and Toshima H (1986), 'The diet and 15-year death rate in the Seven Countries Study', *Am J Epidemiol*, 124, 903–15.

Kris-Etherton PM and Yu S (1997), 'Individual fatty acid effects on plasma lipids and lipoproteins: human studies', *Am J Clin Nutr*, 65 (suppl) 1628S–1644S.

Masson LF, McNeill G, and Avenell A (2003), 'Genetic variation and the lipid response to dietary intervention: a systematic review', *Am J Clin Nutr*, 77, 1098–111.

Mensink RP, Zock PL, Kester AD and Katan MB (2003), 'Effects of dietary fatty acids and carbohydrates on the ratio of serum total to HDL cholesterol and on serum lipids and apolipoproteins: a meta-analysis of 60 controlled trials', *Am J Clin Nutr*, 77, 1146–1155.

© Woodhead Publishing Limited, 2011

Minihane AM, Jofre-Monseny L, Olano-Martin E and Rimbach G (2007), 'ApoE genotype, cardiovascular risk and responsiveness to dietary fat manipulation', *Proc Nutr Soc*, 66, 183–97.

Nestel P, Clifton P and Noakes M (1994), 'Effects of increasing dietary palmitoleic acid compared with palmitic and oleic acids on plasma lipids in hypercholesterolemic men', *J Lipid Res*, 35, 656–62.

Nicholls SJ, Lundman P, Harmer JA, Cutri B, Griffiths KA, Rye K-A, Barter PJ and Celermajer DS (2006), 'Consumption of saturated fat impairs the anti-inflammatory properties of high density lipoproteins and endothelial function', *J Amer Coll Cardiol*, 48, 715–20.

Nkondjock A, Krewski D, Johnson KC, Ghadirian P and the Canadian Cancer Registries Epidemiology Research Group (2005), 'Specific fatty acid intake and the risk of pancreatic cancer in Canada', *Br J Cancer* 92, 971–7.

Oh K, Hu FB, Manson JE, Stampfer MJ, Willett WC (2005), 'Dietary fat intake and risk of coronary heart disease in women: 20 years of follow-up of the nurses' health study', *Am J Epidemiol*, 16, 1672–9.

Öhrvall M, Berglund L, Salminen I, Lithell H, Aro A and Vessby B (1996), 'The serum cholesterol ester fatty acid composition but not the serum concentration of alpha tocopherol predicts the development of myocardial infarction in 50-year-old men: 19 years follow-up', *Atherosclerosis*, 127, 65–71.

Romijn JA, Coyle EF, Sidossis LS, Gastaldelli A, Horowitz JF, Endert E and Wolfe RR (1993), 'Regulation of endogenous fat and carbohydrate metabolism in relation to exercise intensity and duration', *Am J Physiol*, 265, E380–91.

SACN (2007), *Update on Trans Fatty Acids and Health*, London, TSO, 162pp.

Schaefer EJ (2002), 'Lipoproteins, nutrition and heart disease', *Am J Clin Nutr*, 75, 191–212.

Siri-Tarino PW, Sun Q, Hu FB and Krauss RM (2010), 'Meta-analysis of prospective cohort studies evaluating the association of saturated fat with cardiovascular disease' *Am J Clin Nutr*, 91, 535–46.

Skeaff C M and Miller J (2009), 'Dietary Fat and Coronary Heart Disease: Summary of Evidence from Prospective Cohort and Randomised Controlled Trials', *Ann Nutr Metab*, 55, 173–201.

Smith JG, Yokoyama WH and German JB (1998), 'Butyric acid from the diet: Actions at the level of gene expression', *Crit Rev Food Sci*, 38, 259–97.

Sundram K, Karupaiah, T and Hayes KC (2007), 'Stearic acid-rich interesterified fat and trans-rich fat raise the LDL/HDL ratio and plasma glucose relative to palm olein in humans', *Nutr Metab*, 4, 3.

Temme EHM, Mensink RP and Hornstra G (1996), 'Comparison of the effects of diets enriched in lauric, palmitic, or oleic acids on serum lipids and lipoproteins in healthy women and men', *Am J Clin Nutr*, 63, 897–903.

Turpeinen O, Karvonen MJ, Pekkarinen M, Miettinen M, Elosuo R and Paavilainen E (1979), 'Dietary prevention of coronary heart disease: the Finnish Mental Hospital Study', *Int J Epidemiol*, 8, 99–118.

Warensjö E, Sundström J, Vessby B, Cederholm T, and Risérus U (2008), 'Markers of dietary fat quality and fatty acid desaturation as predictors of total and cardiovascular mortality: a population-based prospective study', *Am J Clin Nutr*, 88, 203–209.

Weggemans RM, Zock PL, Urgert R and Katan MB (1999), 'Differences between men and women in the response of serum cholesterol to dietary changes', *Eur J Clin Invest*, 29, 827–34.

West SG (2001), 'Effect of diet on vascular reactivity: an emerging marker for vascular risk', *Curr Atheroscler Rep*, 3, 446–55.

WHO/FAO (2003), *Diet, nutrition and the prevention of chronic diseases. Report of a Joint WHO/FAO Expert Consultation*, Geneva, WHO, 148 pp.

© Woodhead Publishing Limited, 2011

WHO (2006), 'Gaining health: The European strategy for the prevention and control of noncommunicable diseases'. Available at http://www.euro.who.int/__data/assets/pdf_file/0008/76526/E89306.pdf (accessed 3 December 2010).

Zock PL (2006), 'Health problems associated with saturated and *trans* fatty acids intake', in Williams CM and Buttriss J, *Improving the fat content of foods*, Woodhead Publishing Ltd, Cambridge, pp. 3–24.

© Woodhead Publishing Limited, 2011

6

Nutritional characteristics of palm oil

P. Khosla, Wayne State University, USA and K. Sundram, Malaysian Palm Oil Council, Malaysia

Abstract: Palm oil (*Elaeis guineensis*) is the leading edible oil in terms of global production and export, with Indonesia and Malaysia being the leading producers. Palm oil's very high yield per hectare necessitates the use of substantially less arable land than any other edible oil. A balanced fatty acid composition (~ 50% saturated and 50% unsaturated fatty acids) makes it a versatile oil for numerous food applications. Various minor components (pro vitamin A and vitamin E) provide additional avenues for its use in human nutrition. This chapter reviews the nutritional attributes of palm oil, primarily from the standpoint of its fatty acid composition.

Key words: palm oil, fatty acids, saturated fatty acids, blood cholesterol, lipoprotein metabolism.

6.1 Introduction

Palm oil and palm kernel oil, obtained from the pulp and seed, respectively, of the oil palm (*Elaeis guineensis*), accounted for ~30% of global fats and oil production in 2008. Palm oil was the leading edible oil produced, overtaking soybean oil which accounted for ~23% of global production. In terms of exports, palm oil and palm kernel oil accounted for almost 60% of global exports. Furthermore, given that palm oil yield per hectare is roughly ten times the yield of soybean oil, this means that global palm oil output is obtained from less than 5% of the total arable land. These figures alone highlight the key role that palm oil plays in human nutrition today, and is likely to play in the immediate future. This widespread availability means that palm oil is finding ever increasing uses in the food sector. Fractionation procedures (discussed elsewhere in this book) produce an array of products which greatly expand palm oil's usage in diverse food formulations. In addition, the presence of various minor components (micronutrients) in the crude oil, including carotenoids (some with vitamin A activity) and vitamin E (including a high concentration of

© Woodhead Publishing Limited, 2011

tocotrienols), has resulted in palm oil becoming a global player in various public health initiatives. This chapter will discuss some of the nutritional aspects of palm oil and summarize key findings. These will be discussed primarily from the standpoint of palm oil's fatty acid composition and the role of its minor components.

6.2   Serum cholesterol, lipoproteins and dietary fatty acids

Cardiovascular disease (CVD) accounts for a major proportion of chronic-disease-related deaths worldwide. One of the readily measured markers that has been studied extensively is the plasma lipid profile with elevations in total cholesterol (TC) and low-density lipoprotein cholesterol (LDL-C) associated with increased risk, while elevated high-density lipoprotein cholesterol (HDL-C) is protective. Numerous dietary factors can impact the plasma lipid profile including macronutrient quality, fiber, antioxidants, various phytochemicals and alcohol. Of these dietary components, dietary fat has perhaps been subjected to the greatest scrutiny. Historically, epidemiological studies revealed a positive association between serum cholesterol and coronary heart disease (CHD) risk. The fact that serum cholesterol could be affected by dietary fat resulted in a quick and dramatic focus on this dietary component. Initially, studies evaluated the role of dietary fat quantity and quality on total serum cholesterol (TC). The classical studies by Hegsted, Keys and their colleagues (Hegsted *et al.*, 1965, Keys *et al.*, 1965) delineated the cholesterolemic effects of SFA, monounsaturated fatty acids (MUFA) and polyunsaturated fatty acids (PUFA). These studies showed that SFA were twice as effective in raising TC as the PUFA were in lowering it, while stearic acid (18:0) – an SFA – and oleic acid (18:1) – a MUFA – were both neutral. Both groups of workers summarized their findings using simplified mathematical relationships which have been the basis for dietary guidelines with a primary goal of lowering TC concentrations (specifically by decreasing LDL-C) and thereby reducing the risk of CVD. When individual fatty acids were considered, the original regression equations developed by Hegsted revealed that myristic acid (14:0) raised serum cholesterol (SC) four times more than palmitic (16:0), while PUFA (mainly linoleic acid) lowered SC (Hegsted *et al.*, 1965). Thus the simple public health message to emerge from this era was that SFA were to be replaced with unsaturated fatty acids (UFA). Hence food manufacturers invested enormous resources in producing a slew of products with lower fat and saturated fat content.

Based on the above studies, the SFA content of palm oil became the driving force in its being branded a cholesterol-raising fat. Several dietary studies evaluating palm oil's ability to influence blood cholesterol were initially reported. While some studies evaluated the effects of individual SFA and used palm oil as a source of palmitic acid, others compared palm oil *per se* with other dietary oils or fats.

Mattson and Grundy (1985) evaluated 20 hypercholesterolemic men fed liquid formula diets with 40%en from a single fat-source-palm oil, high oleic safflower oil or high linoleic safflower oil. Each diet utilized extreme shifts in fatty acids, which would be difficult to achieve using solid-food diets. Replacing ~15%en

© Woodhead Publishing Limited, 2011

from 16:0 (palm oil) with 18:1 (high oleic safflower oil) lowered TC and LDL-C. When ~22%en from 18:1 was additionally replaced with 18:2 (high linoleic safflower oil), TC and HDL-C was further lowered. Distinct differences were observed between the normotriglyceridemic and hypertriglyceridemic subjects. Although these diets approximated the typical American fat content (40%en), they did not mimic the typical fatty acid distribution. This was probably the first study to show a potent hypercholesterolemic effect of 16:0, which was magnified by the use of hypercholesterolemic subjects.

Bonanome and Grundy (1988) compared the effects of replacing palm oil with either an 18:0 rich or 18:1-rich fat, in 11 mildly hypercholesterolemic male subjects fed liquid formula diets, again in a metabolic ward setting. In order to formulate the diet with a high 18:0 content, fully hydrogenated soybean oil and high oleic sunflower oil were chemically hydrolysed and randomly re-esterified (a process that could have resulted in 'atypical' triglyceride moieties). Replacing 15%en from 16:0 (palm oil) with either 18:0 or 18:1 (high oleic sunflower) lowered both TC and LDL-C. Although neither the 18:0-rich or 18:1-rich diets significantly affected HDL-C concentrations, the 18:0-rich diet significantly improved the LDL-C/HDL-C ratio as compared to the 16:0-rich diet. As with the study by Mattson and Grundy (1985), the baseline TC concentration was lowered by all diets, regardless of fatty acid composition.

Finally, again using cholesterol-free liquid formula diets, Denke and Grundy (1992) compared the effects of 12:0 with either 16:0 (palm oil) or 18:1 in 18 men. The 12:0-rich diet (17.6%en from 12:0) raised TC by 9 mg/dL compared to a diet with 17.4%en from 16:0. The increase occurred exclusively in LDL-C. Both diets supplied 16–18%en from 18:1 and 2.5–4%en from 18:2. In comparison to the 18:1-rich diet (30.3%en 18:1, 0.04%en 12:0) the 12:0-rich diet (17.6%en 12:0, 17.8%en 18:1) increased TC, LDL-C and HDL-C by 28, 15 and 5 mg/dL, respectively. TG levels were unaffected. In the above studies, whether palm oil or palm stearin or a variant fraction was used in the studies was never readily apparent as authors frequently reported a fatty acid composition taken from published data (as opposed to actual measurement).

The above three metabolic-ward studies were characterized by 1) the use of liquid-formula diets, 2) high levels of total fat intake ~40%en, 3) relatively 'older' male subjects with moderate to severe hypercholesterolemia based on their entry level SC concentrations and 4) the feeding of atypical diets (with 16:0 representing ~45% of the total fatty acids in the palmitic-acid enriched diets and 18:1 accounting for ~75–80% of the total fatty acids in the oleic-acid enriched diets) which would be very difficult to achieve in the everyday human experience. However, the above studies were not designed to evaluate palm oil *per se*. The objectives of these studies was to evaluate the ability of UFA to lower cholesterol when they replaced SFA (as predicted by the Hegsted equations), in *hypercholesterolemic* individuals consuming *high-fat diets*.

It is clear that given the above conditions, high concentrations of UFA lower TC relative to high concentrations of SFA, and as palm oil was used as the source of 16:0 the extrapolation was that palm oil was hypercholesterolemic. Whether palm oil

© Woodhead Publishing Limited, 2011

affected cholesterolemia in *normocholesterolemic* individuals or subjects consuming moderate (30% calories) or low levels (20% of calories) of fat was not considered. Based on the above, when solid-food diets were utilized with more realistic fatty acid exchanges and mildly hypercholesterolemic to normocholesterolemic younger subjects were used, the hypercholesterolemia attributed to palmitic acid (the main SFA in palm oil) was either blunted or disappeared.

6.3   Effects of palm olein as part of a low-fat healthy diet

Instead of palm oil, palm olein (a liquid fraction with a higher oleic content), when consumed as part of a low-fat (< 30% calories) diet, has been evaluated for its cholesterolemic effects in several human studies. Marzuki *et al.* (1991) evaluated the effect of consuming foods containing either palm olein or soybean oil in young healthy volunteers and found no significant difference in serum TC and LDL-C. In a similar study (Ng *et al.*, 1991), when volunteers were switched from a coconut oil diet to a palm olein or a corn oil diet, serum TC decreased. Ghafoorunissa *et al.* (1995) substituted palm olein for groundnut oil in the typical Indian diet with 27% calories coming from dietary fat. Although this doubled the SFA content and decreased linoleic acid content, plasma levels of cholesterol and lipoproteins were not affected.

6.3.1   Effects of palm olein in comparison to oleic rich oils

Ng *et al.* (1992) evaluated the effects of palm olein and olive oil on serum lipids and lipoproteins in comparison to a coconut oil diet, with each oil providing two-thirds of the total fat intake. The coconut oil diet significantly raised all lipoprotein parameters while a one-to-one exchange between palm olein (rich in 16:0) and olive oil (rich in 18:1) resulted in similar values. Choudhury *et al.* (1995) managed a 5% energy exchange between palm oil (16:0-rich) and olive oil (18:1-rich) in 21 healthy normocholesterolemic Australian subjects consuming a low-fat (30% energy) and low dietary cholesterol (< 200 mg/day) diet. Under these conditions, TC and LDL-C were not significantly different between the two oils.

Truswell *et al.* (1992) also reported a similar effect between palm olein and canola oil. The above-mentioned studies (Ng *et al.*, 1992, Truswell *et al.*, 1992, Choudhury *et al.*, 1995), showed that in healthy normocholesterolemic humans, palm olein could be exchanged for olive oil (high oleic) without adversely affecting serum lipids and lipoprotein levels. Sundram *et al.* (1995) fed 23 healthy normocholesterolemic male volunteers diets containing canola oil (18:1-rich), palm olein (16:0-rich) or an AHA Step 1 diet, all with ~31% energy as fat and < 200 mg dietary cholesterol/day. The AHA oil blend was obtained by blending soybean oil (50%), palm oil (40%) and canola oil (10%), which resulted in a 1:1:1 ratio of the SFA, MUFA and PUFA. Serum TC, VLDL-C and LDL-C were not significantly affected by these diets. The high 18:1 canola and high 16:0 palm olein resulted in almost identical plasma and lipoprotein cholesterol. Only HDL-C after the AHA diet was significantly raised compared with the other two diets.

© Woodhead Publishing Limited, 2011

Zock *et al.* (1994) reported that replacing 10% energy from 16:0 with 18:1 in normocholesterolemic subjects significantly lowered TC and LDL-C. However, this Dutch study did not use natural fat sources. The 18:1-rich diet was prepared by blending high 18:1 sunflower oil, fully hydrogenated sunflower oil and high 18:2 sunflower oil and interesterified palm oil mixed with other edible oils. The 16:0-rich diet was formulated by blending fractionated palm oil, cottonseed oil and fully hydrogenated sunflower oil. The feeding of fat blends containing atypical triglyceride moieties may have been partially responsible for the observed increases in TC and LDL-C. When Sundram *et al.* (1992) maximally replaced the habitual Dutch diet with palm oil, TC and LDL-C were unaffected.

6.3.2   Effects of palm olein in comparison to saturated fats
The original studies of Hegsted *et al.* (1965) suggested that 18:0 was neutral, while 14:0 was four times more potent than 16:0. However, the simplified public health message was that all SFA were the same. The studies described in the preceding section – in which palm olein gave equivalent plasma lipid concentrations with high 18:1-containing oils – suggested that 16:0 itself may not be as hypercholesterolemic as the other SFA and may under certain instances appear 'neutral'.

Sundram *et al.* (1994) fed 17 normocholesterolemic subjects whole-food diets that exchanged 5% energy between 16:0 and 12:0+14:0 (lauric + myristic, LM). Compared with the latter diet, the 16:0 rich diet showed a 9% lower TC concentration, reflected primarily by a lower LDL-C. Heber *et al.* (1992) evaluated diets enriched with palm oil, coconut oil or hydrogenated soybean oil for three-week test periods in healthy American males. Significant increases in TC and LDL-C were apparent following consumption of the coconut oil diet but not the palm oil and hydrogenated soybean oil diets. In the Ng *et al.* (1991, 1992) studies, coconut oil enriched diets were compared to palm olein. In both populations, coconut oil feeding resulted in significant increases in TC and LDL-C compared with the palm olein feeding. These studies compared the effects of 12:0+14:0 (LM) occurring naturally in coconut oil and palm kernel oil. This suggests that the cholesterolemic effect due to 16:0 (palmitic acid) is significantly lower than that of an LM combination.

Wood *et al.* (1993) compared the effects of butter, hard margarine, sunflower oil and palm oil (crude and refined) on lipoprotein profiles in subjects consuming 38% energy as fat (typical US fat intake at that time). The test fats provided almost 50% of the total fat intake, which was equivalent to 16% energy. Diets containing crude or refined palm oil did not elevate TC relative to the habitual American diet while LDL-C was unaffected relative to all other test diets. However, refined palm oil significantly increased HDL-C and improved the ratio of LDL/HDL-cholesterol.

Studies from Clandinin's group (Cook *et al.*, 1997, Clandinin *et al.*, 1999, Clandinin *et al.*, 2000, French *et al.*, 2002) have evaluated palm olein within the context of prudent diets both in terms of total fat (~30% of total calories) and saturated fatty acid content (~10% of total calories). Under such conditions, stable-isotope studies have revealed no effects on endogenous cholesterol synthesis.

© Woodhead Publishing Limited, 2011

The 'neutral' effect of palm olein typically observed in studies, in which total fat represented ~30% of total calories, may in part be explained by the 'threshold hypothesis' of Hayes (see Hayes, 1995, Hayes and Khosla, 2007, Khosla, 2006, Khosla and Sundram, 1996 for a more detailed discussion). According to this hypothesis any deleterious effects that SFA may have on blood lipids can be blunted or even abolished, if 'threshold' levels of dietary 18:2 are present (~5% of total calories). Below this threshold value, the relative potencies of the individual SFA are readily apparent, whereas above threshold levels of 18:2 the SFA begin to appear 'neutral'. This is believed to reflect, in part, 18:2's ability to maximally express LDL receptors. This is consistent with epidemiological data on the ability of PUFA to decrease CHD risk (discussed in subsequent sections). Thus palm olein, which is essentially devoid of 12:0 and 14:0, appears to have sufficient 18:2 to counter any deleterious effects of 16:0. In the above model, 18:1 is believed to be neutral. The above concept of using 18:2 to essentially balance SFA in the diet is ingrained into most current dietary recommendations, which essentially advocate equivalent amounts of SFA and PUFA, with the remaining fatty acids being derived from MUFA. In this regard it is interesting that the original equations of Hegsted *et al.* (1965) showed that in diets devoid of 14:0, the change in TC was negated by a balance between 16:0 and PUFA.

6.4   Effects of dietary fatty acids on LDL-C/HDL-C ratios

For several years the modulation of LDL-C became the sole criterion for evaluating the efficacy of any dietary intervention, even though evidence was available that LDL-C was not the sole driving force behind CVD. Thus it is known that small dense LDL particles are more atherogenic than large buoyant LDL particles – and SFA decrease small dense LDL (Dreon *et al.*, 1998, Siri-Tarino *et al.*, 2010). Lp(a), an independent predictor of CHD risk, which is generally refractory to dietary perturbations, is decreased by dietary SFA (Clevidence *et al.*, 1997, Hornstra *et al.*, 1991). Risk assessment studies designed to assign 'risk' to various dietary and lifestyle contributors to CHD, although showing beneficial effects of PUFA (specifically n-3 fatty acids), frequently fail to show any contribution to risk from SFA (Barraj *et al.*, 2008, Mente *et al.*, 2009).

With a greater understanding of lipoprotein metabolism, the research focus shifted to delineating the effects of dietary fat (fatty acids) on specific lipoprotein classes – very low-density lipoprotein (VLDL), LDL and HDL. Since humans normally transport two to three times as much cholesterol in LDL as opposed to HDL, the primary focus of attention has been factors that affect LDL-C concentrations. Accordingly, the principal public health message has been targeted towards lowering LDL-C concentration. However, HDL-C is also related to CHD risk, with low levels increasing risk. Thus the ratio of LDL-C/HDL-C (or TC/HDL-C), an easily determined indicator of risk, is a far more valuable CHD risk predictor than either LDL-C or HDL-C.

© Woodhead Publishing Limited, 2011

Mensink *et al.* (2003) compared the effects of fatty acid classes as well as individual SFA on the ratio of TC/HDL-C (in relation to carbohydrate). These authors noted that SFA had no effect on this ratio, while MUFA and PUFA improved it. Amongst individual SFA, lauric acid and stearic acid (18:0) resulted in improvements in the TC/HDL-C ratio (12:0 being the most beneficial), while 14:0 and 16:0 had no effect. These differential effects on TC/HDL-C result by virtue of the fact that 12:0, 14:0 and 16:0 all raise LDL-C and HDL-C to different degrees.

6.4.1   Effects of *trans* fatty acids on plasma lipids and CHD

Since 1990, *trans* MUFA – specifically those produced by partial hydrogenation of liquid vegetable oils (PHVO) – have also been the subject of intense scrutiny. There is now a concordance of evidence from clinical studies as well as epidemiological data showing that of all the fatty acids, *trans* fatty acids (tFA) are the most detrimental in terms of their effects on plasma lipids (TC/HDL-C ratio) as well as actual 'hard' clinical end points in relation to CHD. Thus in the analyses by Mensink *et al.* (2003), isoenergetic replacement of carbohydrate with tFA (or SFA) resulted in increased LDL-C (as compared to isoenergetic exchanges of carbohydrates with cisMUFA or PUFA). In the case of HDL-C, there was no effect when tFA replaced carbohydrate, whereas replacement with SFA, cisMUFA or PUFA all increased HDL-C to varying degrees. As a result of these changes, the ratio of TC/HDL-C was significantly elevated by tFA, while SFA had no effect and cisMUFA and PUFA resulted in improved ratios (Fig. 6.1). In agreement with

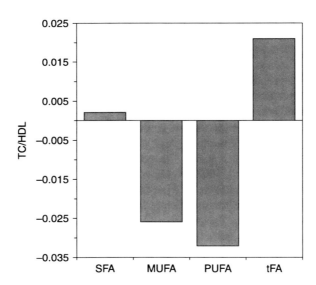

Fig. 6.1   Effects on the TC/HDL-C ratio of replacing isoenergetic amounts of carbohydrates with an equivalent amount of calories from specific fatty acids. Data shows the effects of replacing 1% calories from carbohydrates with either saturated, *cis* monounsaturated, polyunsaturated or *trans* fatty acids. Adapted from Mensink *et al.*, 2003.

© Woodhead Publishing Limited, 2011

these observations palm olein has been shown to produce favorable lipoprotein profiles when compared to tFA (Sundram *et al.*, 1997, Sundram *et al.*, 2007). In the case of the study by Sundram *et al.* (2007), palm olein was also superior to an interesterified 18:0-rich fat.

A 2% increase in tFA has been shown to result in a significant increase in relative risk (RR) for CHD in several epidemiological studies. Using data from the Nurses Health study, Hu *et al.* (1997) showed that, relative to carbohydrate, a 5% en increase in SFA resulted in a 17% non-significant ($p < 0.10$) increase in CHD, while similar increases from MUFA or PUFA were associated with significant reductions in RR of 19% ($p < 0.05$) and 38% ($p < 0.003$), respectively (Fig. 6.2). However, replacing 2% of calories from carbohydrate with transMUFA resulted in a significant doubling of CHD risk (RR 1.93, $p < 0.001$). In a subsequent analysis of data from the same cohort, Salmeron *et al.* (2001) evaluated type II diabetes risk. Again, replacing 5% of calories from carbohydrate with PUFA resulted in a significant reduction in risk (RR 0.63, $p < 0.0001$) while similar exchanges with SFA (RR 0.97, $p = 0.68$) and MUFA (RR 1.05, $p = 0.52$) had no effect. Again, replacing 2% of calories from carbohydrate with transMUFA was associated with the largest increase in risk (RR 1.39, $p = 0.0006$) (Fig. 6.2). Thus the results from these (and other studies) are important drivers in public health messages advocating replacing *trans* and saturates with unsaturated fatty acids.

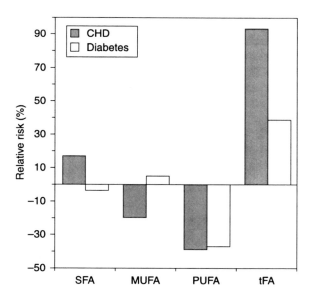

Fig. 6.2   Effects on CHD and type II diabetes risk of replacing isoenergetic amounts of carbohydrates with an equivalent amount of calories from specific fatty acids. Data shows the effects of replacing 5% of calories from carbohydrates with either saturated, *cis* monounsaturated and polyunsaturated fatty acids, while for the *trans* fatty acids the data is for a 2% calorie exchange. Adapted from: (a) CHD data – Hu *et al.*, 1997; and b) Diabetes data – Salmerón *et al.*, 2001.

© Woodhead Publishing Limited, 2011

These data have been largely borne out by longer-term studies. Thus, Oh *et al.* (2005), when evaluating 20-year data from the Nurses Health study noted that the major fatty acid that increased CHD risk was transMUFA while PUFA significantly lowered risk. Of interest was the observation that SFA intake, even at levels greater than the level – 10% of calories – advocated by most health agencies, was not significantly associated with CHD risk.

The above epidemiological data are especially relevant when considering palm oil. The latter has a roughly balanced composition between SFA and UFA. In the data from Hu *et al.* (1997) the increase in CHD risk (17%) attributable to a 5% calorie increase in SFA (at the expense of carbohydrate) is more than offset by a similar decrease in CHD risk (19%) when the exchange is with MUFA. Thus, theoretically, replacement of carbohydrate with palm oil would not be expected to impact CHD. This concept has not been formally tested with CHD end points *per se*.

The above concept is also important from another standpoint. CHD is affected by multiple factors which include, for example, elevated LDL-C, C-reactive protein (CRP), Lp(a), the apoB/apoA1 ratio and low levels of HDL-C. Therefore, focusing on a specific parameter may lead to divergent conclusions. Thus all SFA increase LDL-C (with the exception of 18:0), making them undesirable, while SFA lower Lp(a) and raise HDL-C, making them beneficial. Similarly SFA increase the concentration of large, buoyant LDL particles but decrease the concentration of small, dense atherogenic LDL particles. While these may be important in their own right, the major end point of course is CHD. In this regard the recent study of Mozaffarian and Clarke (2009) is of interest.

In this study, Mozaffarian and Clarke (2009) evaluated the effects on CHD of replacing partially hydrogenated vegetable oils (containing 20%, 30% and 45% of *trans* fatty acids) with specific fats and oils, including palm oil, soybean oil, butter, lard, high oleic safflower oil and canola oil. The authors took the analysis one step further by evaluating CHD risk in relation to the contribution from TC/HDL-C, Lp(a), C-reactive protein and the apoB/ApoA1 ratio. Using this composite analysis, replacing 7.5% of energy from partially hydrogenated vegetable oil (containing 45% transMUFA) with palm oil decreased CHD risk by ~ 30% while the figure for highly unsaturated oils (soybean or canola) was closer to 40%.

6.5   Palm oil minor components

The nutritional properties of palm oil's minor components have also been the focus of intense study. Crude palm oil is one of the richest known sources of biologically active carotenoids (500 to 700 parts per million), of which α- and β-carotene account for ~ 35% and 56%, respectively. However, these are destroyed during conventional refining. Palm oil also contains appreciable amounts of vitamin E (600–1000 ppm) – both the tocopherols and tocotrienols – and is one of the richest natural sources of the latter. The vitamin E content is partially lost during processing, and in some instances less than 50% may be retained as compared to the crude oil. A refined palm oil is available which retains in excess

© Woodhead Publishing Limited, 2011

of 80% of the carotenoids that were originally present in the crude oil. This, red palm oil, has been exploited by nutrition researchers for its pro-vitamin A activity. Additionally, sitosterol, campesterol, stigmasterol and cholesterol constitute the phytosterols in palm oil. Cholesterol content in palm oil is negligible and the phytosterol levels are further reduced on refining.

6.5.1   Palm oil and vitamin A deficiency

Several studies in humans have been reported in which beta-carotene-rich red palm oil has been used effectively in dietary intervention studies to fight vitamin A deficiency without the need to resort to synthetic vitamin A. Children fed traditional Indian sweets made with red palm oil (2.4 mg β-carotene per day for one to two months) increased blood retinol levels, indicative of red palm oil's efficacy as a means for delivering pro vitamin A (Manorama et al., 1997). When school children were fed biscuits baked in a commercialized baking fat containing red palm oil, there was a significant improvement in vitamin A status, as measured by serum retinol levels, which were comparable to that obtained when the children had been fed biscuits with added synthetic β-carotene (van Stuijvenberg et al., 2001). Similarly, higher serum retinol levels were also obtained in school children who were given 5 ml of red palm oil on a daily basis for ten months. The enhancement in serum retinol translated into a significant reduction in Bitot's spot (Sivan et al., 2002). Cooking green leafy vegetables in red palm oil resulted in twice as much β-carotene being made available as compared to cooking in sunflower oil (Hedren et al., 2002). In studies in Burkina Faso, actively promoting red palm oil use (along with other vitamin A rich foods) in certain villages led to a significant reduction in vitamin A deficiency within 24 months of promotion (Zagre et al., 2003). Addition of 15 ml of red palm oil to school meals three times per week for up to one year reduced vitamin A deficiency (Zeba et al., 2006).

6.5.2   Palm oil and vitamin A status in pregnant and lactating women

In addition to the above studies, several studies have also reported on the successful use of red palm oil to improve the vitamin A status of pregnant or lactating women and their offspring. A ten-day dietary supplementation with red palm oil, a total of 90 mg β-carotene, resulted in significant improvement in serum carotenes as opposed to a supplement of synthetic beta carotene in lactating mothers (Canfield et al., 2001). This was accompanied by a significantly higher increase in breast-milk β-carotene of the mothers supplemented with red palm oil, as opposed to those supplemented with synthetic β-carotene. The results suggested, indirectly, that the vitamin A status of the infants would have been improved. Similarly, feeding 8 mL of red palm oil (~ 2.2 mg β-carotene) for the two months prior to delivery resulted in significantly higher serum retinol levels in both the mothers and their infants, as compared to feeding of groundnut oil (Radhika et al., 2003). Finally, in pregnant women in their third trimester, the use of red palm oil in household cooking resulted in higher plasma and breast-milk retinol concentrations

© Woodhead Publishing Limited, 2011

than those observed in women who had been using sunflower oil (Lietz *et al.*, 2001). Thus the above studies illustrate the safety and efficacy of using red palm oil for fighting vitamin A deficiency.

6.5.3   Palm tocotrienols

Unlike the studies on pro vitamin A activity discussed above where palm oil was *fed*, primarily to exploit its β-carotene content, the bulk of the studies exploiting palm oil's vitamin E properties have been conducted using a vitamin E-enriched (primarily, tocotrienol-enriched) fraction *derived* from palm oil. These studies have revealed that, *in vitro*, tocotrienols inhibit cholesterol synthesis (Parker *et al.*, 1993), but studies in humans fed palm-derived tocotrienol supplements have been inconclusive with regards to the use of tocotrienols in managing blood lipid levels (Mensink *et al.*, 1999, Mustad *et al.*, 2002).

Palm tocotrienols have also been touted for their anti-cancer properties. Sundram *et al.* (1989) suggested that crude palm oil was more effective than refined palm oil in increasing the tumour latency period in 7, 12-dimethylbenz [α]anthracene-treated rats. Palm oil devoid of its vitamin E produced more tumours (Nesaretnam *et al.*, 1992). Addition of palm vitamin E to corn oil (500 or 1000 ppm) resulted in a lower tumour incidence and yield compared to rats fed corn oil alone.

Tocotrienols were also effective in inhibiting human breast cancer cells *in vitro* (Guthrie *et al.*, 1997). A palm tocotrienol-rich fraction decreased the severity of hepatocarcinogenesis in rats treated with 2-acetylaminofluorene (Wan Zurinah *et al.*, 1991). Studies from Sylvester's group have delineated the mechanisms for the antiproliferative effects of tocotrienols in breast cancer cells (Shah *et al.*, 2003, Wali *et al.*, 2009, Samant *et al.*, 2010). Recently studies in cell culture and in rodents have provided some exciting insights into the potential therapeutic value of tocotrienols in protecting against neurodegeneration, but these studies are still in their infancy (Sen *et al.*, 2000, Khanna *et al.*, 2005). Although highly promising results have been obtained in animal studies as well as in cell culture models, none of these areas of research have progressed sufficiently for an assessment of their practical use for human populations. One of the problems with the studies with tocotrienols has been the conflicting reports on their absorption rates *in vivo*. However, recent work from Khosla *et al.* (2006) and Fairus *et al.* (2006) has shown that in humans, tocotrienols are indeed transported as part of plasma lipoproteins, albeit with a much shorter half-life than the tocopherols.

6.6   Conclusion and future trends

The current review has traced efforts, primarily over the past three decades, targeted at understanding the nutritional outcomes of palm oil and its products on human health. The outcomes have indeed been a leap forward in this much-needed area since palm oil can be anticipated to continue as one of the two major edible oils consumed around the world. Despite these efforts there are potential gaps that

© Woodhead Publishing Limited, 2011

need to be addressed by future research and these can be illustrated with reference to olive oil – this reference is particularly valid from the standpoint that both olive and palm oil are derived from fruits. A primary reason for olive oil's quick acceptance by the scientific community was the fact that findings from early laboratory and human dietary trials were reinforced through observations from epidemiological data. Thereafter, the acceptances of the benefits of the Mediterranean diet were made apparent. In the case of palm oil, and despite the fact that more than 30 million tonnes are consumed as food annually, there is no epidemiological data from major palm oil-consuming populations that can be used to support the small number of human dietary trials that have been carried out. The results from such well-described epidemiological trials are eagerly awaited and their results could either support or debunk the many scientific observations already cited in this review.

Another important consideration relates to potential alterations in the fatty acid composition of variants of palm oil that can be produced in the future. Faced with increasing concerns for sustainability and environmental management, palm oil producers are already moving ahead to try to achieve the true biological production capacity of the oil palm tree. The current average yields of four tonnes per hectare are likely to be increased to nearly eight tonnes per hectare even in the short term (within the next decade). The scientific tools employed by crop scientists are also likely to result in changes to the overall composition of palm oil.

There have been suggestions, for example, for palm oil of the future to mimic olive oil, with higher levels of oleic acid. Other fatty acid alterations being examined include balancing of the n-6/n-3 ratio in the oil while reducing the overall saturated fatty acid content. Given the nature of palm oil and processing technologies used, these fatty acid alterations would be widespread and geared for applications throughout the global food industry. For example, a higher oleic acid variety palm oil would be an attractive alternative for the frying and fast food industries, taking into consideration that production efficiencies are higher and costs are likely to be lower for palm compared to similar GMO oils. Such huge shifts in fatty acid composition would require a complete re-evaluation of the nutritional end points that are so critical in our benchmarking of a dietary fat.

Fatty acid composition is not the only component that is likely to be altered. Any fatty acid change would invariably be accompanied by alterations in the TAG structure within a fat. In our pursuit to better understand the complexities of fat nutrition, TAG effects including positioning of the fatty acid molecules or *sn* placements are being evaluated. This science is evolving (e.g. through human postprandial studies) and with it our understanding of the complexities of fat nutrition. In this context, palm oil has been less evaluated and, with compositional variations as described above, these new palm oils could emerge as highly interesting materials for scrutiny by future lipid scientists.

In terms of the micronutrient content of palm oil (e.g. tocotrienols, carotenoids, phenolic acids, phytosterols), several human studies have demonstrated the efficacy of crude and red palm oil for delivering pro vitamin A from regular foods in helping to combat vitamin A deficiency. The presence of vitamin E (especially

© Woodhead Publishing Limited, 2011

the high content of tocotrienols) has been the subject of extensive research, especially as different tocotrienols may beneficially impact multiple diseases. Recently the Food and Drug Administration in the United States granted a final notification for GRAS ('generally recognized as safe') status for tocotrienols. As a result tocotrienols (extracted from palm oil) can now be incorporated into food products. These changes, as well as the global dynamics of palm oil trade, will continue to attract considerable attention from nutrition researchers in the years to come.

6.7   Sources of further information and advice

For more detailed information the reader is referred to reviews by Sambanthamurthi *et al.*, 2000, and Hayes and Khosla, 2007, as well as a recent special supplement on palm oil published in the *Journal of the American College of Nutrition* (2010). A new open-access journal – *Journal of Oil Palm and the Environment* – was launched in July 2010 and can be accessed at http://www.jope.com.my.

The following websites also provide information on palm oil-related matters:

Malaysian Palm Oil Board	http://www.mpob.gov.my
Malaysian Palm Oil Council	http://www.mpoc.org.my
Palm Oil World	http://www.palmoilworld.org
Palmoil.com	http://palmoil.com/
Roundtable on Sustainable Palm Oil	http://www.rspo.org

6.8   References

Barraj, L. M., N. L. Tran, *et al.* (2008). 'Perspective: risk apportionment and disease intervention strategies.' Risk Analysis **28**(2): 477–86.

Bonanome, A. and S. M. Grundy (1988). 'Effect of dietary stearic-acid on plasma-cholesterol and lipoprotein levels.' New England Journal of Medicine **318**(19): 1244–8.

Canfield, L. M., R. G. Kaminsky, *et al.* (2001). 'Red palm oil in the maternal diet increases provitamin A carotenoids in breastmilk and serum of the mother–infant dyad.' European Journal of Nutrition **40**(1): 30–8.

Choudhury, N., L. L. Tan, *et al.* (1995). 'comparison of palmolein and olive oil – effects on plasma-lipids and vitamin E in young adults.' American Journal of Clinical Nutrition **61**(5): 1043–51.

Clandinin, M.T., S. L Cook, *et al.* (1999). 'The effect of palmitic acid on lipoprotein cholesterol levels and endogenous cholesterol synthesis in hyperlipidemic subjects.' Lipids **34**(S1): S121–S124.

Clandinin, M.T., S. L Cook, *et al.* (2000). 'The effect of palmitic acid on lipoprotein cholesterol levels.' Int J Food Sci Nutr **51**(6): S61–71.

Clevidence, B. A., J. T. Judd, *et al.* (1997). 'Plasma lipoprotein (a) levels in men and women consuming diets enriched in saturated, cis-, or trans-monounsaturated fatty acids.' Arterioscler Thromb Vasc Biol **17**(9): 1657–61.

Cook, S. L., S. D. Konrad, *et al.* (1997). 'Palmitic acid effect on lipoprotein profiles and endogenous cholesterol synthesis or clearance in humans.' Asia Pacific Journal of Clinical Nutrition **6**: 6–11.

© Woodhead Publishing Limited, 2011

Denke, M. A. and S. M. Grundy (1992). 'Comparison of effects of lauric acid and palmitic acid on plasma lipids and lipoproteins.' American Journal of Clinical Nutrition **56**(5): 895–8.

Dreon, D. M., H. A. Fernstrom, *et al.* (1998). 'Change in dietary saturated fat intake is correlated with change in mass of large low-density-lipoprotein particles in men.' American Journal of Clinical Nutrition **67**(5): 828–36.

Fairus, S., R. M. Nor, *et al.* (2006). 'Postprandial metabolic fate of tocotrienol-rich vitamin E differs significantly from that of alpha-tocopherol.' American Journal of Clinical Nutrition **84**(4): 835–42.

French, M.A., K. Sundram, *et al.* (2002). 'Cholesterolemic effect of palmitic acid in relation to other dietary fatty acids.' Asia Pac J Clin Nutr **11 Suppl 7**: S401–7.

Ghafoorunissa, V. Reddy, *et al.* (1995). 'Palmolein and groundnut oil have comparable effects on blood-lipids and platelet-aggregation in healthy Indian subjects.' Lipids **30**(12): 1163–9.

Guthrie, N., A. Gapor, *et al.* (1997). 'Inhibition of proliferation of estrogen receptor–negative MDA-MB-435 and -positive MCF-7 human breast cancer cells by palm oil tocotrienols and tamoxifen, alone and in combination.' Journal of Nutrition **127**(3): S544–8.

Hayes, K. C. (1995). 'Saturated fats and blood-lipids – new slant on an old story.' Canadian Journal of Cardiology **11**: G39–46.

Hayes, K. C. and P. Khosla (1992). 'Dietary fatty acid thresholds and cholesterolemia.' Faseb Journal **6**(8): 2600–7.

Hayes, K. C. and P. Khosla (2007). 'The complex interplay of palm oil fatty acids on blood lipids.' European Journal of Lipid Science and Technology **109**(4): 453–464.

Hayes, K. C., A. Pronczuk, *et al.* (1991). 'Dietary saturated fatty acids (12–0, 14–0, 16–0) differ in their impact on plasma cholesterol and lipoproteins in nonhuman primates.' American Journal of Clinical Nutrition **53**(2): 491–8.

Heber, D., Ashley, J.M., *et al.* (1992). 'The effects of palm oil enriched diet on plasma lipids and lipoproteins in healthy young men.' Nutrition Research, **12**: 53S–59S.

Hedren E, G. Mulokozi, *et al.* (2002). 'In vitro accessibility of carotenes from green leafy vegetables cooked with sunflower oil or red palm oil.' Int J Food Sci Nutr. **53**(6): 445–53.

Hegsted, D. M., R. B. McGandy, *et al.* (1965). 'Quantitative effects of dietary fat on serum cholesterol in man.' American Journal of Clinical Nutrition **17**(5): 281–25.

Hornstra G., A. C. van Houwelingen, *et al.* (1991). 'A palm oil-enriched diet lowers lipoprotein(a) in normocholesterolemic volunteers.' Atherosclerosis **90**: 91–93.

Hu, F. B., M. J. Stampfer, *et al.* (1997). 'Dietary fat intake and the risk of coronary heart disease in women.' New England Journal of Medicine **337**(21): 1491–9

Keys A, J. T. Anderson, *et al.* (1965). 'Serum cholesterol response to changes in the diet. IV. Particular saturated fatty acids in the diet.' Metabolism **14**: 776–77.

Khanna, S., V. Patel, *et al.* (2005). 'Delivery of orally supplemented alpha-tocotrienol to vital organs of rats and tocopherol-transport protein deficient mice.' Free Radic Biol Med **39**(10): 1310–19.

Khosla, P. (2006). 'Palm oil: a nutritional overview.' Agro Food Industry Hi-Tech **17**(3): 21–23.

Khosla, P., V. Patel, *et al.* (2006). 'Postprandial levels of the natural vitamin E tocotrienol in human circulation.' Antioxidants & Redox Signaling **8**(5–6): 1059–68.

Khosla, P. and K. Sundram (1996). 'Effects of dietary fatty acid composition on plasma cholesterol.' Progress in Lipid Research **35**(2): 93–132.

Lietz, G., C. J. K. Henry, *et al.* (2001). 'Comparison of the effects of supplemental red palm oil and sunflower oil on maternal vitamin A status.' American Journal of Clinical Nutrition **74**(4): 501–9.

Manorama, R., M. Sarita, *et al.* (1997). 'Red palm oil for combating Vitamin A deficiency.' Asia Pac J Clin Nutr **6**(1): 56–9.

© Woodhead Publishing Limited, 2011

Marzuki, A., F. Arshad, *et al.* (1991). 'Influence of dietary fat on plasma lipid profiles of Malaysian adolescents.' American Journal of Clinical Nutrition **53**(4 Suppl): 1010S–1014S.

Mattson, F. H. and S. M. Grundy (1985). 'Comparison of effects of dietary saturated, monounsaturated, and polyunsaturated fatty acids on plasma lipids and lipoproteins in man.' Journal of Lipid Research **26**(2): 194–202.

Mensink, R. P., A. C. van Houwelingen, *et al.* (1999). 'A vitamin E concentrate rich in tocotrienols had no effect on serum lipids, lipoproteins, or platelet function in men with mildly elevated serum lipid concentrations.' American Journal of Clinical Nutrition **69**(2): 213–19.

Mensink, R. P., P. L. Zock, *et al.* (2003). 'Effects of dietary fatty acids and carbohydrates on the ratio of serum total to HDL cholesterol and on serum lipids and apolipoproteins: a meta-analysis of 60 controlled trials.' American Journal of Clinical Nutrition **77**(5): 1146–55.

Mente, A., L. de Koning, *et al.* (2009). 'A systematic review of the evidence supporting a causal link between dietary factors and coronary heart disease.' Arch. Intern. Med. **169**: 659–69.

Mozaffarian, D. and R. Clarke (2009). 'Quantitative effects on cardiovascular risk factors and coronary heart disease risk of replacing partially hydrogenated vegetable oils with other fats and oils.' European Journal of Clinical Nutrition **63**: S22–33.

Mustad, V. A., C. A. Smith, *et al.* (2002). 'Supplementation with 3 compositionally different tocotrienol supplements does not improve cardiovascular disease risk factors in men and women with hypercholesterolemia.' American Journal of Clinical Nutrition **76**(6): 1237–43.

Nesaretnam, K., R. Ambra, *et al.* (2004). 'Tocotrienol-rich fraction from palm oil affects gene expression in tumors resulting from MCF-7 cell inoculation in athymic mice.' Lipids **39**(5): 459–467.

Ng, T. K., K. Hassan, *et al.* (1991). 'Nonhypercholesterolemic effects of a palm-oil diet in Malaysian volunteers.' American Journal of Clinical Nutrition **53**(4): S1015–20.

Ng, T. K., K. C. Hayes, *et al.* (1992). 'Dietary palmitic and oleic acids exert similar effects on serum-cholesterol and lipoprotein profiles in normocholesterolemic men and women.' Journal of the American College of Nutrition **11**(4): 383–90.

Oh, K., F. B. Hu, *et al.* (2005). 'Dietary fat intake and risk of coronary heart disease in women: 20 years of follow-up of the nurses' health study.' American Journal of Epidemiology **161**(7): 672–9.

Parker, R. A., B. C. Pearce, *et al.* (1993). 'Tocotrienols regulate cholesterol production in mammalian cells by post-transcriptional suppression of 3-hydroxy-3-methylglutaryl-coenzyme A reductase.' J Biol Chem. **268**: 11230–8.

Radhika, M. S., P. Bhaskaram, *et al.* (2003). 'Red palm oil supplementation: a feasible diet-based approach to improve the vitamin A status of pregnant women and their infants.' Food Nutr Bull **24**(2): 208–17.

Salmeron, J., F. B. Hu, *et al.* (2001). 'Dietary fat intake and risk of type 2 diabetes in women.' American Journal of Clinical Nutrition **73**(6): 1019–26.

Samant, G. V., V. B. Wali, *et al.* (2010). 'Anti-proliferative effects of gamma-tocotrienol on mammary tumour cells are associated with suppression of cell cycle progression.' Cell Prolif **43**(1): 77–83.

Sambanthamurthi, R., K. Sundram, *et al.* (2000). 'Chemistry and biochemistry of palm oil.' Progress in Lipid Research **39**(6): 507–58.

Sen, C. K., S. Khanna, *et al.* (2000). 'Molecular basis of vitamin E action. Tocotrienol potently inhibits glutamate-induced pp60(c-Src) kinase activation and death of HT4 neuronal cells.' J Biol Chem **275**(17): 13049–55.

Shah, S., A. Gapor, *et al.* (2003). 'Role of caspase-8 activation in mediating vitamin E-induced apoptosis in murine mammary cancer cells.' Nutr Cancer **45**(2): 236–46.

Siri-Tarino, P. W., Q. Sun, *et al.* (2010). 'Meta-analysis of prospective cohort studies evaluating the association of saturated fat with cardiovascular disease.' American Journal of Clinical Nutrition **91**(3): 535–46.

© Woodhead Publishing Limited, 2011

Sivan, Y. S., Y. A. Jayakumar, *et al.* (2002). 'Impact of vitamin A supplementation through different dosages of red palm oil and retinol palmitate on preschool children.' Journal of Tropical Pediatrics **48**(1): 24–8.

Sundram, K., K. C. Hayes, *et al.* (1994). 'Dietary Palmitic Acid Results in Lower Serum-Cholesterol Than Does a Lauric–Myristic Acid Combination in Normolipemic Humans.' American Journal of Clinical Nutrition **59**(4): 841–6.

Sundram, K., K. C. Hayes, *et al.* (1995). 'Both dietary 18/2 and 16/0 may be required to improve the serum LDL/HDL cholesterol ratio in normocholesterolemic men.' Journal of Nutritional Biochemistry **6**(4): 179–87.

Sundram, K., G. Hornstra, *et al.* (1992). 'Replacement of dietary fat with palm oil: effect on human serum lipids, lipoproteins and apolipoproteins.' Br J Nutr **68**(3): 677–92.

Sundram, K., A. Ismail, *et al.* (1997). 'Trans (elaidic) fatty acids adversely affect the lipoprotein profile relative to specific saturated fatty acids in humans.' Journal of Nutrition **127**(3): S514–20.

Sundram, K., T. Karupaiah, *et al.* (2007). 'Stearic acid-rich interesterified fat and trans-rich fat raise the LDL/HDL ratio and plasma glucose relative to palm olein in humans.' Nutr Metab (Lond) **4**: 3–12.

Sundram, K., H. T. Khor, *et al.* (1989). 'Effect of dietary palm oils on mammary carcinogenesis in female rats induced by 7,12-dimethylbenz(a)anthracene.' Cancer Res. **49**: 1447–51.

Truswell, A. S., N. Choudhury, *et al.* (1992). 'Double-blind comparison of plasma-lipids in healthy subjects eating potato crisps fried in palmolein or canola oil.' Nutrition Research **12**: S43–52.

van Stuijvenberg, M. E., M. A. Dhansay, *et al.* (2001). 'The effect of a biscuit with red palm oil as a source of beta-carotene on the vitamin A status of primary school children: a comparison with beta-carotene from a synthetic source in a randomised controlled trial.' European Journal of Clinical Nutrition **55**(8): 657–62.

Wali, V. B., S. V. Bachawal, *et al.* (2009). 'Suppression in mevalonate synthesis mediates antitumor effects of combined statin and gamma-tocotrienol treatment.' Lipids **44**(10): 925–34.

Wan Zurinah, W. N., Zanariah, J., *et al.* (1991). 'Effect of tocotrienols on hepatocarcinogenesis induced by 2-acetylaminofluorene in rats.' Am J. Clin. Nutr **53**: 1076s–1081s.

Wood, R., K. Kubena, *et al.* (1993). 'Effect of palm oil, margarine, butter, and sunflower oil on the serum–lipids and lipoproteins of normocholesterolemic middle-aged men.' Journal of Nutritional Biochemistry **4**(5): 286–97.

Zagre, N. M., F. Delpeuch, *et al.* (2003). 'Red palm oil as a source of vitamin A for mothers and children: impact of a pilot project in Burkina Faso.' Public Health Nutr **6**(8): 733–42.

Zeba, A. N., Y. M. Prével, *et al.* (2006). 'The positive impact of red palm oil in school meals on vitamin A status: study in Burkina Faso.' Nutr J **5**: 17.

Zock, P. L., J. H. de Vries, *et al.* (1994). 'Impact of myristic acid versus palmitic acid on serum lipid and lipoprotein levels in healthy women and men.' Arterioscler Thromb **14**(4): 567–75.

© Woodhead Publishing Limited, 2011

Part II

Food reformulation to reduce saturated fats

© Woodhead Publishing Limited, 2011

7

Reducing saturated fat using emulsion technology

W. G. Morley, Leatherhead Food Research, UK

Abstract: The saturated fat content of a food may be reduced by reducing the total fat content, reducing the saturated fat component of the oil phase, or a combination of both. Most foods that contain oils and fats are emulsions, so it follows that emulsion technology can have an important role in maintaining the product quality while these changes to the oil phase are made. This chapter examines a number of technologies that may be applied to emulsified foods for the reduction of saturated fat. These include the use of fat replacement ingredients, changes to the composition and properties of the oil phase, different methods for the formation of emulsions, manipulation of the aqueous phase behaviour, and use of the intrinsic instability of emulsified oil droplets.

Key words: emulsion, emulsion stability, emulsion droplet aggregation, duplex emulsion, double emulsion, multiple emulsion, fat replacer, interesterification, cryo-crystallisation.

7.1 Introduction

7.1.1 Oil and water in foods

Most foods contain oil or water, and many contain both, with one of these dispersed in the other in the form of an emulsion. The water or aqueous phase typically contains a range of dissolved and dispersed ingredients, ranging from vegetables and herbs to stabilisers, proteins and salts. The oil phase typically contains liquid oil, solid crystalline fat, and oil-soluble ingredients such as colours and vitamins. The oils and fats may be of animal or vegetable origin and are typically blended to give the desired properties. The saturated fat content of a food may be reduced by reducing the total fat content, reducing the saturated fat component of the oil phase, or a combination of both.

© W. G. Morley, 2011

7.1.2   Emulsifiers

The foods that contain oil and water will also contain emulsifiers. Emulsifiers have a structure that comprises a hydrophilic 'head-group' region and a lipophilic or hydrophobic 'tail' region. The hydrophilic head-group preferentially resides in the aqueous phase and the lipophilic tail in the oil phase. This structure allows the emulsifier to typically perform two functions: firstly to facilitate the formation of the emulsion by lowering the interfacial tension, and secondly to stabilise the emulsion to coalescence and phase separation. Food emulsions typically contain a blend of emulsifiers in order to achieve the desired properties.

7.1.3   Oil-in-water emulsions

Oil-in-water (O/W) emulsions comprise a continuous aqueous phase and a dispersed oil phase. The oil content may be as low as 1% w/w in the case of semi-skimmed milk or as high as 80% w/w for full-fat mayonnaise. The emulsifiers will generally be more hydrophilic in nature and have structures with relatively large head-groups. Figure 7.1 is a micrograph of a mayonnaise-type O/W emulsion.

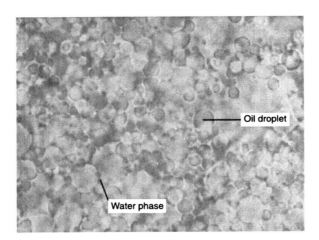

Fig. 7.1   Light micrograph of an O/W emulsion (mayonnaise-type product). Image width approx. 40 µm. Image courtesy of Kathy Groves, Leatherhead Food Research.

7.1.4   Water-in-oil emulsions

Water-in-oil (W/O) emulsions comprise a continuous oil phase and a dispersed aqueous phase. The oil content may be as low as 20% w/w in the case of low-fat spread or as high as 80% w/w for butter. The emulsifiers will generally be more hydrophobic in nature and have structures with relatively small head-groups. Figure 7.2 is a micrograph of a spread-type W/O emulsion.

© W. G. Morley, 2011

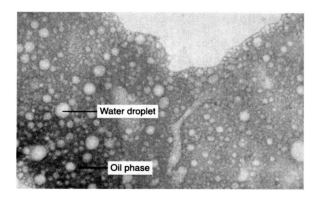

Fig. 7.2 Light micrograph of a W/O emulsion (spread-type product) stained with a red dye to show the oil as a darker colour. Image width approx. 100 μm. Image courtesy of Kathy Groves, Leatherhead Food Research.

7.1.5 Multiple emulsions

Multiple emulsions, sometimes called duplex or double emulsions, may be of the water-in-oil-in-water (W/O/W) or oil-in-water-in-oil (O/W/O) type. They are made by dispersing an emulsion into another continuous phase and require the use of hydrophilic and hydrophobic emulsifiers. Figure 7.3 is a micrograph of a mayonnaise-type W/O/W emulsion, clearly showing the internal aqueous phase droplets.

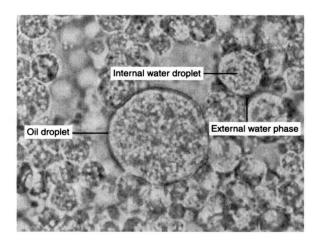

Fig. 7.3 Light micrograph of a W/O/W multiple emulsion (mayonnaise-type product). Image width approx. 40 μm. Image courtesy of Kathy Groves, Leatherhead Food Research.

© W. G. Morley, 2011

7.2   Fat composition

7.2.1   Fat composition changes

Changing the composition of the fat phase of an emulsion is perhaps the most obvious method of reducing the saturated fatty acid content of a food. Changing to an oil or fat with a lower saturated fat level or blending the fat with a lower saturated alternative will achieve the desired aim. The challenge, however, is to maintain the important physical and organoleptic properties with lower levels of saturated fat, and this section will consider some of the more common methods.

Animal feeds

Milk from dairy cows, and derivatives such as cream and butter, are common emulsions that are used in the food industry. Such products, however, are generally considered to be high in saturated fat and the dairy industry can employ modifications to animal feeds to result in milk with reduced levels. The milk that is produced can be used to manufacture other foodstuffs such as cheese, ice cream and butter. For example, in one study (Aigster *et al.*, 2000) early- to mid-lactation Holstein cows were fed calcium salts of high-oleic sunflower oil (>86% oleic acid) as dietary supplements, with the milk that was produced being used to manufacture Latin American white cheese, queso blanco. The saturated fat content of the oil phase was reduced from 65.7% to 53.0% with no reported differences in the firmness or sensory quality of the cheese. In another study (Gonzalez *et al.*, 2003) the diets of Holstein cows were modified to result in milks with higher levels of linoleic acid or oleic acid. In these cases the saturated fatty acid levels of the milk were reduced from 69.3% to 64.1% (high-oleic acid treatment) and 62.2% (high-linoleic acid treatment). Both treatments reduced the viscosities of ice-cream mixes and the firmness of butters when compared to the control milk. There were no significant differences in the sensory firmness of either finished ice cream, based on dipping tests.

Filled emulsions

Another option for changing the composition of the fat phase is the use of filled emulsions. In this process the existing fat phase in a naturally occurring emulsion such as dairy milk or coconut milk is wholly or partially removed and replaced with a lower saturated alternative. This has been particularly applied in the production of cheese products from dairy milk and some examples are summarised in Table 7.1. It can be seen that many of the positive quality attributes can be maintained with significant reductions in the levels of saturated fats using this process. Table 7.1 also contains the key processing steps that were used to prepare the filled emulsions.

Coconut milk has also been adapted in this way with the replacement of some of the coconut oil with sunflower oil (Jittanoonta *et al.*, 1998, pp. 134–9). In a feeding study with rats, decreased levels of blood triglyceride and increased levels of high-density lipoprotein (HDL) cholesterol were observed with increasing levels of sunflower oil.

© W. G. Morley, 2011

Table 7.1   Production of cheese products with reduced levels of saturated fat using filled dairy milk emulsions

Cheese type	Fats and oils used	Attributes maintained	Key processing steps	Ref.
Soft ripened cheese	25% milk fat fraction of low melting point, 50% oleic acid-enriched sunflower oil, 25% soyabean oil	Lipid oxidation. Flavour and shelf-life characteristics.	None. Traditional method of manufacture was used.	During *et al.*, 2000
Low (5%) fat Cheddar cheese	Blends of milk fat and fish oil high in omega-3 fatty acids	Colour, fracture stress and strain, pH, microbial counts, microstructure, body and texture scores (up to 75% replacement of milk fat).	None. Traditional method of manufacture was used.	Aryana, 2007
Various: cheddar-, gouda-, mozzarella-type etc	Preferably wheat germ oil or rice bran oil	Oil retention, meltability, texture, flavour, mechanical properties.	Injection of vegetable oil into skimmed milk to atomise and disperse oil. No emulsifier required	May and Slater, 2003
Cheese (20% milk fat)	Rapeseed oil (17% in cheese)	Reduction of blood serum total and LDL cholesterol levels by 5.0% and 6.4% respectively.	Not stated.	Karvonen *et al.*, 2002

Alternative oils and blends

The manufacture of such products without using either of the processes described above may require novel or modified processing steps in order to maintain the desired quality attributes. Table 7.2 summarises a number of studies in which oil and water continuous food emulsion systems have been produced with lower levels of saturated fat than is normal for the particular food type. A series of positive attributes are claimed and it can be seen that acceptable products can be produced with lower levels of saturated fats than equivalent products. Table 7.2 also contains the key processing steps that were used to prepare the emulsions.

Emulsifiers

Emulsifiers have also been employed to alter the composition of fat blends. An example is the use of polyglycerol esters to act as crystallisation agents in fatty acid mixtures obtained from vegetable oils such as soya bean oil or rapeseed oil

© W. G. Morley, 2011

Table 7.2   Food emulsions with reduced levels of saturated fats

Food type	Fats and oils used	Positive attributes	Key processing steps	Ref.
Dairy cream substitute for frozen dessert	Vegetable, marine and fish oils	Enhanced stability and consistency with alcoholic or acidic ingredients, or at high temperatures.	Protein denaturation step whereby high viscosity sodium caseinate is added to oil phase under controlled temperature and agitation.	St-Jean and Lahaye, 2005
Aqueous dispersion for use in water and fat continuous spreads	Aqueous dispersion contains phytosterols or other high-melting lipid	Formulations do not require conventional thickeners such as xanthan gum or gelatin.	Molten phytosterol and emulsifier dispersed in water under shear. Dispersion less than 10 μm.	Patrick and Traska, 1998
Fat continuous spread	Vegetable oil and free plant sterols	Improved textural properties and mouthfeel.	Mixture of vegetable oil and free plant sterols in elongated crystal form added to W/O emulsion.	Bons *et al.*, 2008
Shortening for use in bakery products	Blend of fully hydrogenated fat and liquid oil	Greater oxidative stability than conventional shortenings.	Cooling and tempering a blend of 11–18% hard fat and 82–89% liquid oil; liquid oil contains 0.1–7% α-linolenic acid.	Unger, 2005
Shortening for use in bakery products	Blend of high stearic, high oleic soybean oil, and a hydrogenated oil	Higher melting range and improved oxidative stability.	Conventional scraped surface heat exchangers.	Kincs *et al.*, 2008.

(Hendree *et al.*, 2003). The process firstly involves fractional distillation to remove most of the palmitic (C16:0) and lower fatty acids, and then fractional crystallisation to remove the stearic (C18:0) fatty acids. The crystallisation agent is preferably triglyceryl monostearate and the process can reduce the total saturated fatty acid level to less than 2%.

7.2.2   Fat level changes

Reducing the fat content of an emulsion with no change in the fat composition has the added benefit of reducing the saturated fat content of the emulsion as a whole. As with changing the fat composition, the challenge is to maintain the desired physical and organoleptic properties with a reduced fat content and it may be necessary to

© W. G. Morley, 2011

increase the saturated fat proportion of the fat blend by changing the composition. This is not ideal and this section considers some alternative techniques.

Oil-in-water emulsions
In a study with fresh cheese, it was discovered that a high pH in combination with a higher salt content produced a creamy product with a lower fat content than standard products (Brown, 2010). The type of fresh cheese is not specified but cottage cheese is listed as an example of the type of product that fits into this category. The fat level of the fresh cheese was reduced from 9% to 3% without affecting the perceived creaminess. Furthermore, it was reported that increasing either the pH or salt content alone did not have the desired effect.

In another study, this time using ewe's milk to manufacture Roncal cheese, a raw ewe's milk cheese, acceptable organoleptic properties were recorded with a shorter ripening time of 60 to 90 days. The fat content of the ewe's milk was reduced from the control 8% to 4%, and apart from the ripening time, conventional procedures were used. However, the quality of the cheese was unacceptable when 2% fat ewe's milk was used (Irigoyen *et al.*, 2004).

A third oil-in-water emulsion example uses oil droplets that are substantially less than 4 μm in diameter in combination with a thickener system to produce dressings compositions that have excellent organoleptic properties (Merolla and Bialek, 2006). The thickener system comprises 1% to 6.5% starch and optionally up to 1% insoluble fibre. The organoleptic properties are claimed to be better than other starch-containing dressings and substantially the same as full-fat, thickener-free compositions.

Other oil-in-water examples in which reduced oil droplet sizes have been employed, but without the addition of thickening systems, are described in section 7.3.2.

Water-in-oil emulsions
The reduction of the fat content for a product normally sold as a bulk fat requires the incorporation of water in the form of an emulsion. An example of this is chocolate and the use of cocoa butter water-in-oil emulsions. Such products were prepared using a high shear mixer with either 2% soybean lecithin or 1% polyglycerol polyricinoleate (PGPR) as the emulsifier (Norton *et al.*, 2009). The water was present in small droplets (<10 μm) with addition levels of up to 20%. A laboratory scale margarine line, comprising a scraped surface heat exchanger followed by a pin stirrer, was also used to prepare cocoa butter water-in-oil emulsions, again with 1% PGPR as the emulsifier (Norton *et al.*, 2009). In this case the water droplet size was around 1 μm with 20% water addition.

Another confectionery application involves the incorporation of water into the filling component while leaving the coating, with a water activity of around 0.2, unchanged (Campbell, 2000). The filling contains around 20% water with a water activity reduced to less than 0.75 with the use of humectants in the form of reduced-calorie sucrose substitutes, and a fat mimetic such as inulin. The inulin is present at levels in the range 20–50% and also acts to emulsify the water.

© W. G. Morley, 2011

A third application is laminating fats that are used for dough products. Such products contain a plurity of thin dough layers that are separated from one another by thin continuous layers of laminating fat. In order to reduce the total fat and saturated fat levels a hydrated laminating fat can be used but the water phase should be properly emulsified in order to prevent it being released into the dough. In one example a hydrated laminating fat containing up to 50% dispersed aqueous phase was prepared using a range of emulsifiers, of which alpha-monoglyceryl stearate was found to perform well (Staeger et al., 2008). The resulting laminated dough products were stable for 75 to 120 days under refrigerated conditions and for two to eight months when frozen.

7.3   Emulsion droplets

7.3.1   Emulsion droplet aggregation

Emulsion systems are thermodynamically unstable and coalescence of the dispersed phase droplets and eventual phase separation will tend to occur in order to minimise the contact area between the two phases. Of course the use of emulsifiers and other stabilising mechanisms such as fat crystals will impart some kinetic stability to the emulsion. In the case of oil-in-water emulsions, coalescence will not occur if the oil droplets have a certain rigidity through the use of crystalline fats, either used alone or in combination with liquid oils. The destabilisation of these emulsions may lead to partial coalescence in which the interfacial film has been ruptured leading to fat–fat contact. Flocculation is a form of dispersed phase droplet aggregation in which the interfacial film has not been ruptured, so in the case of oil-in-water emulsions there will be no fat–fat contact.

Oil droplet aggregation is required for the formation of whipped cream structures but otherwise is generally undesirable because it is difficult to control during the storage of the emulsion. However, such aggregated structures lead to increases in the effective dispersed phase volume due to the incorporation of an interstitial water phase, so may offer scope for the reduction of the total fat level. This section gives some examples of studies that have attempted to produce controlled amounts of aggregation through ingredients and processing modifications.

Ingredients for controlled aggregation
The ability of individual sunflower proteins to form and stabilise emulsions was investigated as a function of pH and ionic strength and after heat treatment (Gonzalez-Perez et al., 2005). Extensive aggregation and coalescence was observed in the emulsions prepared with sunflower albumins, although this was avoided at pH 3. This is believed to be due to sufficiently strong electrostatic repulsion resulting in stable emulsions. In the case of helianthinin, mostly stable emulsions were obtained, except at pH 7, and high ionic strength (100 mM). The addition of $CaCl_2$, however, resulted in significant aggregation except at pH 3. Finally, sunflower protein isolate (SI) emulsions at pH 7 underwent significant aggregation whereas at pH 3 and pH 8 the emulsions were stable at low ionic strength (20 mM).

© W. G. Morley, 2011

The globular protein beta-lactoglobulin was used as the emulsifier in a study of the effect of glycerol and sorbitol on the flocculation stability of n-hexadecane oil-in-water emulsions (Chanasattru *et al.*, 2009). In the absence of glycerol or sorbitol, and without added salt, the emulsions were stable to flocculation following heat treatments in the range 30–90°C. However, with the addition of 150 mM NaCl before heat treatment, flocculation occurred at all temperatures and at 80–90°C the majority of the initial droplets appeared to have aggregated. The addition of glycerol to the salt-containing system led to some improvements in the stability up to 70°C whereas for sorbitol this was the case at all temperatures.

Another example requires a combination of ingredients and processing effects to result in the aggregation of oil droplets and thickening of the emulsion. In this case the aggregation mechanism is not partial coalescence since the thickening is reversible and does not result in increased oil droplet sizes on reheating (Benjamins *et al.*, 2006). Specifically, the thickening occurs when the emulsion is cooled such that the secondary emulsifier is present in a mesomorphic (liquid crystalline) or solid state. The preferred primary emulsifiers are milk, whey and soy proteins, and secondary emulsifiers are saturated mono- and/or di-glycerides and mixtures thereof. This example also applies in the case of fat-phase compositions that contain little or no saturated fat.

Processing for controlled aggregation
In some cases the processing of specific ingredients or of complete products may be used to control the aggregation of emulsion droplets. In one example soya protein isolate (SPI)-dextran mixtures were incubated at 60°C for one week and then used to prepare 20% oil-in-water emulsions (Diftis and Kiosseoglou, 2006). The stability to oil droplet aggregation was assessed by heating the emulsions to 100°C in boiling water. Such samples exhibited no signs of an increase in droplet size, even after 30 minutes of heating. However, the emulsions prepared with non-incubated SPI-dextran mixtures underwent significant aggregation. The formation of a SPI-dextran hybrid following incubation is postulated to inhibit aggregation when adsorbed at the emulsion droplet surface.

Characterisation of aggregated structures
A number of techniques are available for the study of aggregated structures and in particular for measuring the size distributions. The measurement by laser light scattering may result in a bimodal distribution with the peak at smaller sizes attributed to the original droplets, whereas the peak at larger sizes may be due either to aggregated structures or to coalesced droplets. Microscopy can also be a valuable tool in assessing the extent of aggregation.

Further techniques for characterising aggregated structures are now being developed. For example the spin-echo small-angle neutron scattering (SESANS) technique was used to investigate the structure of droplet aggregates by measuring the normalised polarisation of the neutron beam (P/Po), and the density correlation function, as a function of the spin echo length in the region 100 nm to 10 µm (Bot *et al.*, 2007). This technique is useful in that the shape of the P/Po vs. spin echo

© W. G. Morley, 2011

length plot can indicate the homogeneity of the emulsion gels, in particular the presence of large droplets or aggregates. In this study, model emulsion gels containing 30% vegetable oil and 4% whey protein concentrate as the emulsifier were prepared, and characterised by SESANS, pulsed-field gradient nuclear magnetic resonance (PFG-NMR) to measure the oil droplet size ($d3,3$), firmness, and confocal scanning laser microscopy. It was found that temperature cycling had the biggest effect on the structure of the emulsion gels, followed by acidification. By contrast, the differences between one- and two-stage homogenisation processes were relatively modest.

7.3.2   Emulsion droplet size changes

The formation of an emulsion results in an increase in the total surface area of the dispersed phase. Reducing the size of the emulsion droplets will result in an increased number of droplets, which may alter the physical and organoleptic properties of the food product via enhanced droplet–droplet interactions. The further increase in surface area may also lead to the enhanced release of dispersed phase soluble ingredients such as flavours.

The size of the dispersed phase droplets in an emulsion depends on the equilibrium between the droplet break-up and coalescence processes in the emulsification device and beyond. The droplet break-up is a function of the energy input from the emulsification device and the reduction in interfacial tension from the emulsifier, and the coalescence is controlled mainly by the ability of the emulsifier to stabilise the emulsion. Therefore attempts to reduce the emulsion droplet size to below the standard levels require either the use of a modified emulsification device with increased energy input, or an alternative emulsifier that has a greater ability to reduce coalescence.

An example of such an emulsification device is described as a pipe which is partially obstructed by one or more transversally arranged plates. The pipe has a diameter in the range 20 to 80 mm, and the plates contain at least one opening of diameter 0.5 to 3 mm. The device is supplied with a pre-emulsion at a pressure of 10 to 50bar. It has been used to process mayonnaise-type products with reduced fat contents in the range 55 to 75%, which have viscosity values in the range normally expected for 80% full-fat mayonnaise (Oberacker and Schroeder, 2001). This was achieved with oil droplets that have a size below those in standard products, and without the use of additional thickening agents.

In another study an ultra-high-pressure homogeniser was used to produce very fine oil-in-water emulsions from sunflower oil (20%), with 1.5% whey protein concentrate as the emulsifier. Homogenisation pressures of up to 350 MPa were used in this study, significantly higher than those commonly used in the food industry (typically up to around 60 MPa) (Desrumaux and Marcand, 2002). The results indicate that the average emulsion droplet size, $d3,2$, decreased with increasing pressure from 50 to 90 MPas, with an accompanying increase in viscosity. However, at higher pressures a more complex picture emerged with minimum $d3,2$ values at 100, 250 and 350 MPa. Various mechanisms are proposed,

© W. G. Morley, 2011

including 'over processing' of the emulsion from 100 to 210 MPa, and protein conformation changes above 210 MPa.

7.4   Phase structuring and emulsions

7.4.1   Fat phase structuring

As stated earlier, the fat phase of a food emulsion may comprise a blend of liquid oil and hardstock in the form of crystalline fat. The crystals impart rigidity to the fat phase, which is important for the desirable physical and organoleptic properties of the food. In foods with lower levels of saturated fats it may be necessary to introduce alternative methods of structuring the fat phase or to enhance the structuring provided by fat crystals using formulation or processing changes.

A comprehensive review of alternatives to fat crystal networks for structuring unsaturated oils is given in Rogers (2009). In particular the use of the L_α liquid-crystalline lamellar phase, inverse bilayers forming rod-shaped tubules (sorbitan monostearate gels and lecithin gels), crystal platelets, and self-assembled fibrillar networks are discussed. The L_α liquid-crystalline lamellar phase is formed by monoglycerides such as monopalmitin and monostearin, and arises because of the ability to self-assemble into various structures. Examples of materials that form inverse bilayers are sorbitan monostearate and lecithin, and of crystal platelets are long-chain fatty acids and alcohols, waxes, and sorbitan tristearate. Finally, fibrillar networks are formed by many materials including hydroxylated fatty acids, phytosterols and oryzanols, and ceramides.

A fat-phase composition comprising a combination of a recrystallisation agent and a saturated fat source has been claimed to improve the physical stability of an oil or fat component without the need for hydrogenated fats and oils (Ringhouse and Sinclair, 2006). The recrystallisation agent was selected from carnauba wax, beeswax or paraffin wax, and examples of the saturated fat source include palm stearin, tallow, butter, lard and cocoa butter. The composition was added as a pre-blended powdered ingredient in a number of butter and spread-type products, and reduced or substantially eliminated the oil or fat separation.

Emulsifiers

An emulsifier composition comprising monoglycerides and diglycerides, an alpha-tending emulsifier, an ionic coemulsifier, and their mixtures, has been applied in a shortening system with an unsaturated vegetable oil such as soya bean oil, sunflower oil or corn oil (Doucet, 2005). The basis of the preparation is to maintain the monoglyceride in the α-form such that when mixed with water it spontaneously swells into the α-gel phase. This can build viscosity in its own right as well as adhering to oil. The α-tending emulsifiers include propylene glycol esters, lactic acid esters and acetic acid esters, and the ionic coemulsifiers include sodium stearoyl lactylate (SSL) and diacetylated tartaric acid esters of monoglycerides (DATEM). The emulsifier blend is claimed to facilitate meltdown

© W. G. Morley, 2011

and flavour release, and has been applied in sheeted, extruded and laminated baked products such as cookies, crackers, fillings and tortillas.

The use of diglycerides is described in a further example but in this case other emulsifiers are not required. A glyceride emulsifier containing a high diglyceride content was prepared by the interesterification or glycerolysis of triglycerides with glycerol. The preferred diglyceride content of 74% was then obtained by vacuum distillation. The high diglyceride emulsifier was used at levels in the range 10–16% to prepare a puff pastry margarine containing 55–65% vegetable oil and 13–25% saturated fat (Skogerson *et al.*, 2006). This margarine was finally used to prepare puff pastry products that were of equal quality to that of standard commercial products produced with partially hydrogenated fat. Typical examples of saturated fat reduction were from 46% in the commercial margarine to 41% and 38% in those prepared with the high-diglyceride emulsifier.

Selected emulsifiers have also been used in combination with specific hardstocks to result in reductions in saturated fat levels when compared to standard products. For example, beta-promoting palm oil hardstock and an emulsifier blend containing propylene glycol monostearate (PGMS) and distilled monoglyceride was successfully applied in a liquid shortening for cake batter formulations (Wassell, 2006).

7.4.2   W/O/W emulsions

Water-in-oil-in-water (W/O/W) multiple emulsions are of considerable interest in reducing the fat contents of foods because the internal water phase may be considered to be part of the dispersed phase of the emulsion. Such emulsions, however, have not found a wide applicability in foods for two main reasons. Firstly, they can be relatively unstable with coalescence of the internal and external water phases resulting in the transition to an O/W emulsion and a reduction in the effective dispersed phase volume. Secondly, it is generally accepted that the most effective W/O emulsifier in these systems is polyglycerol polyricinoleate (PGPR). This emulsifier is considered to be not particularly 'label-friendly' and has a limited legal usage in foods (European Parliament and Council Directive 95/2/EC). It can also be difficult to characterise W/O/W emulsions, in particular the size of the internal water droplets. This section will review some of the recent work to address these issues.

An example of the application of W/O/W emulsions is in reduced-fat cheese-like products. In one example such products were prepared from blends of skimmed milk and 27 g of different W/O/W emulsions per litre, and compared to a control white fresh cheese that was made from milk containing 27 g of milk fat per litre and skimmed milk (Lobato-Calleros *et al.*, 2008). The resulting total fat contents of the reduced-fat cheese-like products were in the range 11–13% compared to the control white fresh cheese at 15%. Firstly the 20% W_1/O emulsion was prepared with 0.1% gellan gum and diacetylated tartaric acid esters of monoglycerides (DATEM)/PGPR as the emulsifiers. This was then emulsified at 20% into five different biopolymer solutions. The results of this work are that

© W. G. Morley, 2011

carboxymethyl cellulose resulted in products with similar textural behaviour to the control, gum arabic contributed to a higher yield and fat content in comparison to carboxymethyl cellulose and low-methoxy pectin, and gum arabic and low-methoxy pectin contributed to increased values of hardness and chewiness.

Stability of W/O/W emulsions
Protein-polysaccharide complexes have been used to increase the stability of $W_1/O/W_2$ emulsions containing ferrous bisglycinate in the internal water phase (Jiminez-Alvardo *et al.*, 2009). In this study a primary ferrous bisglycinate aqueous solution (50%) in mineral oil W_1/O emulsion was prepared with 5% PGPR:DATEM (6:4 ratio) as the emulsifier. This was then emulsified at 20% into aqueous solutions of whey protein concentrate and polysaccharide (2:1 ratio, total concentration 5%). Finally the pH was adjusted using 0.1N HCl in order to allow the formation of a biopolymeric complex at the outer oil–water interface. The stability of the $W_1/O/W_2$ emulsions was determined by measuring the release of ferrous bisglycinate from W_1 to W_2, and it was found that mesquite gum was better in this regard than gum arabic or low methoxy pectin.

The influence of the oil type on the stability of W/O/W emulsions and the release of encapsulated magnesium has also been studied (Bonnet *et al.*, 2009). In this case the $W_1/O/W_2$ emulsions contained 4% W_1, 6% oil, and 90% W_2, with PGPR and sodium caseinate as the emulsifiers. The internal W_1 phase contained magnesium chloride and the leakage of magnesium into the external W_2 phase was studied as a function of oil type (rapeseed oil, olive oil, milk fat olein and Miglyol® 812 – C8:0/C10:0 saturated fatty acids). It was found that higher leakage occurred for the oils that were characterised by a lower viscosity and a higher proportion of saturated fatty acids. It is postulated that the leakage was not due to water droplet coalescence but to diffusion and/or permeation mechanisms involving the oil phase.

A mixture of emulsifiers was used to prepare a stable W/O/W emulsion with organoleptic properties similar to those of full-fat O/W systems. The internal W/O emulsion was preferably prepared with a mixture of a low molecular weight emulsifier and a high molecular weight emulsifier. Glycerol monooleate (GMO) and PGPR respectively are reported to be especially suitable. The internal water phase in addition contained solutes such as salts, polyols and sugars, that initially created an osmotic pressure gradient between the inner and outer aqueous phases, which caused a swelling of the former (Folmer *et al.*, 2008). The external water phase comprised a hydrophilic polymer or polymer aggregates as the emulsifier. Some examples of the preferred hydrophilic polymers include whey protein isolate and egg yolk. The W/O/W emulsion was prepared in the standard manner by combining a W/O emulsion with an external water phase.

The potential of whey protein isolate (WPI) for stabilising W/O emulsions has been investigated, as well as the use of these W/O emulsions to form stable W/O/W emulsions. In particular it was postulated that gelled internal water droplets, such

© W. G. Morley, 2011

as those produced by heating WPI solutions, would result in increased stability (Surh *et al.*, 2007). The initial 20% W/O emulsions with PGPR as the emulsifier were prepared without WPI, with WPI but with no heating, and with WPI and heating to 80°C for 20 minutes to gel the protein. These emulsions were then emulsified at 20% into an aqueous phase with polyoxyethylene sorbitan monolaurate as the emulsifier. Both premix membrane emulsification and high-pressure homogenisation processes were used. The emulsions generally displayed good stability during the second emulsification step with little loss of the internal aqueous phase. In addition the W/O emulsions were stable during shearing, thermal processing and extended ambient storage tests. Overall there was little impact of gelation of the internal water phase on the stability of the W/O/W emulsions, although the emulsions containing WPI (gelled or not) had larger mean droplet diameters than those with no WPI.

A novel emulsification technique has been used to produce acidic W/O/W emulsions. A first acidic W/O emulsion was mixed with a second acidic O/W emulsion, instead of the standard technique of mixing a W/O emulsion with an external water phase. Both emulsions contained oil, fat and vinegar, but the emulsifiers differed in that egg albumin was used for the W/O emulsion, and egg yolk for the O/W emulsion (Wakamatsu, 2004). In addition the O/W emulsion had a much smaller droplet size than the W/O emulsion.

Alternatives to polyglycerol polyricinoleate (PGPR)
The work to identify alternatives to PGPR has generally centred around lecithin and lecithin derivatives, as these are generally considered to be 'label friendly' W/O emulsifiers. One example is a de-oiled fractionated powder soybean lecithin which was used as the W/O emulsifier in a dairy-type W/O/W emulsion in which the hydrophilic emulsifier was sodium caseinate (Akhtar and Dickinson, 2001). The emulsions were characterised by measuring the droplet size of the primary W/O emulsions and both the droplet size and retained yield of the W/O/W emulsions. The results were very positive in that the retained yield of the lecithin-containing emulsion was around 78% compared to the PGPR emulsion at 48%, indicating a greater stability. It is also reported that the lecithin-containing emulsion had a creamier mouthfeel when compared to the one containing PGPR.

Characterisation of W/O/W emulsions
The characterisation of W/O/W multiple emulsions is important but difficulties are often encountered in identifying the roles of the internal water phase and the dispersed oil phase. In particular it is important to measure the droplet size distributions of the inner and outer emulsions as they can affect the rheological and sensory attributes of the food products. In one study PFG-NMR was used to characterise W/O/W emulsions (Wolf *et al.*, 2009). The $W_1/O/W_2$ emulsions were prepared using 7% PGPR as the W_1/O emulsifier and polyoxyethylene-20-sorbitan monolaurate as the O/W_2 emulsifier. Firstly the PFG-NMR technique was used to characterise the initial $\overset{\cdot}{W}_1/O$ emulsion and the results were comparable

© W. G. Morley, 2011

with those obtained with laser light scattering. Following this an analysis of the PFG-NMR data for the $W_1/O/W_2$ multiple emulsion resulted in a median droplet size for the W_1 droplets that was similar to that in the W_1/O primary emulsion, when the possible exchange of water molecules between the W_1 and W_2 phases was taken into account. This technique therefore appears to offer potential for characterising the internal water phases of W/O/W emulsions.

Another study compared the rheological properties and microstructure of reduced-fat cheeses obtained by substituting milk fat by W/O/W emulsions stabilised with hydrocolloids, with those of full-fat white fresh cheese. The emulsions were made by firstly preparing a W_1/O emulsion by adding a water phase containing gellan gum and the hydrophilic emulsifier DATEM to an oil phase containing the hydrophobic emulsifier PGPR. This W_1/O emulsion was then emulsified into a second aqueous phase containing different biopolymers to result in the final $W_1/O/W_2$ multiple emulsion. The multiple emulsions contained 11 to 13% fat compared to the control full-fat white fresh cheese (WFC) at 15.3%.

The storage and loss moduli, G' and G'', were measured as a function of strain and all cheeses had a linear viscoelastic region which occurred up to a strain % of 1.2 for the WFC but up to 3.99 for the reduced-fat cheeses. In all cases the G' was higher than G'', indicating a dominant elastic character, and the actual G' and G'' values were higher for the WFC than for the reduced-fat cheeses. The microstructures of the cheeses were also compared using scanning electron microscopy and a detrended fluctuation analysis (DFA) of the micrographs, which indicated that they all displayed a hierarchical configuration, from well-ordered particles in the small scale range to randomly dispersed particles in the high scale range.

7.4.3   O/W/O emulsions

The use of oil-in-water-in-oil (O/W/O) multiple emulsions may not be an obvious choice for the reduction of the saturated fat content of a food product since it involves the addition of oil to the dispersed water phase. However, it can be of value in improving the functionality of a fat continuous product at a constant composition by moving some of the oil or fat from the continuous phase to the internal W/O emulsion phase, thus increasing the effective dispersed phase volume.

In one study of the stability of O/W/O emulsions, the primary O/W emulsions were prepared using a microfluidiser and a high-pressure homogeniser, with stabiliser blends of gum arabic and maltodextrin (Cho and Park, 2003). The stability of the emulsions was shown to be enhanced with the higher ratios of gum arabic. O/W emulsions containing gum arabic were then used to prepare the O/W/O multiple emulsions with different secondary emulsifier blends. The blend of sorbitan monooleate and PGPR resulted in the greatest stability, better than PGPR alone. Sorbitan monooleate alone had no emulsifying capability and blends of polyoxyethylene sorbitan monooleate and PGPR appeared to result in phase inversion.

© W. G. Morley, 2011

7.4.4 O/W/W emulsions

O/W/W emulsions are systems in which an oil-in-water (O/W_1) emulsion has subsequently been dispersed in a second water phase (W_2). Of course the two water phases must be phase separated such that one of them remains dispersed in the other. The use of such $O/W_1/W_2$ emulsions offers another technical route for the reduction of the fat content by increasing the effective dispersed phase volume of a water continuous food system.

In one study the phase behaviour of aqueous systems of heat-denatured whey protein isolate (HD-WPI) and high methoxy pectin were studied, and it was found that under certain conditions a two-phase system was formed. The HD-WPI-enriched lower phase (W_1) and the pectin-enriched upper phase (W_2) were then used to prepare water-in-water emulsions (W_1/W_2 or W_2/W_1) (Kim et $al.$, 2006). Interestingly it was then possible to combine the various phase-separated biopolymer solutions with an oil-in-water emulsion comprising 10% oil and 1% native whey protein isolate as the emulsifier. This resulted in either oil-in-water-in-water ($O/W_1/W_2$) multiple emulsions or mixed oil-in-water/water-in-water (O/W_1- W_2/W_1) systems, depending on the initial biopolymer composition. However, the work also demonstrated that the W/W and O/W/W systems had limited stability due to coalescence of the dispersed water droplets, so further work is required before they can be exploited in real food-based systems.

7.4.5 Water phase structuring (ice)

Many of the studies described in this chapter include the use of hydrocolloids in the water phase to improve the functionality and to reduce the negative impact of reducing the total or saturated fat level. Such methods are employed in frozen products such as ice cream and water ices but in addition the manipulation of ice crystal formation offers much potential. In this case, structured ice, via an enhanced ice crystal network, can offer an alternative to structuring by fat.

Ice structuring proteins (ISP) influence the formation of ice crystals during ice cream manufacture and the recrystallisation of ice during storage. By binding to ice crystals they limit the growth rate of the ice and influence the morphology of the ice structure. The presence of ISP does not result in an increase in the quantity of ice, but rather in the formation of an enhanced ice crystal network. As a result, improvements in texture have been obtained in low-fat or even fat-free products (Watson, 2006, and Crilly, 2007).

7.5   Fat replacers

One of the simplest methods for reducing the total fat level of an emulsion is to replace some of the fat with an ingredient that has similar properties. In such a way it may be possible to avoid complex changes to the manufacturing process. In extreme cases of fat replacement the emulsification step may be dramatically reduced or even removed altogether. The maintenance of the physical and

© W. G. Morley, 2011

organoleptic properties of the food material can be difficult when replacing fat with other ingredients and this section describes some of the materials and techniques that have been studied.

7.5.1   Fat replacement ingredients

Many fat replacement ingredients are commercially available on the market and have claimed applications in a range of food products. A number of these are summarised in Table 7.3. Beta-glucan, a soluble fibre present in oats, appears to be the active component in a number of fat replacement ingredients. It has been applied at the naturally occurring level of ~5% in hydrolysed oat flour as a replacement for butter in baked desserts and for coconut cream in Thai desserts (Inglett et al., 2000). The hydrolysed oat flour was used as a 25% gel (with 75% water) and as a 15% suspension (85% water). Beta-glucan was applied at a concentrated level in thermo-mechanically processed oat bran as an ingredient in beverages (Zammer, 2002) and again as a replacement for coconut cream in Thai desserts (Inglett et al., 2005). In the latter case the material was applied as 5% gel (95% water). The oat bran gel was also used as an ingredient in low-fat beef patties (Pinero et al., 2008).

Oat bran has also been used as a component in a hydrocolloid blend with soya bean flour as a replacement for coconut milk in Asian foods (Inglett et al., 2003). In this case the blend was prepared by mixing equal quantities of soya bean flour and oat bran and then subjecting the mixture to a thermo-mechanical process.

Other fibre and bran materials with claimed applications as fat replacers include rice bran, which was applied at 10% in emulsified pork meatballs (Huang et al., 2005), citrus pulp fibre (Anon., 2005), and inulin, fruit (peach, apple, orange) fibres, and cereal (wheat, oat) fibres in dry fermented sausages (Muguerza et al., 2004). Further details are given in Table 7.3.

Xanthan gum and guar gum have been applied as fat replacers in low-fat cake products. The cakes with 25% substitution of the fat were statistically equivalent to the standard, and at 50% substitution there was no effect on the firmness or elasticity of the cakes (Zambrano et al., 2004). At this higher level the cakes produced with xanthan gum were more acceptable than those produced using guar gum.

So-called non-digestible lipids have been used to formulate fillings for biscuit sandwich products that have reduced total or saturated fat contents when compared to control products. Such lipids comprise polyol fatty acid polyesters such as sucrose polyesters and have been used at levels above 20% (Trout and Kirkpatrick, 2001, and Trout et al., 2001a) in order to reduce the total fat level by at least 20%. At polyol fatty acid polyester levels below 20% it is reported that the saturated fat level may be reduced by at least 20% (Trout et al., 2001b). The compositions may also contain crystallising lipids such as partially or fully hydrogenated vegetable oils (Trout and Kirkpatrick, 2001, and Trout et al., 2001b). In the case of cheese fillings, further ingredients are dehydrated cheese powder and a bulking agent such as corn syrup solids or polydextrose.

© W. G. Morley, 2011

Table 7.3   Examples of fat replacers

Fat replacer	Application	Results	Refs.
Enzyme hydrolysed oat flour (contains ~5% beta-glucan) (Oatrim)	Replacement for butter in baked desserts, and for coconut cream in Thai desserts	Up to 50% substitution of butter in baked desserts with 25% gel	Inglett *et al.*, 2000
Thermo-mechanically processed oat bran with beta-glucan concentrated to ~10% (8.6% in Inglett *et al.*, 2005) (Nutrim)	Ingredient in beverage formulations (Zammer, 2002), replacement for coconut cream in Thai desserts (Inglett *et al.*, 2005), and ingredient in low fat beef patties (Pinero *et al.*, 2008)	60–100% substitution of coconut cream in various Thai desserts with 5% gel (Inglett *et al.*, 2005), 13.45% addition of gel to low fat (~8%) beef patties compared to control (~17% fat) patties (Pinero *et al.*, 2008)	Zammer, 2002, Inglett *et al.*, 2005, Pinero *et al.*, 2008
Thermo-mechanically processed soyabean flour and oat bran (contains 22–27% beta-glucan) (Soytrim)	Replacement of coconut milk in Asian foods such as Thai green curry	Up to 50% substitution of coconut milk in various Asian foods	Inglett *et al.*, 2003
Rice bran (various kinds)	Ingredient in 'Kung-wan' – emulsified pork meatballs	Up to 10% addition to reduce total fat content	Huang *et al.*, 2005
Citrus pulp fibre (Citri-Fi)	Baked goods	Addition or substitution levels not stated	Anon., 2005
Inulin, fruit fibres, cereal fibres	Lower fat dry fermented sausages	Addition of 11.5% inulin or 1.5% cereal/ fruit fibre to improve acceptability	Muguerza *et al.*, 2004
Guar gum and xanthan gum	Low fat cakes	Up to 50% substitution of fat with gum. Xanthan gum more acceptable than guar gum	Zambrano *et al.*, 2004
Collagen hydrolysate (Instant Gel Schoko)	Milk chocolate	39% replacement of cocoa butter with 5% collagen hydrolysate	Anon., 2006
Sucrose polyesters	Biscuit sandwich fillings, for example cheese-based	Around 20% reduction in fat	Trout and Kirkpatrick, 2001, Trout *et al.*, 2001a, Trout *et al.*, 2001b

© W. G. Morley, 2011

Finally a collagen hydrolysate, a special protein generated in a dedicated enzymatic process, has been applied as a replacement for cocoa butter in milk chocolate (Anon., 2006, and Anon., 2007).

7.5.2   Fat replacement structures

An alternative approach to fat replacement ingredients is the formation of fat replacement structures using some of the ingredients normally found in emulsions. Such an example is a cellular solid matrix that provides oil-based products with a fat-like consistency yet contain low levels of saturated fatty acids. The cellular solid contains non-ionic surfactant, ionic surfactant, oil and water (Marangoni and Idziak, 2004). A preferred composition is 4 to 7% monoglyceride as the non-ionic surfactant, 0.2 to 0.35% ionic surfactant such as sodium stearoyl lactylate (SSL), 40 to 60% oil, and 20 to 60% water. The oil can be virtually any edible type, and those low in saturates are preferred. The process for making the cellular solid structure is to heat the surfactants and oil to above the melting temperature of the surfactants, add the heated aqueous solution, vigorously mix the composition and then cool. The cellular solid matrix can also be used as a component in other food products such as ice cream, soft cheeses and cream substitutes.

An alternative edible granular structuring composition has been prepared from a non-glyceride edible solid material and a glyceride composition with non-lauric or semi-hard fat and crystallised fat. Examples of the non-glyceride material include powdery products such as sugar, starch, wheat flour, skimmed milk and their combinations (Cleenewerck and Ushioda, 2006). The glyceride compositions preferably include at least 50% SUS triglycerides where S denotes a saturated fatty acid chain and U an unsaturated fatty acid chain. Suitable examples include StUSt and PUSt, where St denotes stearic acid and P denotes palmitic acid. The unsaturated fatty acid is preferably oleic acid. A simple blending process is used to prepare the granular material.

Finally, proteins have been used to prepare fat replacement particles. In one example microparticulated protein particles (MPPPs) were prepared from mung bean protein, a by-product of mung bean starch production (Sirikulchayanont et al., 2007). The MPPPs were prepared by thermal aggregation and/or chemical precipitation under high shear conditions. For example, a 5% solution of mung bean protein concentrate was heated at 83°C (the denaturation temperature as determined by differential scanning calorimetry) for 15 minutes in the presence of calcium chloride while being stirred with a homogeniser at 17 000 rev/min, and then homogenised at 23 000 to 27 000 rev/min. This resulted in particles mostly in the range 0.1 to 3.0 μm. To precipitate particles larger than 3 μm the suspension was centrifuged at 1000 to 4000g for ten minutes. The mung bean protein microparticulated particles are reported to have characteristics similar to those of other proteins and therefore appear to have potential as fat replacers.

Another application of proteins in fat replacement particles is in combination with fats, whereby the liposome-like structure comprises a protein core and a fatty coat. In one example the protein core is a charged and denatured supramolecular

© W. G. Morley, 2011

structure which is in the form of a gel, rod, micelle or aggregate (Pouzot *et al.*, 2007). The first step in preparing this is the denaturation of a native protein in order to induce aggregation or gelation. The protein is preferably not casein-based. The second step is altering the pH of the solution such that the supramolecular structure is positively charged, and finally the third step is ionic complexation with negatively charged lipids. Examples of such lipids are sulphated butyl oleate, DATEM, and sodium lauryl sulphate (SLS). The liposome structure was used in applications as diverse as yoghurt, ice cream, biscuits and margarine.

In another example casein was used to prepare a microcapsule which when aggregated was filled into fat droplets (Poortinga, 2006). This was prepared by adding a coagulant to a solution of calcium caseinate at a low temperature, emulsifying this in oil with a low hydrophilic–lipophilic balance emulsifier such as sorbitan trioleate or sorbitan monooleate, and then heating the mixture to form the network. The capsules so formed can be transferred to an aqueous solution or used directly with the oil. Furthermore, if the capsules are made without using an emulsifier in the oil phase, and are then subsequently emulsified in water, then an O/W emulsion is created in which the fat droplets are filled with aggregated casein capsules.

7.6   Processing

The processing of oils and fats that are relatively low in saturated fat, such that the performance in foods is similar to those with higher levels of saturated fat, is an attractive option. This is especially the case if the food material can be manufactured according to the same procedures and using the same equipment, since the modified fat is simply a replacement ingredient. A number of methods of processing oils and fats have been studied over the years and two examples are given in this section.

7.6.1   Interesterification

Interesterification is the process whereby one or more of the fatty acid residues present in a triglyceride molecule is replaced by another fatty acid residue from the same or another fat source.

A chemical interesterification process using sodium methoxide as catalyst was used to produce shortenings from blends of palm oil (PO) with either sunflower oil (SFO) or soybean oil (SBO) (Mayamol *et al.*, 2008). It was found that the interesterified blends containing 80 to 90% PO and 10 to 20% SFO or SBO had higher solid fat contents than the respective non-interesterified blends. This could be due to the higher levels of triglycerides such as PPP and PPSt. In another study a hard structural fat for margarines and spreads was produced from a blend of a selectively fractionated non-hydrogenated palm oil fraction with a lauric fat such as dry-fractionated non-hydrogenated palm kernel fraction (Sahasranamam, 2001). The structural fat contains less than 20% of tripalmitin and longer trisaturated fatty acids and was used at levels of up to 40% in the margarine and spread products.

© W. G. Morley, 2011

7.6.2   Cryo-crystallisation

Cryo-crystallisation is a process whereby atomised liquid fats and oils come into contact with a liquid cryogen such as liquid nitrogen. The atomised feed particles then solidify instantly into free-flowing particles that have increased solid fat contents when compared to standard processes (Brooker, 2001). The process has been successfully applied to a smooth peanut butter formulation containing vegetable oil (unspecified type) and hydrogenated rapeseed oil.

Cryo-crystallisation has also been used to produce short-crust pastry fats that were subsequently used to produce doughs and then baked. Two examples of short-crust pastry fats that were diluted with rapeseed oil to saturated fat contents of 3.9% and 5.0%, and then cryo-crystallised were found to result in doughs and baked pastries that had properties similar to those of a commercially available product containing over 10% saturated fat (Titoria and Clarke, 2009).

7.7   Applications

7.7.1   Aerated products

The use of oil blends with reduced levels of saturated fat can have a detrimental impact on the whippability of water continuous emulsions. In the whipping of dairy cream, for example, air is incorporated into the structure and stabilised by the adsorption of fat droplets onto the air bubble surface. This is most effective with oil droplets that are solid in character, containing relatively high levels of crystallised fat, such that oil droplet aggregation in the form of partial coalescence occurs. Figure 7.4 is an electron micrograph of a whipped cream showing aggregated oil droplets at the air bubble surface.

If the oil blend contains too much liquid oil then coalescence can occur, leading to lower air contents and softer structures. The production of whippable emulsions

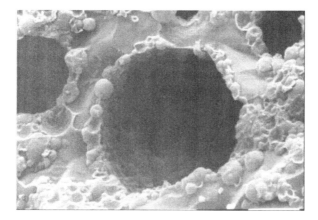

Fig. 7.4   Cryo-scanning electron micrograph of a whipped cream. Image width approx. 100 μm. Image courtesy of Kathy Groves, Leatherhead Food Research.

© W. G. Morley, 2011

with reduced levels of saturated fats is thus a real challenge. In one study a proportion of anhydrous milk fat was replaced by an olein-rich fraction and this resulted in increased incorporation of air and a more uniform size distribution for the air bubbles (Bazmi *et al.*, 2007). A commercially available whipping agent based on sunflower oil claims to be suitable in a wide range of creamy desserts and can generate very high volumes at low dosage levels (Montague-Jones, 2009).

Protein aggregation (gelation) has been used to produce stable foams from casein-based liquid oil emulsions (Allen *et al.*, 2006). A range of caseinate-stabilised groundnut oil emulsions were acidified with glucono-δ-lactone (GDL) and whipped when the pH reached different known values in the range 5.1 to 5.6. It was found that the overrun (air incorporation) was maximised when the starting pH was higher. This was attributed to a greater time for air incorporation during the gradual process of gelation as the pH was reduced. These casein emulsion foams had longer whipping times and much higher overruns than standard whipping cream.

7.7.2   Frozen products

The incorporation of air into food products can reduce the intake of saturated and total fats for those products that are sold by volume rather than by weight. The challenges, however, in retaining the air in the structure and in delivering acceptable organoleptic properties when compared to non-aerated foods may be considerable. It is likely that employing aeration in frozen structures may be more successful than in ambient systems due to the formation of a rigid matrix that can stabilise the air.

Frozen aerated confections with low saturated fat contents have been prepared by carefully selecting the fat according to specific criteria. In one example of products containing 5 to 12% fat and with an overrun of at least 40%, the fat component contained less than 55% saturated triglycerides and less than 8% long-chain SSS triglycerides, where S denotes a saturated fatty acid (Dilley *et al.*, 2005). The ratio of the solid fat content at 5°C to the percentage of the fatty acids that are saturated is greater than 1 and the fat content comprises less than 60% cocoa butter or shea nut oil. Furthermore, it is preferred that the sum of the SSU and SUU (where U denotes an unsaturated fatty acid) triglycerides is greater than 60% and the ratio of the percentage of SSU to SUU triglycerides is greater than 1.

7.8   Future trends

7.8.1   Fat replacers

Fat replacement ingredients and structures have attracted much attention and this is likely to continue as product developers look for solutions that can be easily implemented in existing manufacturing processes. This will result in more complex blends of hydrocolloids, as the search continues for aqueous-based ingredients that have similar mouthfeel characteristics to fats. This approach will

© W. G. Morley, 2011

probably achieve more success if fat is included, for example as part of an encapsulated structure. Success in this area may be achieved by the development of novel co-processing techniques for blends of fats and hydrocolloids.

7.8.2   Controlled aggregation of O/W emulsions

The factors that influence the stability of oil-in-water emulsions have been extensively studied and are well known. It is also clear that the aggregation of oil droplets leads to the incorporation of a portion of the water phase into the three-dimensional structure and an increase in the effective dispersed phase volume.

The controlled aggregation of oil droplets therefore has potential for the reduction of fat levels in O/W emulsions. While in general terms aggregation behaviour has not been studied for this purpose, this may change as researchers look to technological approaches that do not require the addition of ingredients that are unfamiliar to the product types in question.

7.8.3   W/O/W multiple emulsions

W/O/W multiple emulsions have been studied for many years and have been shown in numerous studies to be effective in allowing reductions in fat content to be made. While the legislative position regarding the usage of PGPR may not change, it is likely that work will continue to evaluate novel W/O emulsifiers, and to improve the stability of the internal water droplets.

These two aspects of W/O/W emulsion science will be combined rather than being studied separately. Success in this area will require the application of novel hydrocolloid aqueous phase behaviour, and new techniques for the manipulation of the W/O and O/W interfaces.

7.8.4   Cryo-crystallisation of oils and fats

The cryo-crystallisation of oils and fats appears to have great potential for the reduction of saturated fat levels, but there has been limited work so far on food systems. This is likely to change as the equipment and technology become more widely available.

The main challenges in implementing the technology may be in the inclusion of cryo-crystallised fats into foods, especially when the current processing methods involve the melting and recrystallisation of the fat phase. In such cases novel processing methodologies may be required in order to maintain the functionality of the cryo-crystallised fat.

7.9   Sources of further information and advice

Emulsion science has been the subject of many publications over the years and many excellent textbooks give comprehensive overviews of the formation and

© W. G. Morley, 2011

properties of both O/W and W/O systems. See for example Sherman, 1968, and Friberg and Larsson, 1997. Such texts include details on the factors that control emulsion stability, considering the roles of fat crystals, emulsifiers and aqueous phase hydrocolloids, as well as salts, acids and so on. The developments in emulsion science have also been reported in conference proceedings such as those in Dickinson, 1986, and Dickinson and Rodriguez Patino, 1999.

Multiple emulsions are also covered in these general texts but more comprehensive overviews are available in selected chapters such as those in Dickinson and McClements, 1995. These cover all aspects of multiple emulsion science, especially the factors that control the stability, and have tended to focus mainly on the W/O/W multiple emulsion type.

Many texts are available on fat replacement ingredients and structures, giving comprehensive overviews of the different types that are available and the applications. In some cases information on the labelling, nutritional claims, and regulatory aspects of these systems are also covered; see for example Swanson, 2006.

7.10   References

Aigster A, Sims C, Staples C, Aschmidt R and O'Keefe S F (2000), 'Comparison of cheeses made from milk having normal and high oleic fatty acid compositions', *J Food Sci*, 65(5), 920–4.

Akhtar M and Dickinson E (2001), 'Water-in-oil-in-water multiple emulsions stabilized by polymeric and natural emulsifiers', in Dickinson E and Miller R, *Food colloids: fundamentals of formulation: proceedings of a conference, Potsdam, April 2000*, Cambridge, RSC, 78–83.

Allen K E, Dickenson E and Murray B (2006), 'Acidified sodium caseinate emulsion foams containing liquid fat: a comparison with whipped cream', *Lebensmittel-Wissenschaft und –Technologie*, 39(3), 225–34.

Anon. (2005), 'Citri-Fi from Fiberstar Inc.', *Snack Food and Wholesale Bakery*, 94(7), 47.

Anon. (2006), 'Instant Gel Schoko fat replacer from Gelita', *World Food Ing*, Oct–Nov, 113.

Anon. (2007), 'Chocolate with less fat. More than evolution, it's innovation', *Food Marketing Tech*, Feb, 13–14.

Aryana K J (2007), 'Cheddar cheese manufactured with oil high in omega-3 fatty acids', *Milchwissenschaft*, 62(2), 167–70.

Bazmi A, Duquenoy A and Relkin P (2007), 'Aeration of low fat dairy emulsions: effects of saturated-unsaturated triglycerides', *Int Dairy J*, 17(9), 1021–7.

Benjamins J, Zoet F D and van Aken R H (2006), 'Thickened emulsions and methods for the preparation thereof', *PCT Patent Application*, WO 2007/004882.

Bonnet M, Cansell M, Berkaoui A, Ropers M H, Anton M and Leal-Calderon F (2009), 'Release profiles of magnesium from multiple W/O/W emulsions', *Food Hydrocolloids*, 23(1), 92–101.

Bons J R, Diks R M M, Garbolino C, Huizinga H and Zuiderwijk M A (2008), 'Edible fat continuous spreads', *PCT Patent Application*, WO 2008/125380.

Brooker B E (2001), 'Preparation of food products', *European Patent Application*, 1 114 674.

Bot A, Duval F P, Duif C P and Bouwman W G (2007), 'Probing the droplet cluster structure in acidified temperature-cycled O/W emulsion gels by means of SESANS', *Int J Food Sci Tech*, 42(6), 746–52.

© W. G. Morley, 2011

Brown H (2010), 'Arla reduces cheese fat but keeps it creamy', *American Dairy Products Institute news article*, available at http://www.adpi.org/tabid/74/mid/419/newsid419/562/Arla-Reduces-Cheese-Fat-but-Keeps-it-Creamy/Default.aspx. Accessed 6 December 2010.

Campbell B E (2000), 'Reduced calorie coated confections', *United States Patent*, 6 387 422.

Chanasattru W, Decker E A and McClements D J (2009), 'Influence of glycerol and sorbitol on thermally induced droplet aggregation in oil-in-water emulsions stabilized by beta-lactoglobulin', *Food Hydrocolloids*, 23(2), 253–61.

Cho Y-H and Park J (2003), 'Evaluation of process parameters in the O/W/O multiple emulsion method for flavour encapsulation', *J Food Sci*, 68(2), 534–8.

Cleenewerck B and Ushioda T (2006), 'Structuring granular composition', *PCT Patent Application*, WO 2006/136536.

Crilly J (2007), 'ISP: a breakthrough for better ice cream', *New Food*, 10(3), 40–4.

Desrumaux A and Marcand J (2002), 'Formation of sunflower oil emulsions stabilized by whey proteins with high-pressure homogenization (up to 35MPa): effect of pressure on emulsion characteristics', *Int J Food Sci Tech*, 37(3), 263–9.

Dickenson E (1986), *'Food emulsions and foams*, London, RSC.

Dickinson E and McClements D J (1995), 'Water-in-oil-in-water multiple emulsions', in Dickinson E and McClements D J, *'Advances in food colloids'*, Glasgow, Blackie, 280–300.

Dickinson E and Rodriguez Patino J M (1999), *'Food emulsions and foams. Interfaces interactions and stability'*, Cambridge, RSC.

Diftis N and Kiosseoglou V (2006), 'Stability against heat-induced aggregation of emulsions prepared with a dry-heated soy protein isolate-dextran mixture', *Food Hydrocolloids*, 20(6), 787–92.

Dilley K M, Greenacre J, Smith K W and Underdown J (2005), 'Frozen aerated confections', *PCT Patent Application*, WO 2006/066979.

Doucet J (2005), 'Emulsifier composition for shortening', *PCT Patent Application*, WO 2005/089568.

During A, Mazette S, Combe N and Entressangles B (2000), 'Lipolysis and oxidative stability of soft ripening cheeses containing vegetable oils', *J Dairy Res*, 67(3), 461–6.

European Parliament and Council Directive 95/2/EC of 20 February 1995 on food additives other than colours and sweeteners (OJ L 61, 18.3.1995, p. 1).

Folmer B, Michel M, Gehin-Delval C, Acquistapace S, Leser M, Syrbe A and Marze S (2008), 'Stable double emulsions', *PCT Patent Application*, WO 2009/003960.

Friberg S E and Larsson K (1997), *Food emulsions*, New York, Marcel Dekker.

Gonzalez S, Duncan S E, O'Keefe S F, Sumner S S and Herbein J H (2003), 'Oxidation and textural characteristics of butter and ice cream with modified fatty acid profiles', *J Dairy Sci*, 86(1), 70–7.

Gonzalez-Perez S, van Koningsveld G A, Vereijken J M, Merck K B, Gruppen G and Voragen A G J (2005), 'Emulsion properties of sunflower (Helianthus annuus) proteins', *J Ag Food Chem*, 53(6), 2261–7.

Hendree G, Martin S, Breuer T E and Walker K (2003), 'Process for separating saturated fatty acids from fatty acid mixtures by aid of polyglycerol esters', *PCT Patent Application*, WO 2004/033409.

Huang S C, Shiau C Y, Liu T E, Chu C L and Hwang D F (2005), 'Effects of rice bran on sensory and physico-chemical properties of emulsified pork meatballs', *Meat Sci*, 70(4), 613–19.

Inglett G E, Maneepun S and Vatanasuchart N (2000), 'Evaluation of hydrolysed oat flour as a replacement for butter and coconut cream in bakery products', *Food Sci Tech Int*, 6(6), 457–62.

Inglett G E, Carriere C J, Maneepun S and Boonpunt T (2003), 'Nutritional value and functional properties of a hydrocolloid soybean and oat blend for use in Asian foods', *J Sci Food Agriculture*, 83(1), 86–92.

© W. G. Morley, 2011

Inglett G E, Carriere C J and Maneepun S (2005), 'Health-related fat replacers prepared from grain for improving functional and nutritive values of Asian foods, in Shi J, Ho C-T and Shahidi F, *Asian functional foods*, Boca Raton, CRC Press, 103–27.

Irigoyen A, Oneca M, Ortigosa M, Ibanez F C and Torre P (2004), 'Elaboration and acceptability of a Roncal-type fat-reduced ewe's milk cheese', *Milchwissenschaft*, 59(5–6), 270–3.

Jiminez-Alvardo R, Beristain C I, Medina-Torres L, Roman-Guerrero A and Vernon-Carter E J (2009), 'Ferrous bisglycinate content and release in W1/O/W2 multiple emulsions stabilized by protein-polysaccharide complexes', *Food Hydrocolloids*, 23(8), 2425–33.

Jittanoonta P, Cuptapun Y, Hengsawadi D, Mesomya W and Na-Thalang V (1998), 'Application of reconstituted coconut milk in staple foods: nutritional qualities and health aspects', in Kong L K and Seng L Y, *Proceedings of the 6th Asean Food Conference, Singapore, November 1997*, Singapore, SIFST, 134–9.

Karvonen H M, Tapola N S, Uusitupa M I and Sarkkinen E S (2002), 'The effect of vegetable oil-based cheese on serum total and lipoprotein lipids', *European J Clinical Nut*, 56(11), 1094–101.

Kim H-J, Decker E A and McClements D J (2006), 'Preparation of multiple emulsions based on thermodynamic incompatibility of heat-denatured whey protein and pectin solutions', *Food Hydrocolloids*, 20(5), 586–95.

Kincs F R, Narine S and Teran P (2008), 'High stearic high oleic oil blends', *PCT Patent Application*, WO 2008/137871.

Lobato-Calleros C, Sosa-Perez A, Rodriguez-Tafoya J, Sandoval-Castilla O, Perez-Alonso C and Vernon-Carter E J (2008), 'Structural and textural characteristics of reduced-fat cheese-like products made from W1/O/W2 emulsions and skim milk', *Lebensmittel-Wissenschaft und – Technologie*, 41(10), 1847–56.

Marangoni A G and Idziak S H J (2004), 'Food product', *United States Patent Application*, 2005/0249856.

May S and Slater N K H (2003), 'Cheese alternative product and process for preparing a cheese alternative product', *PCT Patent Application*, WO 2004/056188.

Mayamol P N, Thomas S, Sukumar D, Saritha S S, Balachandran C and Sundaresan A (2008), 'Process for zero-trans shortening using palm oil, sunflower oil and soybean oil through interesterification', *J Food Sci Tech*, 45(4), 305–11.

Merolla T V and Bialek J M (2006), 'Reduced oil dressing composition and method for making the same', *PCT Patent Application*, WO 2007/065505.

Montague-Jones G (2009), 'Cognis launches first sunflower oil-based whipping agent', *Decision News Media news article*, http://www.foodnavigator.com/Financial-Industry/Cognis-launches-first-sunflower-oil-based-whipping-agent, accessed 22 July 2009.

Muguerza E, Gimeno O, Ansorena D and Astiasaran I (2004), 'New formulations for healthier dry sausages: a review', *Trends Food Sci Tech*, 15(9), 452–57.

Norton J E, Fryer P J, Parkinson J and Cox P W (2009), 'Development and characterisation of tempered cocoa butter emulsions containing up to 60% water', *J Food Eng*, 95(1), 172–78.

Oberacker T and Schroeder V (2001), 'Oil-in-water foodstuff emulsion of the mayonnaise type having a reduced fat level, and a process for its preparation', *PCT Patent Application*, WO 02/39833.

Patrick M and Traska E W (1998), 'Aqueous dispersions or suspensions', *European Patent Application*, 1 197 153.

Pinero M P, Parra K, Huerta-Leidenz N, Arenas de Moreno L, Ferrer M, Araujo S, and Barboza Y (2008), 'Effect of oat's soluble fibre (beta-glucan) as a fat replacer on physical, chemical, microbiological and sensory properties of low-fat beef patties', *Meat Sci*, 80(3), 675–80.

Poortinga A T (2006), 'Microcapsules', *PCT Patent Application*, WO 2006/091081.

Pouzot M, Schmitt C and Mezzenga R (2007), 'Food protein and charged emulsifier interaction', *PCT Patent Application*, WO 2008/025784.

© W. G. Morley, 2011

Ringhouse T A and Sinclair A E (2006), 'Composition for reducing fat migration in food products', *PCT Patent Application*, WO 2007/035933.

Rogers M A (2009), 'Novel structuring strategies for unsaturated fats – meeting the zero-trans, zero-saturated fat challenge: a review', *Food Res Int*, 42(7), 747–753.

Sahasranamam U M (2001), 'Trans free hard structural fat for margarine blend and spread', *European Patent Application*, 1 552 751.

Sherman P (1968), *Emulsion Science*, London, Academic Press.

Sirikulchayanont P, Jayanta S, Pradipasena P and Miyawaki O (2007), 'Characteristics of microparticulated particles from mung bean protein', *Int J Food Prop*, 10(3), 621–30.

Skogerson L, Boutte T, Robertson J and Zhang F (2006), 'Non-hydrogenated vegetable oil based margarine for puff pastry containing an elevated diglyceride emulsifier composition', *PCT Patent Application*, WO 2007/078311.

St-Jean M and Lahaye P (2005), 'Emulsion food ingredient', *PCT Patent Application*, WO 2006/045180.

Staeger M A, Folstad J E, Enz J, Mandl K and Olson E (2008), 'Hydrated fat compositions and dough articles', *PCT Patent Application*, WO 2008/091842.

Surh J, Vladisavavljevic G T, Mun S and McClements D J (2007), 'Preparation and characterisation of water/oil and water/oil/water emulsions containing biopolymer-gelled water droplets', *J Ag Food Chem*, 55(1), 175–84.

Swanson B G (2006), 'Fat replacers: mimetics and substitutes', in Shahidi F, '*Neutraceutical and speciality lipids and their co-products*', Boca Raton, CRC, 329–40.

Titoria P M and Clarke M R (2009), 'Reducing the level of saturated fats in short crust pastry', *Leatherhead Food Research report*, No. 938.

Trout J E and Kirkpatrick D P (2001), 'Reduced fat lipid-based fillings', *PCT Patent Application*, WO 02/34056.

Trout J E, Kirkpatrick D P and Romanach B A (2001a), 'Low-moisture, reduced fat lipid-based fillings', *PCT Patent Application*, WO 02/34057.

Trout J E, Kirkpatrick D P and Romanach B A (2001b), 'Reduced saturated fat lipid-based fillings', *PCT Patent Application*, WO 02/34055.

Unger E H (2005), 'Fat products containing little or no trans-fatty acids', *PCT Patent Application*, WO 2006/014322.

Wakamatsu T (2004), 'Multiple emulsion-type acidic oil-in-water emulsified food', *Japanese Patent Application*, JP2005-261233.

Wassell P (2006), 'Investigation into the performance of emulsified liquid shortenings containing palm-based hard stocks', *Palm Oil Dev*, 45, 1–11.

Watson E (2006), 'Anti-freeze', *Food Ingredients and Analysis Int*, Sept–Oct, 6–8.

Wolf F, Hecht L, Schuchmann H P, Hardy E H and Guthausen G (2009), 'Preparation of W1/O/W2 emulsions and droplet size distribution measurements by pulsed-field gradient nuclear magenetic resonsance (PFG-NMR) technique', *European J Lipid Sci Tech*, 111(7), 730–42.

Zambrano F, Despinoy P, Ormenese R C S C and Faria E V (2004), 'The use of guar and xanthan gums in the production of 'light' low fat cakes', *Int J Food Sci Tech*, 39(9), 959–66.

Zammer C M (2002), 'Drink to your heart's content', *Food Processing, Chicago*, 63 supplement 'Wellness Foods', 31 & 33–34.

© W. G. Morley, 2011

8

Diacylglycerol oils: nutritional aspects and applications in foods

O. M. Lai, Universiti Putra Malaysia, Malaysia and S.-K. Lo, Sime Darby Research Sdn. Bhd., Malaysia

Abstract: Diacylglycerols (DAG) have been shown to have beneficial effects on obesity and weight-related disorders. The reduction on the body fat accumulation shown by DAG in both animal and human studies is believed to be attributed to its metabolic pathway, which is different from triacylglycerol (TAG) metabolism. In this chapter, we highlight the differences in the physicochemical properties and the metabolic pathway between DAG and TAG. Various patented processes for the production of DAG oil from different reaction routes are discussed. A review of patent literature of the commercial products based on DAG fats and oils and the regulatory and safety aspects of these products is also provided.

Key words: diacylglycerol, obesity, physiochemical properties, metabolic pathway, health benefits, animal and human trials, production processes, products, regulatory aspects, safety.

8.1 Introduction

There is a common misconception that all fats and oils are bad for health, when in actuality the right types of oils and fats will provide an effective energy source for the body, as well as enhance the texture, taste and aroma of many foods. Various types of oils and fats are commonly used in the preparation of many types of foods by methods such as cooking, baking and frying, and are also an important component in fillings, icings, toppings and coatings. The key to a healthy diet is to stay away from foods and oils with high levels of *trans* and hypercholesterolemic fats.

Unfortunately, a high-fat diet is often linked to obesity, which is subsequently related to various diseases (Krawczyk, 2000). In the past two decades, the image of fats and oils has shifted from bad to healthful (Kennedy, 1991). As is often the

© Woodhead Publishing Limited, 2011

case in the field of nutrition, there are always new products and new developments to stay on top of. One recent commercial development in functional edible oils and fats is a product named 'Healthy Econa Cooking Oil', developed and patented by Kao Corporation (Japan) in 1999. This novel oil contains at least 80% diacylglycerols (DAG), predominantly the 1,3-isoform, and can be used in the same way as conventional edible oils. The most important feature of this product is its ability to reduce and prevent fat accumulation in the body. This functional oil was a hit in the Japanese market when it was first launched in February 1999, with demand outstripping production. Currently, the oil is used as a key component in a variety of products such as phytosterol-enriched cooking oil, salad dressings, margarine, canned products and bread. Sales of 'Healthy Econa Cooking Oil' account for 80% of premium oils, which constitutes around 14% of the total Japanese edible oil market worth around ¥10 billion (Sakaguchi, 2001). Being designated as GRAS (generally recognised as safe) by the US Food and Drug Administration, the functional oil reached the US market at the end of 2002 through a joint venture with Archer Daniels Midland Co. called ADM Kao LLC (Decatur, Illinois). The patented process for the production of DAG in this oil involves hydrolysis of triacylglycerols in refined edible oils, followed by 1,3-position selective esterification using 1,3-position selective lipases (Yamada *et al.*, 1999).

Diacylglycerols (DAG) or diglycerides are commonly used in different degrees of purity as non-ionic emulsifiers in the food, cosmetics and pharmaceutical industries in addition to their utilisation as synthetic intermediates in the chemical industry (Giacometti *et al.*, 2001). Often mixtures of monoacylglycerols (MAG) and DAG are used in these applications since they are cheap and perform well. DAG are also reported to have a large potential use as building blocks for organic synthesis of products such as phospholipids (van Deenen and de Haas, 1963) and glycolipids (Wehrli and Pomeranz, 1969). DAG can also be utilised as a starting material for synthesis of various prodrugs such as 1,3-DAG conjugated chlorambucil for treatment of lymphoma (Garzon-Aburbeh *et al.*, 1983) and 1,2-DAG conjugated (S)-(3,4-dihydroxyphenyl)alanine (L-Dopa) for treatment of Parkinson's disease (Garzon-Aburbeh *et al.*, 1986).

8.1.1   Basic chemistry of diacylglycerols (DAG)

DAG are esters of the trihydric alcohol glycerol in which two of the hydroxyl groups are esterified with fatty acids. They can exist in three isomers, namely 1,2-, 2,3- and 1,3-DAG (Fig. 8.1). These isomers will undergo acyl migration to form equilibrium at a ratio of 3–4:7–6 between 1,2-(2,3-) and 1,3-DAG (Takano and Itabashi, 2002), often assisted by the presence of an acid, alkali or heat (Sedarevich, 1967). 1,3-DAG is more thermodynamically stable due to the steric effect of the molecule.

In general, the melting temperature of 1,3-DAG is approximately 10°C higher than that of TAG, and that of 1,2-DAG is approximately 10°C lower than that of 1,3-DAG of the same fatty composition (Benson, 1967; Formo, 1979; Bockish, 1998).

© Woodhead Publishing Limited, 2011

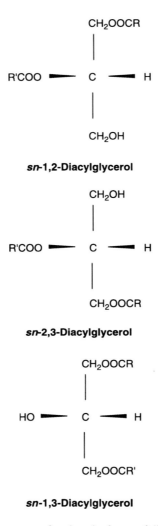

Fig. 8.1   Structures of various isoforms of diacylglycerol.

These melting point differences are due to the strength of hydrogen bonding of the hydroxyl group and fatty acid chain arrangement of the DAG isomers. 1,3-DAG has a V-shaped fatty acid chain arrangement, while 1,2-DAG has a hairpin-shaped conformation (Fig. 8.2). The type of molecular arrangement of the DAG isomer is related to its polymorphic form. Unlike TAG polymorphism, DAG exhibits two types of polymorphic forms. 1,2-DAG exhibits the α- and β'-forms but has no β-form; while 1,3-DAG has no α-form, but exhibits two types of β-form, $\beta 1$ and the more unstable $\beta 2$ (Nakajima *et al.*, 2004).

© Woodhead Publishing Limited, 2011

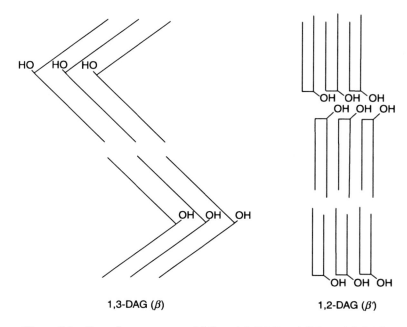

1,3-DAG (β)   1,2-DAG (β')

Figure 8.2   Crystal arrangement of β-form 1,3-DAG and β'-form 1,2-DAG.

8.2   Digestion, absorption and metabolism of DAG

DAG can be digested by the same gastrointestinal enzymes that hydrolyse TAG. However, upon digestion, DAG does not follow the resynthetic pathway of TAG, which includes the 2-monoacylglycerol (2-MAG) pathway and the glycerol-3-phosphate (GP) pathway (Friedman and Nylund, 1980). In TAG digestion, the human pancreatic lipase hydrolyses fatty acids from the 1- and 3- positions of the TAG molecule to form 1,2- and 2,3-DAG as intermediate products. These intermediate products can be further hydrolysed by the pancreatic lipase to form 2-MAG. As such, the pancreatic lipase can also hydrolyse 1,3-DAG to form 1(3)-MAG and free fatty acids (Kondo et al., 2003). The key characteristic of DAG metabolism lies in the formation of 1(3)-MAG rather than 2-MAG as found in TAG metabolism.

In TAG absorption, 2-MAG will undergo re-esterification with fatty acids via the 2-MAG pathway to reform TAG, which will then be transported as a chylomicron complex into the bloodstream via the lymphatic system. In the case of DAG, however, 1(3)-MAG is poorly re-esterified via the 2-MAG pathway, and thus has an insignificant contribution towards TAG resynthesis (Lehner et al., 1993). Instead, substantial amounts of 1(3)-MAG are further hydrolysed to free fatty acids and glycerol, which are precursors of the GP pathway, while some are reesterified to 1,3-DAG (Mansbach and Nevin, 1998). The efficiency of DAG digestion products to convert into TAG in the small intestines was also found to be low. Another important difference between DAG and TAG metabolism is the

© Woodhead Publishing Limited, 2011

substrate specificity of the diacylglycerol acyltransferase (DGAT) enzymes, DGAT-1 and DGAT-2, in the small intestines (Cases *et al.*, 1998, 2001). DGAT is involved in the final synthetic step of TAG by catalysing the acylation of 1,2(2,3)-DAG, which are products from the 2-MAG pathway (Bell and Coleman, 1980; Lehner and Kuksis, 1996). However, DGAT has low substrate specificity towards 1,3-DAG and therefore does not significantly convert 1,3-DAG to TAG (Lehner and Kuksis, 1993). Conclusions from these findings on the nature of DAG digestion and absorption may explain the reduction of postprandial TAG levels in the blood.

Numerous animal (Murata *et al.*, 1997; Watanabe *et al.*, 1997; Murase *et al.*, 2002a and 2002b; Meng *et al.*, 2003) and clinical (Kamphuis *et al.*, 2003) studies have all shown that ingestion of DAG oil, in comparison with TAG oil, increases the rate of β-oxidation of fatty acids. Additionally, the activities of enzymes involved in fatty acid synthesis, such as glucose-6-phosphate dehydrogenase (G6PD), malic enzyme (ME) and fatty acid synthetase (FAS), were observed to significantly decrease in subjects fed with DAG oil (Murata *et al.*, 1997). On the other hand, hepatic enzymes involved in the β-oxidation pathway, such as acyl-CoA dehydrogenase, acyl-CoA oxidase, enoyl-CoA hydratase, carnitine palmitoyltransferase, 3-hydroxyacyl-CoA dehydrogenase, 2,4-dienoyl-CoA reductase and $\delta 3, \delta 2$-enoyl-CoA isomerase, were found to increase in activity in a dose-dependent manner with DAG intake (Murata *et al.*, 1997). In a clinical study (Kamphuis *et al.*, 2003), it was interesting to note that the increase in β-oxidation occurred even without any change in daily energy expenditure resulting from resting activity or activity related to physical exertion. It is believed that the increase in β-oxidation of DAG metabolism relates to the corresponding reduction in body fat and serum TAG levels.

8.2.1   Health benefits of DAG

The ingestion of DAG oil has been shown to reduce body fat accumulation (Nagao *et al.*, 2000; Murase *et al.*, 2001, 2002a and 2002b; Maki *et al.*, 2002; Meng *et al.*, 2003) and lower serum TAG levels (Hara *et al.*, 1993; Murata *et al.*, 1994; Taguchi *et al.*, 2000; Tada *et al.*, 2001; Yamamoto *et al.*, 2001; Kondo *et al.*, 2003; Yanagisawa *et al.*, 2003; Yamamoto *et al.*, 2005). Murase *et al.* (2001) reported a 70% reduction in body weight of mice after five months on a diet containing 30% DAG oil. Significant fat reductions surrounding the epididymal, mesenteric, retroperitoneal and perirenal areas were observed. However, other animal tests (Sugimoto *et al.*, 2003a and 2003b) revealed that the effect of DAG oil on reducing body weight was not found at low intakes (10% or less) of DAG.

In order to compare the effects of DAG and TAG oil ingestion on human body fat, Nagao *et al.* (2000) conducted a 16-week double-blind study on 38 healthy men with an average body mass index (BMI) of approximately 24 kg/m². The subjects were randomly provided with food products that contain either DAG or TAG oil at a dosage of 10 g/day during the treatment period. The results revealed that reductions in body weight, body mass index (BMI), waist circumference and total fat area were more distinct in subjects consuming the DAG oil diet than that of TAG oil (Nagao

© Woodhead Publishing Limited, 2011

et al., 2000). In another related study, Maki *et al.* (2002) observed similar findings in a six-month investigation on the effect of diets rich in DAG and TAG oils on obese men and women with BMI of approximately 34 kg/m^2. On the other hand, several studies did not find any significant change in body fat reduction of the subjects after the treatment period (Flatt, 1988; Schutz, 1995; Nagao *et al.*, 2000).

Studies investigating the effect of DAG oil on serum TAG levels in animals and humans also showed inconsistent results. Reductions in serum TAG levels were observed in some studies (Hara *et al.*, 1993; Murata *et al.*, 1994; Taguchi *et al.*, 2000; Tada *et al.*, 2001; Yamamoto *et al.*, 2001; Kondo *et al.*, 2003; Yanagisawa *et al.*, 2003; Yamamoto *et al.*, 2005), while in others, there was no change in serum TAG levels (Nagao *et al.*, 2000; Meguro *et al.*, 2001; Soni *et al.*, 2001; Maki *et al.*, 2002; Kamphuis *et al.*, 2003; Sugimoto *et al.*, 2003a and 2003b). Hara *et al.* (1993) investigated the effect of feeding diets containing 10% DAG oil to rats and concluded that DAG has an ability to reduce serum TAG levels. Murata *et al.* (1994) suggested that the ingestion of DAG oil decreased serum TAG levels by retarding the chylomicron assembly that is essential for TAG transportation. In another study, Kondo *et al.* (2003) reported that TAG synthesis in DAG-infused rats was less pronounced than in TAG-infused rats. On the other hand, Taguchi *et al.* (2002) did not find any decrease in serum TAG levels of rats fed with diets containing 30% DAG oil. Interestingly, it was found that the DAG oil suppressed the hepatic activity of microsomal TAG transfer protein (MTP) and MTP mRNA. MTP is an important component for the transportation of TAG from the site of synthesis to the site of assembly with apolipoprotein B (ApoB) at the endoplasmic reticulum (ER). In a study using obesity-prone mice, the effect of a DAG diet on reducing serum TAG level was shown after eight months of treatment (Murase *et al.*, 2001). Murase *et al.* (2001) suggested that the up-regulation of lipid metabolism and β-oxidation may be partially responsible for the lower serum TAG levels. Murase *et al.* (2001) also observed that significant reductions in serum cholesterol levels were observed in these obesity-prone rats. Other studies (Murase *et al.*, 2002a and 2002b) suggest that DAG stimulates intestinal lipid metabolism by changing the mucosal lipid profile, which, in turn, affects the regulation of gene expression in the small intestine.

Similar discrepancies were also observed in various clinical studies, where some trials confirmed that DAG intake was able to decrease serum TAG levels (Taguchi *et al.*, 2000; Tada *et al.*, 2001; Yamamoto *et al.*, 2001; Yanagisawa *et al.*, 2003; Yamamoto *et al.*, 2005), while others reported otherwise (Nagao *et al.*, 2000; Meguro *et al.*, 2001; Maki *et al.*, 2002; Kamphuis *et al.*, 2003). However, DAG intake was shown to be beneficial in reducing serum TAG levels in young women with hyperlipidemia-prone variants of fatty acid binding protein 2 and MTP (Yanagisawa *et al.*, 2003) and in type 2 diabetic patients (Yamamoto *et al.*, 2001). Additionally, the consumption of DAG oil also reduces glycosylated haemoglobin (HbA$_{1c}$) concentrations in these diabetic patients (Yamamoto *et al.*, 2001). The level of HbA$_{1c}$ is an accurate indication of the recent overall blood glucose concentration in diabetic patients. However, no significant reductions in serum TAG levels were noted in studies involving overweight and obese subjects (Nagao *et al.*, 2000; Maki *et al.*, 2002). These inconsistent results may be attributed

© Woodhead Publishing Limited, 2011

to different quantities of DAG in the study diets, as well as different physiological condition of the subjects, e.g. healthy, hyperlipidemic, diabetic, overweight and obese. DAG oil is also beneficial in reducing remnant-like lipoprotein particles (RLP) (Tada *et al.*, 2001). RLPs are atherogenic metabolites of TAG-rich lipoproteins such as chylomicrons and very low-density lipoproteins (VLDL). However, in another study, high-density lipoprotein (HDL) cholesterol was found to increase with DAG ingestion (Teramoto *et al.*, 2004). In spite of these inconsistencies, DAG oil has proved to be beneficial for reducing body fat accumulation in both animal and human subjects.

8.3   Production process patents

Various routes for the production of DAG oil have been reported in patent literature. In general, DAG oil can be produced via glycerolysis between TAG and glycerol, esterification of fatty acids or its derivatives to glycerol, hydrolysis of TAG, or a combination of these methods. These processes often involve either a chemical or an enzyme catalyst. Apart from these methods for the production of DAG, other related technologies, such as DAG separation and purification methods, that complement DAG production have also been patented. In this section, patent literature on processes related to DAG oil is reviewed.

There are a number of patents for the production of DAG oil via esterification of fatty acids or their derivatives such as fatty acid anhydrides and fatty acid methyl esters. Mazur and Hiler's (1992) process involves the esterification of 3–40% of fatty acid anhydride with 3–40% of glycerol in the presence of a water-immiscible hydrocarbon or chlorinated hydrocarbon solvent such as methylene chloride. The reaction is catalysed by a 1,3-position specific immobilised lipase. DAG yield of 41% (w/w) is reported. This method involves the use of chlorinated solvents, which may pose a problem in waste management. Additionally, the use of such solvents may not be an attractive marketing option for DAG oil. Lo and Baharin (2001) reported on a solvent-free method for the production of DAG from fatty acid deodoriser distillates obtained from edible oil refineries. In this method, DAG oil is produced by esterification of free fatty acids present in the deodoriser distillates with glycerol which is added into the reaction. Similarly, the process is catalyzed by a 1,3-position specific immobilised lipase. A yield of 60% (w/w) of DAG oil can be obtained. The advantage of this process is in its use of a lower cost raw material compared with refined fatty acids, and thus may positively reflect on the production cost of the DAG oil. However, since the process requires the use of an immobilised enzyme as catalyst, the process cost may not be low. In order to provide a solution to the high cost of enzymes, Lai *et al.* (2007) reported on the use of a strongly acidic cation exchange resin as a chemical catalyst for the synthesis of DAG oil from free fatty acids. The application of the heterogeneous catalyst will allow for easy separation of the catalyst from the reaction products. The cost of the ion exchange resins is also significantly cheaper than that of commercial immobilised lipases. Another advantage of this process involves the use of relatively lower temperatures as compared to other

© Woodhead Publishing Limited, 2011

chemically catalysed synthetic processes. However, one major drawback of this process is the use of more expensive free fatty acids compared with TAG as raw materials. Yoon *et al.* (2004) disclosed a process for the production of DAG oil containing conjugated linoleic acids, comprising of esterifying monoacylglycerols (MAG) with free fatty acids in the presence of a lipase. A similar process for DAG production involving transesterification between MAG and TAG has been invented by Toshinori *et al.* (2000). These processes utilising MAG as raw materials for DAG production may not be industrially attractive as the cost of MAG is relatively high.

DAG oil can also be produced from partial hydrolysis of TAG. Lai *et al.* (2006) disclose an enzymatic process for partial hydrolysis of TAG to produce DAG. A commercial immobilised lipase was used to catalyse the hydrolysis of TAG under controlled conditions to produce DAG oil. The advantage of this process lies in the single-step hydrolytic reaction of TAG without further addition of other substrates such as glycerol. However, precise control of water content in the reaction system is required for optimal DAG yield.

Sugiura *et al.* (2002a) demonstrated a glycerolysis process to produce DAG from TAG and glycerol, in the presence of small quantities of water and lipase to assist catalysis. The glycerolysis reaction is conducted at relatively lower temperatures (0–25°C). The DAG product is removed by crystallisation during the course of the reaction. This method of DAG separation may not be cost effective in large-scale production as longer reaction times are required (20 to 100 hours). Jacobs *et al.* (2003) reported on a glycerolysis process for producing DAG oil from TAG and glycerol using potassium acetate as a catalyst. The process is claimed to provide a crude DAG product with good colour. However, the process requires a relatively high reaction temperature of 190–240°C, and therefore may translate to a significant energy cost. Nevertheless, the economics of this process are compensated by the use of low-cost raw materials and catalyst.

Another process for the production of DAG oil involves a combination of hydrolysis and esterification reactions (Yamada *et al.*, 1999). The process comprises hydrolysing TAG oil to obtain free fatty acids, followed by esterification of these free fatty acids, without further purification, with glycerol to produce DAG. The hydrolysis step may be performed using steam or in the presence of a lipase. For the esterification step, an immobilised lipase is required for catalysis. In comparison with other enzymatic processes for DAG oil production, this process has potential for industrial feasibility. As a follow-up to this process, Sugiura *et al.* (2002b) up-scaled this process into a production plant setting and described how high-purity DAG oil can be produced at high yields and in a short time by carrying out an esterification reaction of fatty acids with glycerol in an immobilised enzyme-packed tower. Sugiura *et al.* (2002b) explained that the residence time for the reaction substrates in the enzyme-packed tower should not be more than 120 seconds so as to minimise TAG formation. From an engineering viewpoint, the superficial velocity of the substrate is preferably not lower than 1 mm/s so as to minimise mass transfer resistance between solid and liquid and reduction in reaction rate. Based on Kozeny–Carman's equation, Sugiura *et al.* (2002b) determined that the ratio between the packing thickness of the immobilised lipase, L, and the squared average particle

© Woodhead Publishing Limited, 2011

diameter of the immobilised lipase, d^2, defined as L/d^2, should be controlled between a value of 3–25 to maintain a pressure drop of 20 kg/cm^2 or less. Lower pressure drop is desirable in minimising plant cost. In addition, water formed during the reaction is simultaneously removed under reduced pressure. The effects of various process parameters on the yields of DAG and TAG are shown in Table 8.1. Based on this method, a DAG yield of 65% (w/w) is reported.

Table 8.1   Effects of various process parameters on yields of DAG and TAG

	Run number						
	1	2	3	4	5	6	7
Batch size (kg)	100	100	100	100	100	100	1
Oleic acid (kg)	86	86	86	86	86	86	0.86
Glycerol (kg)	14	14	14	14	14	14	0.14
Immobilised lipase	Lipozyme IM	Lipozyme IM	Lipozyme IM	Lipozyme IM	Lipozyme IM	Lipozyme IM	Lipozyme IM
Average particle diameter, d (mm)	0.43	0.43	0.43	0.43	0.43	0.08	0.43
Amount (kg)	5	5	5	5	20	5	0.1
Packing thickness, L (m)	0.18	0.18	0.18	0.18	0.7	0.18	0.33
Superficial velocity, U (mm/s)	4.4	2.2	4.4	1.1	3.7	0.5	2.0
Residence time (s)	40	79	40	158	190	351	164
L/d^2	0.95	0.95	0.95	0.95	3.80	27.50	1.80
Pressure loss, P (kg/cm^2)	2.6	1.5	2.6	0.7	9.5	8.5	2.5
Reaction time (h)	3.5	3.5	3.5	3.5	3.5	3.5	7.0
Oleic acid residue (wt. %)	14.1	15.4	16.4	43.1	11.6	47.8	12.4
Glycerol residue (wt. %)	0.3	0.7	0.5	2.1	0.4	2.7	0.1
Monoacylglycerol (MAG) product (wt. %)	14.1	18.3	16.8	15.3	15.0	16.4	9.3
Diacylglycerol (DAG) product (wt. %)	65.6	58.1	59.5	32.8	55.7	26.8	63.0
Triacylglycerol (TAG) product (wt. %)	5.9	7.5	6.8	6.7	17.3	6.3	15.2
Yield (DAG+TAG)	71.5	65.6	66.3	39.5	73.0	33.1	78.2

Source: Sugiura *et al.*, 2002b

© Woodhead Publishing Limited, 2011

Another interesting method of producing DAG oil was revealed by Choo *et al.* (2007). According to their account, an end product with high DAG content of at least 8% (w/w) can be produced from TAG oil of vegetable origin by subjecting the vegetable oil to short-path distillation (SPD) under vacuum of not more than 0.01 Torr and at a temperature of 300°C and below, where the DAG oil is obtained as the distillate. As mentioned earlier, vegetable oils generally do not contain more than 10% (w/w) of DAG. Due to the relatively low DAG content in vegetable oils, the DAG oil yield obtained from this process will be at most 10% (w/w). The low DAG yield will translate to a high production cost of DAG oil, making this process industrially unattractive.

8.4   Product application patents

The versatility of DAG oil is evident as numerous applications are reported in patent literature; for example as a cooking oil, frying oil, salad oil, salad dressing and mayonnaise, in shortenings and margarines, chocolates, ice-cream fats, confectioner's fats, specialty oils with enriched essential fatty acids, fried and baked food products, beverages, formulations with phytonutrients, and products with specific physiological benefits. The following is a summary of product applications comprising DAG oil as the functional component.

8.4.1   DAG oil composition for specific physiological benefits

The main physiological benefit of DAG oil is its ability to reduce body fat and therefore prevent or treat obesity. Koike *et al.* (2003) disclosed an oil composition for such a purpose which comprises 5–100% (w/w) of a MAG and/or a DAG with a fatty acid composition of 15–90% (w/w) of ω-3 unsaturated fatty acids based on MAG and/or DAG content. Additionally, the oil composition contains an antioxidant to prevent oxidation. Another DAG oil composition claimed to exhibit an excellent inhibitory effect on body fat accumulation while having good flavour, colour, hydrolytic and oxidative stabilities was invented by Takase *et al.* (2003). The oil is comprised of 15–70% (w/w) of DAG in which less than 15% (w/w) of the fatty acids are ω-3 unsaturated fatty acids, and 30–85% (w/w) of TAG in which at least 15% (w/w) of the fatty acids are ω-3 unsaturated fatty acids. This composition also contains a small amount of an antioxidant.

Masui *et al.* (2001) described a DAG oil composition capable of reducing arteriosclerotic factors in the blood and thereby lowering the risks of arteriosclerosis and other degenerative diseases. The authors have described an oil composition comprised of at least 35% (w/w) of DAG, wherein the constituents of the fatty acids of the DAG oil satisfy the following equation:

Amount of *cis*-form unsaturated fatty acid/amount of saturated
fatty acid + amount of *trans*-form unsaturated fatty acid ≥ 6,
wherein the amount of *trans*-form fatty acid is not exceeding
5% (w/w) based on fatty acids of DAG oil.   [8.1]

© Woodhead Publishing Limited, 2011

According to the authors, the intake of DAG oil with such composition will increase HDL cholesterol level and reduce the activity of plasminogen activator inhibitor type 1 (PAI-1), which controls the production of plasmin in the blood. A lower activity of PAI-1 is essential for the prevention of arteriosclerosis. Another oil composition for the prevention of arteriosclerosis was invented by Koike *et al.* (2001). The inventors claim an oil composition containing 10–40% (w/w) of DAG, in which at least 55% (w/w) of the fatty acids are unsaturated and 15–100% (w/w) of these fatty acids are ω-3 unsaturated fatty acids with at least 20 carbon atoms; and 40.1–89.8% (w/w) of TAG, in which at least 70% (w/w) of the fatty acids are unsaturated and 5–80% (w/w) of these fatty acids comprise linoleic acid. In addition to being antiarteriosclerotic, it is also claimed that such an oil composition has excellent oxidation stability and good flavour. Another very similar oil composition was again invented by Koike *et al.* (2002a). The authors describe an oil or fat with excellent visceral fat and body fat burning properties and stability against autoxidation. According to this invention, the oil comprises 60–100% (w/w) of DAG, wherein the fatty acid composition of the oil consists of 15–90% (w/w) of an ω-3 unsaturated fatty acid having less than 20 carbon atoms and the weight ratio of *cis* ω-3 unsaturated fatty acid to the sum of *cis* ω-6 unsaturated fatty acid, saturated fatty acid and *trans* unsaturated fatty acid is from 1 to 6.

Koike *et al.* (2002b) subsequently revealed another DAG oil composition with a specific physiological effect. As described in this account, the consumption of an oil or fat with a composition comprised of 5–99.9% (w/w) MAG having a fatty acid composition of 15–90% (w/w) of an ω-3 unsaturated fatty acid of less than 20 carbon atoms, 1–80% (w/w) of an ω-9 unsaturated fatty acid and 2–50% (w/w) of an ω-6 unsaturated fatty acid; and 0.1–49.9% (w/w) DAG, wherein the weight ratio of DAG to MAG is below 1, and the content of polyunsaturated fatty acid (PUFA) with four double bonds is 20% (w/w) or less based on total fatty acid composition, has a beneficial effect of lowering glutamic oxaloacetic transaminase (GOT) and glutamic pyruvic transaminase (GPT) levels in the blood. High levels of GOT and GPT are often released into the blood when there is a liver or heart malfunction. This formulation is claimed to be useful in pharmaceutical products and foods for the prevention of hepatic function disturbances and obesity.

Another DAG oil formulation for inhibition of platelet aggregation and reduction of body fat, while simultaneously having excellent oxidative stability, flavour and flowability, was again invented by Koike *et al.* (2002c). According to their report, the oil formulation is made up of 0.1–59.8% (w/w) TAG, 40–99.7% (w/w) DAG, 0.1–10% (w/w) MAG, and 0–5% (w/w) FFA, wherein the DAG consists of 15–89.5% (w/w) of ω-3 unsaturated fatty acids with at least 20 carbon atoms and 10–84.5% (w/w) of monounsaturated fatty acids.

DAG oil is also formulated to lower blood sugar level, improve insulin resistance and reduce the effect of leptin, in addition to resisting the accumulation of body and visceral fat (Koike *et al.*, 2002d). Serum leptin levels are reported to be closely linked to the amount of fat in the body (William *et al.*, 2001). In this invention, an oil or fat composition comprising of 10.1–94.9% (w/w) TAG, 0.1–30% (w/w) MAG, and 5–59.9% (w/w) DAG which consists of 15–90% (w/w) of

© Woodhead Publishing Limited, 2011

an ω-3 unsaturated fatty acid with less than 20 carbon atoms is described to possess such properties.

8.4.2   Oil-in-water type emulsion foods

Oil-in-water type emulsion (O/W) food products are commonly represented by mayonnaise and salad dressings. In general, mayonnaise and salad dressings contain oil, egg yolk, vinegar and seasonings (salt, sugar, spices, flavours, etc.). The major difference between mayonnaise and salad dressings is in the oil content. Mayonnaise has an oil content of 65–85% (w/w), while salad dressing has less than 60% (w/w) oil. The application of DAG oil in O/W products was first patented by Nomura *et al.* (1992). They created an O/W product in which the oil phase comprises 30–100% (w/w) DAG with a melting point of 20°C or less. The O/W composition is claimed to exhibit a rich fatty savour even at a low fat content. Several years later, Kawai and Konishi (2000) described an O/W composition that has excellent storage stability combined with good appearance, taste and physical properties. The composition has an oil phase which is comprised of 30% (w/w) or greater of DAG oil and a yolk wherein the ratio of lysophospholipids to the whole phospholipids is at least 15% (w/w) based on phosphorous content. Shiiba *et al.* (2002) provided further improvements by developing an O/W composition that has excellent shelf stability at low temperatures comprising at least 20% (w/w) of the O/W emulsion and 0.5– 5% (w/w) of a crystallisation inhibitor. The crystallisation inhibitor is a polyglycerol fatty acid ester, sucrose fatty acid ester or sorbitan fatty acid ester.

8.4.3   Water-in-oil type emulsion foods

The other form of emulsified food product has a water-in-oil type emulsion (W/O). Examples of such products are margarine, spreads, buttercream fillings and icings used in baking and confectionery industry. Mori *et al.* (1999a) invented a W/O emulsified fat composition that has good stability and spreadability, and is suitable for use as a margarine. The W/O composition is made up of 40% to less than 95% (w/w) of DAG and 5% to less than 60% (w/w) of TAG, wherein the DAG comprises 0.5% to less than 20% (w/w) DAG containing two saturated C14:0-C22:0 fatty acid groups, 20% to less than 55% (w/w) DAG containing one saturated C14:0-C22:0 fatty acid group and one unsaturated C14:0-C22:0 fatty acid group, and 25% to less than 70% (w/w) DAG containing two unsaturated C14:0-C22:0 fatty acid groups, and the weight ratio of total C14:0 and C16:0 saturated fatty acid groups in DAG to total C18:0, C20:0 and C22:0 saturated fatty acid groups in DAG is in the range of one to eight. Another W/O composition claimed to have excellent flavour release during the time of ingestion was invented by Masui and Konishi (2001), who claimed that 30% (w/w) of the W/O oil or fat composition is able to reverse in phase within one minute after coming into contact with water at 36°C, thereby releasing the flavour component. The W/O composition comprises of water as the aqueous phase, 15% (w/w) or more of DAG as the oil phase, and a demulsifier, which comprises at least a polyglycerol

© Woodhead Publishing Limited, 2011

fatty acid ester having a hydrophilic-lipophilic balance (HLB) value of 8 or more, a water-soluble decomposed protein, lysolecithin having HLB value of 8 or more, a sucrose fatty acid ester having HLB of 5 or more, a MAG organic acid ester having HLB of 8 or more, and a sorbitan fatty acid ester having HLB of 8 or more. A W/O composition by Masui and Yasunaga (2001) describes a W/O product that is stable in spite of containing a high water content and has good storage and mouthfeel. The product composition comprises of water as the aqueous phase, 35–95% (w/w) of DAG having a melting point of below 20°C, and the remainder as TAG, which is composed of 13–60% (w/w) palmitic acid and 5% (w/w) or less of fatty acid having 12 carbons or lower, as the oil phase. Additionally, the TAG has to possess a stable polymorphic form of β'.

8.4.4   DAG oil composition containing phytosterols

Phytosterols are lipid compounds that have been shown to lower serum cholesterol levels in humans (Ling and Jones, 1995; Jones *et al.*, 1997). Due to their limited solubility in oil (approx. 1% w/w) and insolubility in water, normal intakes of phytosterols are not efficiently absorbed by the intestines, and are therefore ineffective in lowering serum cholesterol levels. Efforts were made to increase solubility of phytosterols in oil by converting them into phytosterol fatty acid esters (Hendriks *et al.*, 1999). However, Meguro *et al.* (2001) reported that phytosterols can achieve higher solubility in DAG oil without a need for esterification. Several patents were based on DAG oil composition containing dissolved phytosterols.

Goto *et al.* (2000a and 2000b) claimed that the solubility of phytosterol can be increased by 1.2–20% (w/w) when 15% (w/w) or more of DAG oil is used as solvent. Additionally, the authors claimed that 80% (w/w) or more of DAG oil can dissolve 0.05–20% (w/w) of phytosterols. However, 55% (w/w) or more of unsaturated fatty acids have to be present in the DAG oil for effective solubilisation of the phytosterols. In another patent (Goto *et al.*, 2001), an oil composition containing 15% (w/w) or more of DAG and up to 2000 ppm of tocopherol was reported to effectively dissolve 1.2–20% (w/w) of phytosterols. The DAG component is comprised of at least 70% (w/w) unsaturated fatty acids. Nakajima *et al.* (2002) made further improvements to phytosterol solubility in DAG oil in a process whereby an oil composition containing 15–95% (w/w) is used to dissolve 2–10% (w/w) of phytosterol and the resultant oil composition remains a transparent liquid at temperatures of 0–30 °C.

8.4.5   Shortenings

DAG also finds an application in the formulation of shortenings. Doucet and Olathe (1999a) invented a shortening composition comprising a non-hydrogenated vegetable oil and a stearine fraction containing 50–60 mol % of DAG. It is claimed that the shortening formulation has a synergistic amount of solids and crystal matrices that imparts superior organoleptic properties to the food product, without the incorporation of *trans* fatty acids commonly found in partially hydrogenated fats. Concomitantly, Doucet *et al.* (1999b) claimed that the above effects can also

© Woodhead Publishing Limited, 2011

be made possible with the addition of MAG composed predominantly of saturated fatty acids.

8.4.6   Frying applications

Since DAG has a lower molecular weight than TAG, DAG oil has a significantly lower smoke point (30–40 °C) than TAG oil with similar fatty acid compositions. Therefore, frying applications with DAG oil will be problematic. Several DAG compositions suitable for use as frying oil have been reported. Sakai *et al.* (2002a) reported a fat composition containing at least 15% (w/w) of DAG, a fatty acid L-ascorbic ester and a component such as catechin or a natural plant extract such as rosemary, sage and turmeric extracts. The authors claimed that the DAG composition has excellent stability towards oxidation, while providing good flavour and appearance. Another DAG composition reported by Sakai *et al.* (2002b) contains 15% (w/w) or more of DAG and 70 ppm or more of one or more types of organic carboxylic acids such as 2 to 8 carbon hydroxycarboxylic or dicarboxylic acids and their derivatives. The composition is claimed to resist thermal oxidation or hydrolysis after prolonged heating or storage, as well as to reduce smoking when the oil composition is used for frying purposes.

8.4.7   Foods containing DAG oil

Foods which are prepared with or contain DAG oil are summarised in this section. Mori *et al.* (1999b) reported on a fried food with a fat composition containing 55% to less than 95% (w/w) of DAG which was composed of 55% to less than 93% (w/w) of unsaturated fatty acids. The authors claimed that when the food is fried with DAG oil of such composition, the resultant fried food will have a low water content and is unlikely to get moist and reduce in crispness over a prolonged period of time. The fried foods that are covered in this patent are fried cakes, French fried potatoes, fried chicken and doughnuts. A disclosure from Mori and Watanabe (2000) describes a food which is comprised of 0.5–85% (w/w) DAG with C2:0–C10:0 fatty acids. When ingested, the food composition is claimed to possess good organoleptic properties, as well as to reduce body fat accumulation and provide energy at times of exhaustion and fatigue.

Another DAG-containing food product, reported by Kudo *et al.* (2002), is fried or baked potatoes, which comprise of 3–50% (w/w) of oil or fat, wherein the DAG content is 15% to less than 50% (w/w). The fatty acids of the DAG oil are composed of 15–100% (w/w) of ω-3 unsaturated fatty acids of less than 20 carbon atoms. Similar to the findings of Mori *et al.* (1999b), potatoes fried or baked in such a DAG oil composition were reported to provide a product that has low water content, favourable texture and taste, as well as good storage stability.

8.4.8   Ice-cream coating fats

Ice-cream coating fats are generally TAG of medium-chain fatty acids, such as lauric acid-rich coconut oil. The first use of DAG as an ice-cream coating fat was

© Woodhead Publishing Limited, 2011

reported by Cain *et al.* (1999). The fat composition is comprised of 50–90% (w/w) DAG and 10–50% (w/w) TAG of vegetable origin. The DAG oil is composed of 75–90% (w/w) diunsaturated DAG, less than 5% (w/w) disaturated DAG and 10–25% (w/w) DAG with one unsaturated and one saturated fatty acid. The TAG composition in this fat composition is such that the sum of triunsaturated and diunsaturated TAG is at least 50% (w/w). According to this invention, the ice-cream coating fat resulted in a product that was softer and less brittle, but had quicker and smoother meltdown, than cocoa butter-based coating fats.

8.5   Regulatory status

DAG oil has been available in the Japanese market since February 1999. The Ministry of Health and Welfare of Japan has approved DAG oil as Food for Specified Health Use (FOSHU) since 1999, indicating to consumers that the Ministry of Health in Japan has granted a 'healthy' status to this product. Two other products containing DAG oil have also been given the FOSHU labelling since then, namely DAG oil containing phytosterols and DAG mayonnaise-type. All the three products had officially approved 'less likely to become body fat' or 'lowering serum cholesterol' claims attached.

In the US, the Food and Drug Administration (FDA) has approved DAG as a 'Generally Recognised As Safe' (GRAS) substance. On the ingredients statement, the FDA has ruled that the common name to be used is 'diacylglycerol oil'. DAG oil is approved for the European market under the Novel Foods regulation of 2006. Food categories approved include home cooking oil, fat spreads/margarines, mayonnaise, salad dressings, health drinks as meal replacements, yoghurt and baked goods (Empie, 2008). Similarly, Canada, Australia and New Zealand approved DAG oil as a Novel Food in 2004. Also in 2004, Brazil approved the use of DAG oil as an ingredient in foods without claims. It is believed that other countries in Latin America will follow suit.

8.5.1   Safety of DAG

The safety of DAG oils has been tested in both animal and human studies. In one of the animal studies, groups of beagle dogs were fed with diets containing low (1.5% DAG oil), mid (5.5%) and high (9.5%) doses of DAG oil for one year (Chengelis *et al.*, 2006). There were no reported effects on clinical condition, body weights, feed consumption or DAG-related haematology in any of the dogs. There were also no dose-dependent, statistically significant DAG-treated adverse effects in the dogs fed with the doses of up to 9.5% DAG oil in their diet. Additionally, Ichihara *et al.* (2008) conducted a 24-week trial on male F344 rats, which were fed with various edible oils including DAG oil after the administration of known carcinogens. The trial was designed to determine the modifying potential of DAG oil on tumour development. At the end of the 24 weeks, ingestion of DAG oil showed no difference from the TAG oil controls in terms of body weights, feed consumption, clinical

© Woodhead Publishing Limited, 2011

condition, organ weights or survival. Incidences and the severity of neoplastic lesions were found to be comparable across all treatment groups and the authors concluded that the DAG oil did not exert any modifying potential on tumour development. In human clinical trials with healthy adults, ingestion of doses as high as 450 mg DAG oil/kg body weight/day for eight weeks also did not show any adverse effects (Hasegawa, 2000). In genotoxicity tests, Kasamatsu et al. (2005) concluded that both unheated and heated DAG oil did not exhibit any genotoxic effects. Studies were also conducted on physiologically compromised volunteers. In adults with hyperlipidemia and undergoing dialysis treatment, DAG oil was given as a replacement for their normal cooking oil (Teramoto et al., 2000). The mean DAG oil ingested was ~9000 mg/person/day. Results at the end of the trial showed that there was an increased concentration of serum fatty acids which remained above the baseline after the washout period. There were no changes in the total or HDL cholesterol reported. There were no other statistically significant findings in this study. Additional studies involving children and volunteers with diabetes (Yamamoto et al., 2006) or uremic conditions (Teramoto et al., 2004) showed no signs of adverse effects when DAG oil was ingested during the study period.

8.6   Future trends

In the past decade the number of fat or obese people worldwide has risen at an alarming rate. Doctors, scientists and nutritionists are now investigating the role of genetics, metabolism and drugs in contributing to this weight-related problem, as well as new methods to treat it. This, in turn, has directly or indirectly enhanced the very lucrative global anti-obesity market, which currently is worth in excess of USD 240 billion. At this rapidly growing rate, obesity may soon bankrupt national health organisations of certain countries, if appropriate measures to reduce obesity levels are not implemented.

The United States of America has the largest proportion of obese people. In 2008, the US Centers for Disease Control and Prevention (CDC) reported that 26.5% of the US population were obese. However, a collaborative report published by the United Health Foundation, the American Public Health Association and Partnership for Prevention has forecast that the obesity population in the US will hit 47.5% in 2018. At these alarming rates, obesity will certainly place a heavy financial burden on public health care. In order to prevent enormous future health care costs, early steps should be taken to slow down the current obesity rates.

The healthful and functional oils and fats market has certainly benefited from all this publicity. Rising consumer awareness of obesity and mandatory governmental legislations on unhealthful fats has led to a surge in the sales volume of functional oil and fat products. The future trend of edible oils and fats has been gradually shifting towards healthfulness and positive functionality. As DAG has a higher melting point than TAG of the same fatty acid composition, as described above, DAG obtained from certain sources, especially from palm oil, will find suitable applications in solid fat products while having a higher unsaturated fatty

© Woodhead Publishing Limited, 2011

acid content as compared to its corresponding TAG oil. As such, the use of palm-based DAG will give the industry and consumer the benefit of a higher melting fat similar to a conventional solid TAG fat with a higher saturated fatty acid content but without the negative effects of the conventional TAG fat comprising a higher saturated fatty acid content. This unique feature is one of the inherent advantages of DAG. Therefore a strong demand for healthful oils such as DAG oil is anticipated in the future.

8.7   Source of further information

Diacylglycerol Oil by Katsuragi *et al.*, published by AOCS Press, IL, USA (2008)

8.8   References

Bell, R. M. and R. A. Coleman (1980) Enzymes of glycerolipid synthesis in eukaryotes. *Annu. Rev. Biochem.* 49: 459–87.

Benson, F. R. (1967) Polyol surfactants. In *Nonionic surfactants*, ed. Shick, M. J., pp 247–299. New York: Marcel Dekker.

Bockish, M. (1998) Composition, structure, physical data, and chemical reactions of fats and oils, their derivatives, and their associates. In *Fats and oils handbook*, pp 53–120, Illinois: AOCS Press.

Cain, F. W., H. G. A. Manson, P. T. Quinlan and S. R. Moore (1999) Ice-cream coating fats. *United States Patent.* No US5891495.

Cases, S., S. J. Smith, Y. W. Zheng, H. M. Myers, S. R. Lear, E. Sande, S. Novak, C. Collins, C. B. Welch, A. J. Lusis, S. K. Erickson and R. V. Jr. Farese (1998) Identification of a gene encoding an acyl CoA:diacylglycerol acyltransferase, a key enzyme in triacylglycerol synthesis. *Proc. Natl. Acad. Sci. USA.* 95: 13018–23.

Cases, S., S. J. Stone, P. Zhou, E. Yen, B. Tow, K. D. Lardizabal, T. Voelker and R. V. Jr. Farese (2001) Cloning of DGAT2, a second mammalian diacylglycerol acyltransferase, and related family members. *J. Biol. Chem.* 276: 38870–6.

Chengelis, C. P., Kirkpatrick, J.B., Marit, G.B., Morita, O., Tamaki, Y. and Suzuki, H. (2006) A chronic dietary toxicity study of DAG (Diacylglycerol) in beagle dogs. *Food. Chem. Toxicol,* 44: 81–97.

Choo, Y. M., C. W. Puah, A. N. Ma and Y. Basiron (2007) Production of edible oil. *United States Patent Application.* No US20070021625.

Doucet, J. and K. Olathe (1999a) Shortening system, products therewith, and methods for making and using the same. *United States Patent.* No US5908655.

Doucet, J., K. Olathe, C. E. Rethwill, K. McHugh and C. L. Willhelm (1999b) Shortening system. *European Patent Application.* No EP1057887.

Empie, M.W (2008) Regulatory status of diacylglycerol oil in North America, the European Union, Latin America, Australia/New Zealand, and Japan. In *Diacylglycerol Oil*, 2nd edn. ed. Katsuragi *et al.*, pp 173–80. AOCS Press, Urbana IL.

Flatt, J. P. (1988) Importance of nutrient balance in body weight regulation. *Diabetes/Metab. Rev.*, 4: 571–81.

Formo, M. W. (1979) Physical properties of fats and fatty acids. In *Bailey's industrial oil and fat products*, vol. 1, 4th edn, ed. Swern D., pp 177–232. New York: John Wiley & Sons.

Friedman, I. H. and B. Nylund (1980) Intestinal fat digestion, absorption, and transport. *Am. J. Clin. Nutr.* 33:1108–39.

© Woodhead Publishing Limited, 2011

Garzon-Aburbeh, A., J. H. Poupaert, M. Claesen and P. Dumont (1986) A lymphotrophic prodrug of L-Dopa: Synthesis, pharmacological properties, and pharmacokinetic behaviour of 1,3-dihexadecanoyl-2-[(S)-2-amino-3-(3,4-dihydroxyphenyl)propanoyl] propane-1,2,3-triol. *J. Med. Chem.* 29: 687–91.

Garzon-Aburbeh, A., J. H. Poupaert, M. Claesen, P. Dumont and G. Atassi (1983) 1,3-Dipalmitoylglycerol ester of chlorambucil as lymphotrophic, orally administrable anticoplastic agent. *J. Med. Chem.* 26: 1200–3.

Giacometti, J., F. Giacometti, M. Cedomila and D. Vasic-Racki (2001) Kinetic characterization of enzymatic esterification in a solvent system: adsorptive control of water with molecular sieves. *J. Mol. Cat. B*, 11: 921–8.

Goto, N., T. Nishide, Y. Tanaka and T. Yasukawa (2000a) Oil and fat composition containing phytosterol. *United States Patent.* No US6025348.

Goto, N., T. Nishide, Y. Tanaka, T. Yasukawa and K. Masui (2000b) Phytosterol-containing fat composition. *European Patent Application.* No EP0990391.

Goto, N., T. Nishide, Y. Tanaka, T. Yasukawa and K. Masui (2001) Oil or fat composition containing phytosterol. *United States Patent.* No US6326050.

Hasegawa, K. (2000) Long term DAG intake study with young females (*Unpublished Office Report, Kao Corporation, Japan.*)

Hara, K., K. Onizawa, H. Honda, K. Otsuji, T. Ide and M. Murata (1993) Dietary diacylglycerol-dependent reduction in serum triacylglycerol concentration in rats. *Ann. Nutr. Metab.*, 37: 185–91.

Hendriks, H. F. J., J. A. Weststrate, A. T. van Vliet and G. W. Meijer (1999) Spread enriched with three different levels of vegetable oil sterols and the degree of cholesterol lowering in normocholesterolaemic and mildly hypercholesterolaemic subjects. *Eur. J. Clin. Nutr.*, 53: 319–27.

Ichihara, T., Yoshino H. Doi, Y., Nabae, K., Imai, N., Hagiwara, A., Tamano, S., Morita, O., Tamaki, Y. and Suzuki, H. (2008) No enhancing effects of diaclyglycerol oil on tumor development in medium-term multi-organ carcinogenesisi bioassay using male F344 rats. *Food Chem. Toxicol.* 46: 157–67.

Jacobs, L., I. Lee and G. Poppe (2003) Chemical process for the production of 1,3-diglyceride oils. *PCT International Patent.* No WO03029392.

Jones, P. J. H., D. E. MacDougall, F. Ntanious and C. A. Vanstone (1997) Dietary phytosterols as cholesterol-lowering agents in humans. *Can. J. Physiol. Pharmacol.*, 75:217–27.

Kamphuis, M. M., D. J. Mela and M. S. Westerterp-Plantenga (2003) Diacylglycerol affects substrate oxidation and appetite in humans. *Am. J. Clin. Nutr.*, 77: 1133–9.

Kasamatsu, T., R. Ogura, N. Ikeda, O. Morita, K. Saigo, H. Watabe, Y. Saito and H. Suzuki (2005) Genotoxicity studies on dietary diacylglycerol (DAG) oil. *Food Chem. Toxicol.* 43: 253–60.

Kawai, S. and Y. Konishi (2000) Acid oil-in-water emulsified composition. *PCT International Patent Application.* No WO0078162.

Kennedy, J. P. (1991) Structured lipids: Fats of the future. *Food Technology.* 45: 76–83.

Koike, S., N. Hosaya and T. Yasumasu (2001) Oil composition and use thereof. *European Patent Application.* No EP1135991.

Koike, S., T. Yasumasu, T. Hase, T. Murase, T. Yasukawa, Y. Katsuragi and A. Takei (2002a) Oil/fat composition. *PCT International Patent Application.* No WO0211552.

Koike, S., T. Yasumasu, T. Hase, T. Murase and T. Yasukawa (2002b) Oil/fat composition. *PCT International Patent Application.* No WO0211551.

Koike, S., N. Hosoya and T. Yasumasu (2002c) Fat compositions. *European Patent Application.* No EP1211305.

Koike, S., T. Yasumasu, T. Hase, T. Murase, T. Yasukawa, Y. Katsuragi and A. Takei (2002d) Oil/fat composition. *PCT International Patent Application.* No WO0211550.

Koike, S., T. Murase and T. Hase (2003) Oil or fat composition. *United States Patent Application.* No 2003/0054082.

© Woodhead Publishing Limited, 2011

Kondo, H., T. Hase, T. Murase and I. Tokimitsu (2003) Digestion and assimilation features of dietary DAG in the rat small intestine. *Lipids*. 38: 25–30.

Krawczyk, T. (2000) The spreading of obesity. *INFORM*. 11: 160–71.

Kudo, N., Y. Kameo and W. Mizuno (2002) Oil-cooked or baked potatoes. *European Patent Application*. No EP1203534.

Lai, O. M., M. S. A. Yusoff, S. K. Lo, K. Long, C. P. Tan, J. Y. Lim, S. Tahiruddin and K. Hashim (2006) Process for the production of diacylglycerol. *PCT International Patent Application*. No PCT/MY2006/000034.

Lai, O. M., M. S. A. Yusoff, S. K. Lo, K. Long, C. P. Tan, S. Tahiruddin and K. Hashim (2007) Production of acylglycerol esters. *PCT International Patent Application*. No PCT/MY2007/000025.

Lehner, R. and A. Kuksis (1993) Triacylglycerol synthesis by *sn*-1,2(2,3)-diacylglycerol transacylase from rat intestinal microsomes. *J. Biol. Chem.* 268: 8781–6.

Lehner, R. and A. Kuksis (1996) Biosynthesis of triacylglycerols. *Prog. Lipid Res.* 35: 169–201.

Lehner, R., A. Kuksis and Y. Itabashi (1993) Stereospecificity of monoacylglycerol and diacylglycerol acyltransferases from rat intestine as determined by chiral phase high-performance liquid chromatography. *Lipids*. 28: 29–34

Ling, W. H. and P. J. H. Jones (1995) Dietary phytosterols: a review of metabolism, benefits and side effects. *Life Sc.*, 57: 195–206.

Lo, S. K. and B. S. Baharin (2001) Process for producing phytonutrient-enriched diacylglycerols. *Malaysian Patent Application*. No PI20014817.

Maki, K. C., M. H. Davidson, R. Tsushima, N. Matsuo, I. Tokimitsu, D. M. Umporowics, M. R. Dicklin, G. S. Foster, K. A. Ingram, B. D. Anderson, S. D. Frost and M. Bell (2002) Consumption of diacylglycerol oil as part of a reduced-energy diet enhances loss of body weight and fat in comparison with consumption of a triacylglycerol control oil. *Am. J. Clin. Nutr.* 76: 1230–6.

Mansbach, C. M. II and P. Nevin (1998) Intracellular movement of triacylglycerols in the intestine. *J. Lipid Res.* 39: 963–8.

Masui, K. and Y. Konishi (2001) Water-in-oil type emulsified fat and/or oil composition. *PCT International Patent Application.* No WO0101787.

Masui, K. and K. Yasunaga (2001) Water-in-oil type emulsified fat and/or oil composition. *PCT International Patent Application.* No WO0115542.

Masui, K., Y. Katsuragi, T. Toi and T. Yasukawa (2001) Fat or oil composition. PCT International Application No WO0113733.

Mazur, A. W. and G. D. Hiler (1992) Regioselective synthesis of 1,3-disubstituted glycerides. *Canadian Patent.* No CA2106316.

Meguro, S., K. Higashi, T. Hase, Y. Honda, A. Otsuka, Y. Tokimitsu and H. Itakura (2001) Solubilization of phytosterols in diacylglycerol versus triacylglycerol improves the serum cholesterol lowering effect. *Eur. J. Clin. Nutr.*, 55: 513–17.

Meng, X., D. Zou, Z. Shi, Z. Duan and Z. Mao (2003) Dietary diacylglycerol prevents high-fat diet-induced lipid accumulation in rat liver and abdominal adipose tissue. *Lipids*, 39: 37–41.

Mori, H. and T. Watanabe (2000) Food containing fat or oil. *European Patent.* No EP0970615.

Mori, H., H. Sakai, Y. Tanaka and T. Yasukawa T (1999b) Fried food and shortening. *PCT International Patent Application.* No WO9959424.

Mori, H., K. Masui, Y. Tanaka and T. Yasukawa (1999a) Water-in-oil emulsified fat composition. *PCT International Patent Application.* No WO9959422.

Murase, T., M. Aoki, T. Wakisaka, T. Hase and I. Tokimitsu (2002a) Anti-obesity effect of dietary diacylglycerol in C57BL/6J mice: dietary diacylglycerol stimulates intestinal lipid metabolism. *J. Lipid Res.* 43:1312–19.

Murase, T., A. Nagasawa, J. Suzuki, T. Wakisaka, T. Hase and I. Tokimitsu (2002b) Dietary α-linolenic acid-rich diacylglycerols reduce body weight gain accompanying the

© Woodhead Publishing Limited, 2011

stimulation of intestinal β-oxidation and related gene expressions in C57BL/KsJ-db/db mice. *J. Nutr.* 132: 3018–22.

Murase, T., T. Mizuno, T. Omachi, K. Onizawa, Y. Komine, H. Kondo, T. Hase and I. Tokimitsu (2001) Dietary diacylglycerol suppresses high fat and high sucrose diet-induced body fat accumulation in C57BL/6J mice. *J. Lipid Res.*, 42: 372–8.

Murata, M., K. Hara and T. Ide (1994) Alteration by diacylglycerols of the transport and fatty acid composition of lymph chylomicron in rats. *Biosci. Biotechnol. Biochem.* 58: 1416–19.

Murata, M., T. Ide and K. Hara (1997) Reciprocal responses to dietary diacylglycerol of hepatic enzymes of fatty acid synthesis and oxidation in the rat. *Br. J. Nutr.* 77: 107–21.

Nagao, T., H. Watanabe, N. Goto, K. Onizawa, H. Taguchi, N. Matsuo, T. Yasukawa, R. Tsushima, H. Shimasaki and H. Itakura (2000) Dietary diacylglycerol suppresses accumulation of body fat compared to triacylglycerol in men in a double-blind controlled trial. *J. Nutr.* 130: 792–7.

Nakajima, Y., J. Fukasawa and A. Shimada (2004) Physicochemical properties of diacylglycerol. In *Diacylglycerol oil*, eds. Katsuragi, Y., T. Yasukawa, N. Matsuo, B. D. Flickinger, I. Tokimitsu and M. G. Matlock, pp 182–96. Illinois: AOCS Press.

Nakajima, Y., T. Nishide and T. Sakuma (2002) Edible oil and production process thereof. *United States Patent Application.* No US20020045000.

Nomura, M., S. Koike, K. Yamashita, K. Okisaka, Y. Sano, H. Omura, Y. Irinatsu, K. Masui and T. Yasumasu (1992) Edible oil-in-water emulsion. *United States Patent.* No US5160759.

Sakaguchi, H. (2001) Marketing a healthy oil. *Oils & Fats Intl.* 16: 18–19.

Sakai, H., M. Ishibashi and J. Kohori (2002a) Fat compositions. *European Patent Application.* No EP1186648.

Sakai, H., M. Katada and M. Ishibashi (2002b) Oil or fat composition. *European Patent Application.* No EP1249173.

Schutz, Y. (1995) Macronutrients and energy balance in obesity. *Metabolism.* 44: 7–11.

Sedarevich, B. (1967) Glyceride isomerisation in lipid chemistry. *J. Am. Oil Chem. Soc.* 44: 381–93.

Shiiba, D., Y. Asabu, S. Kawai and Y. Nakajima (2002) Acidic oil-in-water type emulsion composition. *United States Patent Application.* No US20020119239.

Soni, M. G., H. Kimura and G. A. Burdock (2001) Chronic study of diacylglycerol oil in rats. *Food Chem. Toxicol.* 39: 317–29.

Sugimoto, T., H. Fukuda, T. Kimura and N. Iritani (2003a) Dietary diacylglycerol-rich oil stimulation of glucose intolerance in genetically obese rats. *J. Nutr. Sc. Vitaminol.*, 49: 139–44.

Sugimoto, T., T. Kimura, H. Fukuda and N. Iritani N (2003b) Comparisons of glucose and lipid metabolism in rats fed diacylglycerol and triacylglycerol oils. *J. Nutr. Sc. Vitaminol.*, 49: 47–55.

Sugiura, M., M. Shimizu, Y. Yamada, K. Mine, E. Maruyama and N. Yamada (2002a) Process for producing partial glyceride. *United States Patent.* No US 6337414.

Sugiura, M., H. Yamaguchi and N. Yamada N (2002b) Preparation process of diglyceride. *United States Patent.* No US6361980.

Tada, N., H. Watanabe, N. Matsuo, I. Tokimitsu and M. Okazaki (2001) Dynamics of postprandial remnant-like lipoprotein particles in serum after loading of diacylglycerols. *Clin. Chim. Acta.* 311: 109–17.

Taguchi, H., T. Omachi, T. Nagao, N. Matsuo, I. Tokimitsu and H. Itakura (2002) Dietary diacylglycerol suppresses high fat diet-induced hepatic fat accumulation and microsomal triacylglycerol transfer protein activity in rats. *Journal of Nutritional Biochemistry*, 13: 678–83.

Taguchi, H., H. Watanabe, K. Onizawa, T. Nagao, N. Goto, T. Yasukawa, R. Tsushima, H. Shimasaki and H. Itakura (2000) Double-blinded controlled study on the effects of

© Woodhead Publishing Limited, 2011

dietary diacylglycerol on postprandial serum and chylomicron triacylglycerol responses in healthy humans. *J. Am. Coll. Nutr.* 19: 789–96.

Takano, H and Y. Itabashi (2002) Molecular species analysis of 1,3-diacylglycerols in edible oils by HPLC/ESI-MS. *Bunseki Kagaku.* 51: 437–42.

Takase, H., S. Koike, H. Sakai, T. Nishide, T. Hase and T. Murase (2003) Oil composition. *PCT International Patent Application.* No WO03024237.

Teramoto, T., Nagao, T., Watanabe, H., Ito, K., Omata, Y., Furukawa, T., Shimoda, H. and Hoshino, M. (2000) Effect of diacylglycerol on the hyperlipidemia of hemodialysis patients. *J. Jpn. Soc. Clin. Nutr.* 21: 35–8.

Teramoto, T., H. Watanabe, K. Ito, Y. Omata, T. Furukawa, K. Shimoda, M. Hoshino, T. Nagao and S. Naito (2004) Significant effects of diacylglycerol on body fat and lipid metabolism in patients on hemodialysis. *Clin. Nutr.* 23: 1122–6.

Toshinori, I., N. Yasuharu, H. Shinichi and K. Shoichi (2000) Production of diglyceride-containing fat and oil composition and fat and oil composition using the same. *Japanese Patent.* No JP2000345189.

van Deenen, L. L. M. and G. H. de Haas (1963) The substrate specificity of phospholipase A. *Biochim. Biophys. Acta.* 70: 538–53.

Watanabe, H., K. Onizawa, H. Taguchi, M. Kobori, H. Chiba, S. Naito, N. Matsuo, T. Yasukawa, M. Hattori and H. Shimasaki (1997) Nutritional characterisation of diacylglycerols in rats. *J. Jpn. Oil Chem. Soc.* 46: 301–8.

Wehrli, H. P. and Y. Pomeranz (1969) Synthesis of galactosyl glycerides and related lipids. *Chem. Phys. Lipids.* 3: 357–70.

William, C. L., M. T. Gulli and R. J. Deckelbaum (2001) Prevention and treatment of childhood obesity. *Curr. Atheroscler. Rep.*, 3: 486–97.

Yamada, Y., M. Shimizu, M. Sugiura and N. Yamada (1999) Process for producing diglycerides. *PCT International Patent.* WO9909119.

Yamamoto, K., H. Asakawa, K. Tokunaga, H. Watanabe, N. Matsuo, I. Tokimitsu and N. Yagi (2001) Long-term ingestion of dietary diacylglycerol lowers serum triacylglycerol in Type II diabetic patients with hypertriglyceridemia. *J. Nutr.* 131: 3204–7.

Yamamoto, K., H. Asakawa, K. Tokunaga, S. Meguro, H. Watanabe, I. Tokimitsu and N. Yagi (2005) Effects of diacylglycerol administration on serum triacylglycerol in a patient homozygous for complete lipoprotein lipase detection. *Metabolism*, 54: 67–71.

Yamamoto, K., K. Tomonobu, H. Asakawa, K. Tokunaga, T. Hase, I. Tokimitsu and N. Yagi (2006) Diet therapy with diacylglycerol oil delays the progression of renal failure in type 2 diabetic patents with nephropathy. *Diabetes Care*, 29: 417–19.

Yanagisawa, Y., T. Kawabata and K. Hasegawa (2003) Improvement in blood lipid levels by dietary sn-1,3-diacylglycerol in young women with variants of lipid transporters 54T-FABP2 and -493g-MTP. *Biochem. Biophys. Res. Comm.*, 302: 743–50.

Yoon, D.-H., G.-W. Han, S-G. Hong and Y.-H. Lee (2004) Preparation method of conjugated linoleic acid diglycerides. *PCT International Application* No WO2004096748.

© Woodhead Publishing Limited, 2011

9

Saturated fat reduction in milk and dairy products

E. S. Komorowski, Dairy UK, UK

Abstract: Although health benefits from reducing dairy saturated fats in the diet are not clear-cut, the dairy industry offers consumers products which have reduced fat or are virtually fat-free. Legislation protects consumers' interests by preventing non-dairy products, or products where some of the dairy part has been replaced by a non-dairy component, being passed off as dairy. This poses particular challenges when making saturated fat reductions. The legal constraints are discussed in detail for each of the products under consideration. The approaches that can be taken to produce reduced saturated fat products are described. The possibility of reducing saturates in cows' milk by feed modifications is discussed briefly.

Key words: saturated fats, dairy, legislation, milk, yogurt, cheese, processed cheese, butter, feed modifications.

9.1   Introduction

Dairy products are products produced from milk, and in the UK and most countries this milk is cows' milk. Most of this chapter relates to cows' milk, but the composition of milk from other species such as sheep, goats or buffaloes is similar to that of cows' milk, and the same principles would apply, though legislation would require that where consumers would otherwise be misled the species must be given.

For many consumers, dairy products are an important part of their diet and this is recognised in many countries throughout the world by dairy products being included in dietary guidelines. For example, the Food and Agriculture Organisation of the United Nations (FAO, 2010) publish the dietary guidelines from many countries around the world and these include dairy products. In the UK the Food Standards Agency's Eatwell Plate (Eatwell Plate, 2010) is used to indicate that

© Woodhead Publishing Limited, 2011

about one-sixth of food intake should be dairy. This emphasis is placed on the benefits of dairy products particularly on account of the useful contribution from the calcium and protein in milk. The UK 'National Diet and Nutrition Survey: adults aged 19 to 64 years' (NDNS, 2004) indicates that on average adults obtain about ten per cent of their energy needs from milk and milk products. Although the fat content of whole milk is only about four per cent, the relatively high consumption of dairy products, together with the fact that about two-thirds of dairy fats is saturated, results in dairy products accounting for a significant part of UK consumers' dietary saturated fat intake. It is estimated (NDNS, 2002) that milks contribute approximately nine per cent of daily saturated fat intakes, cheese ten per cent and butter six per cent.

Health benefits from reducing saturated fats in the diet are being increasingly challenged, with a recent meta-analysis concluding that there is no significant evidence that dietary saturated fat is associated with increased risk of heart disease (Siri-Tarino et al., 2010). For dairy products there is good evidence that whole milk is heart protective (Elwood et al., 2005; Elwood et al., 2010) and the consumption of milk and dairy foods provides a survival advantage (Elwood, et al., 2008). For cheese there is also little evidence that full-fat cheese can be harmful as part of a balanced diet. The reasons for this situation are still the subject of scientific research but may include the detailed composition of dairy fat, where many of the fatty acids present have been shown not to raise LDL-cholesterol (German et al., 2009). Even for the fatty acids which do raise LDL-cholesterol, such as palmitic acid, the presence of certain unsaturated fatty acids such as conjugated linoleic acid naturally present in dairy fat, together with the presence of other micronutrients in milk which may have a protective action, can lead to the situation where dairy products taken as a whole are beneficial to the diet.

Although the role of dairy products and dairy fat in the diet are the subjects of much current research, the dairy industry, while eagerly awaiting its results, is also engaged in offering consumers a range of products ranging from the traditional full-fat versions to products which have reduced dairy fat or are virtually fat-free. These reduced fat products are the subject of this chapter.

The nutritional importance of dairy products, together with their relative expense, has resulted in legislation to protect consumers' interests by preventing non-dairy products, or products where some of the dairy part has been replaced by a non-dairy component, being passed off as dairy. This poses particular challenges to manufacturers seeking to reduce the dairy fat content of dairy products. The legal constraints, which are a feature of food legislation in most countries, are discussed in more detail in the next section.

Manufacturers of non-dairy products can get round this situation by producing imitation or analogue products. These are perfectly legal so long as they are correctly labelled with an appropriate name and list of ingredients, and they do not attempt to present themselves as dairy products. These imitation products are discussed briefly, particularly for certain spreadable fats in which blends of dairy and non-dairy fats are used in order to give the desired spreadability, and incidentally also reduce the saturated fat content of the product.

© Woodhead Publishing Limited, 2011

What is also briefly discussed in this chapter is the possibility of modifying the composition of dairy fat by altering the cows' diet. In many parts of the world cows, if fed on grass, are also fed on supplements and these supplements can be chosen to produce milk with reduced levels of saturated fat. These supplements are natural feedstuffs, and the current research is investigating the changes to dairy fat composition resulting from various feeds, the economics, the properties of the resultant products, and whether diets containing these products will be beneficial to consumers' health. The latter requires study, particularly with the absence of evidence that traditional dairy products are harmful.

9.1.1   Legislative background

As explained above, legislation exists in most countries to protect consumers' interests by requiring that milk and dairy products are produced from milk or milk constituents, and that where other ingredients are added these do not replace in whole or in part any dairy constituent.

At the international level, the Codex Alimentarius Commission sets standards for many dairy products. The Codex General Standard for the Use of Dairy Terms (CODEX, 1999) defines milk, milk product, and composite milk product, with the latter definition stating that the milk constituent must be an essential part in terms of quantity in the final product and that the constituents not derived from milk must not take the place in part or in whole of any milk constituent.

In addition, foods must be described or presented in such a manner as to ensure the correct use of dairy terms intended for milk and milk products, to protect consumers from being confused or misled and to ensure fair practices in the food trade. Furthermore, in respect of a product which is not milk, a milk product or a composite milk product, no label, commercial document, publicity material or any form of point of sale presentation shall be used which claims, implies or suggests that the product is milk, a milk product or a composite milk product, or which refers to one or more of these products.

In the European Union the designation of milk and milk products is protected through Annex XII of Council Regulation (EC) No 1234/2007. 'Milk products' are defined as products derived exclusively from milk, but other substances necessary for their manufacture may be added provided that those substances are not used for replacing, in whole or in part, any milk constituent. This European Regulation goes even further by listing specific products exclusively as milk products, including cream, butter, cheese and yogurt, though traditional products whose exact nature is clear and which use dairy terms are exempt.

The UK, as a Member State of the European Union, enforces the EU legislation. Its guidance (FSA, 2010) makes clear that the restrictions in the Regulation cover labelling, presentation and advertising, and also prohibit direct or indirect suggestion of a dairy association for dairy product alternatives or analogues, since such products compete directly with dairy products and, by trading on the dairy image, may mislead the consumer.

© Woodhead Publishing Limited, 2011

9.2   Milk

9.2.1   Drinking milk

Cows' milk contains about four per cent fat, and this fat contains approximately 65% of saturated fatty acids. The most straightforward means of producing drinking milks with reduced levels of saturated fat is by reducing the level of total fat in the milk. Indeed, for many consumers their interest is in reducing their energy (calorie) consumption from milk, rather than their saturated fat intake, and lower fat milks, rather than lower saturated fat milks, deliver this.

Milk from the cow, if left undisturbed, will separate out with the cream rising to the top. Traditionally this cream layer could be skimmed off manually, and the resultant milk was called skimmed milk. Milk which was approximately half whole milk and half skimmed milk was semi-skimmed milk. In many countries, including the UK, these traditional names have been retained, though the technology has become much more efficient than manual skimming.

Methods for producing both whole and semi-skimmed milks have been described by Earley (1998). The current technology for producing reduced fat milks involves separating the whole milk using high-speed centrifugal separators, producing a skimmed milk stream at less than 0.1% fat, and a cream stream. Some of the cream stream is then re-combined with the skimmed milk stream to give milk of the desired fat content, and this milk is then homogenised, to ensure that the cream is uniformly distributed in fine globules throughout the milk. This fine emulsion of fat in milk remains stable for the shelf-life of the product, obviating any need for the consumer to have to shake the product at the time of use.

Until relatively recently the legislation in most Member States of the European Union restricted the milks which could be marketed to whole milk, semi-skimmed milk and skimmed milk. In the UK consumers increasingly opted for semi-skimmed milk, leading to the situation in 2009 where approximately 65% of the drinking milk sold was semi-skimmed. The reason for this choice was that consumers wanted to reduce their dietary fat (or calorie) intake, and found that semi-skimmed milk gave them a product which was very similar in taste to whole milk. Indeed, in so far as consumers could distinguish semi-skimmed milk from whole milk (in tea, for example) they gradually developed a preference for semi-skimmed milk. In the UK skimmed milk tended to be the choice of determined dieters or people with specific needs, who were prepared to accept the product despite its rather thin and watery taste and appearance. Whole milk was still the preferred choice for traditionalists, people who had no specific dietary needs, and growing children.

The growing acceptance of semi-skimmed milk, together with different milk grades being marketed in the newer Member States, led to the legislation in the European Union being modified in 2008 to permit milk of any fat content to be marketed (Council Regulation (EC) No 361/2008). The legislation stipulates that whole milk, semi-skimmed milk and skimmed milk must be designated as such, to avoid misleading consumers, but milks of other fat contents can be marketed, labelled with their fat content.

© Woodhead Publishing Limited, 2011

The result in the UK has been the marketing of milks at one per cent fat and below, which appear to be enjoying a high level of consumer acceptability, possibly on account of consumers having previously becoming accustomed to semi-skimmed rather than whole milk. The taste difference between semi-skimmed (about 1.6% fat) and one per cent fat milk appears to be relatively small and generally acceptable.

Although consumers seem to find these low-fat milks acceptable it is also possible to formulate products with added ingredients such as stabilisers, emulsifiers or skimmed milk powder to compensate for the reduced level of fat (Komorowski, 1987). The added ingredients improve the mouthfeel by increasing the viscosity to compensate for the rather thin and watery texture of skimmed milk. These are milk-based drinks rather than true milks.

A further type of milk, which has been marketed in the UK but has had limited success, is that of 'filled' milk, or analogue milk. This product can be made by combining skimmed milk with vegetable fat. By choosing an appropriate vegetable fat, it is possible to produce products low in saturates. Of course the products cannot be labelled as 'milk', but possible names include 'blend of skimmed milk and vegetable fat'. To date these products have had most success in catering outlets as tea or coffee whiteners, where their advantage appears to be mainly cheaper cost, rather than their lower saturate content.

For the future it is possible that consumers will increasingly opt for milks with fat contents of semi-skimmed (1.6% fat) and below, as their palates become used to these lower fat products.

9.2.2   Yogurts and fermented milks

Fermented milks are products made by fermenting (i.e. culturing) milks with suitable microorganisms to reduce the pH, with or without coagulation. These starter microorganisms must be viable, active and abundant in the product to the end of its shelf-life. If the product is heat treated after fermentation the requirement for viable microorganisms in the final product does not apply. The milk used may be modified, in terms of its fat content or by the addition of other milk products. Certain fermented milks may be characterised by specific starter cultures used in the fermentation.

Not all countries have national legislation defining yogurts and fermented milks but there is a Codex Standard for Fermented Milks (CODEX, 2003). In the UK, although there is no national legislation there is a Code of Practice for Yogurt, produced jointly by Dairy UK and the Provision Trade Federation and endorsed by LACORS (DairyUK, 2009). According to this Code yogurt is made using *Streptococcus thermophilus* and/or *Lactobacillus delbrueckii* subsp. *bulgaricus*.

The fat content of yogurt arises from the fat content of the milk and milk products used in the manufacture, and according to CODEX STAN 243–2003 must be less than 10% in fermented milk and less than 15% in yogurt. In the current UK market products range from virtually fat-free to indulgence products at up to 10% fat. All are clearly labelled with their fat content, allowing consumers

© Woodhead Publishing Limited, 2011

to opt for the product of their choice. The manufacture of various types of yogurt has been described in detail by Tamime and Robinson (2004).

The addition of various ingredients has been investigated in reduced-fat yogurts in order to produce eating qualities closer to the standard product. Guven et al (2005) report that a product made with 1% inulin had similar eating properties to the whole-milk product. Gelatin and starch have also been found to improve the sensory characteristics of low-fat yogurts (Ares *et al.*, 2007). Different cultures and incubation temperatures of low-fat yogurts have been investigated (Abbasi *et al.*, 2009).

Most yogurts on the UK market are composite milk products which contain a maximum of 50% of non-dairy ingredients (such as nutritive and non-nutritive sweeteners, fruits and vegetables as well as juices, purees, pulps, preparations and preserves derived from these, cereals, honey, chocolate, nuts, coffee, spices and other harmless natural flavouring foods) and/or flavours. The non-dairy ingredients can be mixed in prior to or after fermentation.

9.3   Cheese

Cheese is the dairy product made by coagulating milk or milk products followed by draining of whey, such that the whey protein/casein ratio does not exceed that of milk. The Codex General Standard for Cheese (CODEX, 1978) gives as raw materials milk, skimmed milk, partly skimmed milk, cream, whey cream or buttermilk.

Coagulation is generally carried out by the action of rennet or other suitable coagulating agents, and the essential requirement is that the cheesemaking process results in a concentration of milk protein, or more precisely the casein portion, so that consequently the protein content of the cheese will be distinctly higher than the protein level of the blend of dairy materials that the cheese was made from. Alternative processing techniques which also result in coagulation of the protein and give similar physical, chemical and organoleptic characteristics, are also permitted.

This is a very broad definition, and it becomes even broader when account is taken that the cheese may be unripened or ripened, and also may be of a firmness that ranges from soft to extra-hard. Unripened cheese, including fresh cheese, is cheese which is ready for consumption shortly after manufacture. Ripened cheese is cheese which is not ready for consumption shortly after manufacture but which must be held for such time, at such temperature, and under such other conditions as will result in the necessary biochemical and physical changes characterising the cheese in question. One category of ripened cheese is mould ripened, which is cheese in which the ripening has been accomplished primarily by the development of characteristic mould growth throughout the interior and/or on the surface of the cheese.

Traditionally most countries developed their own cheesemaking techniques and individual cheeses, but since many cheeses have a relatively long shelf-life cheeses

© Woodhead Publishing Limited, 2011

are important in international trade, and these cheeses are often manufactured in many countries in addition to the country where the cheese originated.

Cheeses fall into certain broad categories with individual Codex Standards, including Cheeses in Brine (CODEX, 1999a) and Unripened Cheese (CODEX, 2001). Many cheeses are sufficiently well known and important in international trade to have their own Codex standard, for example the standard for Cheddar cheese is CODEX STAN 263–1966 (CODEX, 1966).

Although in principle reduced fat cheeses are possible since the permitted raw materials include both milk and skimmed milk, in any proportion, there are many challenges. Different varieties of cheese have different fat contents. Table 9.1 illustrates this for some common cheeses.

For a named variety of cheese, it is necessary that the resultant cheese possesses the characteristics of the named variety, such as its flavour, texture and other organoleptic qualities. In addition many named variety cheeses have compositional constraints to prevent fraud and ensure that consumers obtain the intended product. These compositional constraints are generally a maximum moisture and a minimum fat content. To take into account that traditional ripening of cheese results in moisture loss, fat contents are generally given not as percentages of the product, as is the case for most other foods, but as a percentage of the dry matter in the cheese.

In order to permit reduced fat cheeses the Codex Standards define the compositional ranges permitted for the standard named cheese, but also give compositional ranges intended to allow cheeses to be manufactured which retain the essential characteristics of the cheese. These modified cheeses must be labelled in such a way as to ensure that the consumer is aware of the true nature of the product (e.g. 'reduced fat Cheddar'). Current UK legislation does not give this flexibility, though at the time of writing (2010) changes to the legislation to permit this are under consideration.

Fat reductions are obtained by replacing the whole milk used in the traditional cheese by partly skimmed milk, and this partly skimmed milk may be obtained directly by skimming using high-speed centrifugal separators as for drinking milk, or by reconstituting skimmed milk from skimmed milk powder and water.

Table 9.1 Typical fat contents of certain named varieties of cheese

Cheese	Fat content (g per 100 g)
Brie	29.1
Camembert	22.7
Cheddar	34.9
Danish blue	28.9
Edam	26.0
Gouda	30.6
Stilton	35.0

Source: Food Standards Agency, 2002

© Woodhead Publishing Limited, 2011

Fat reductions in cheese must of course be compensated for by some increases, and the two possibilities are moisture or protein, and cheesemakers use one or both of these to develop reduced fat cheese with characteristics as similar as possible to the traditional cheese. Moisture addition leads to a softer cheese while protein addition gives a harder cheese. The addition of whey proteins has been investigated (Punidadas *et al.*, 2000), as has protein concentrate (Shakeel-Ur-Rehman *et al.*, 2003).

In addition, the manufacturing conditions may be modified in order to produce reduced fat cheese closer to the eating qualities of the traditional product. For example, for Cheddar the pasteurisation temperature and pH at milling may be modified (Guinee *et al.*, 1998). Other processing changes are reductions in scald temperature and cheddaring time to increase the moisture content and produce a texture closer to the standard product (Banks *et al.*, 1989). The scald temperature is the temperature to which the curd is heated following the renneting process and which selectively stops the growth of certain types of bacteria and alters the degree of syneresis. The cheddaring time is the time at which the whey is partially drained and the cut curd stacked. Different starter cultures can also be used to modify the properties of the reduced fat Cheddar (Fenelon *et al.*, 2002).

For ripened cheeses, salt (sodium chloride) plays a very important role in regulating the microbiological, biochemical and physical changes which occur as the cheese ripens and which lead to the final product having its required characteristics. The key parameter is not the absolute salt content but the percentage of salt-in-moisture since this influences the water activity (Guinee and Fox, 2004), and it is recognised for Cheddar for example (Lawrence and Gilles, 1980) that this percentage must be in the range 4 to 6. Mild (relatively short ripening) Cheddar will be at the lower end of this range, and mature (relatively long ripening) Cheddar at the higher end. A consequence is that if a reduced fat Cheddar has a higher moisture content than the traditional Cheddar the absolute salt content will need to be increased to maintain the desired salt-in-moisture percentage.

When reduced fat cheeses were first produced they were often considered to be less acceptable by consumers on account of both their flavour and texture, but found favour as cheese toppings on pizzas, for example, and in cheese sauces. Some cheesemakers have now successfully modified their recipes and cheesemaking processes to produce reduced fat ripened cheeses which are very close to the traditional cheese in eating properties. Although these reduced fat ripened cheeses are a relatively small part of the market at present, as consumers are encouraged to try these cheeses it is expected that the market will grow significantly.

9.3.1   Processed cheese

Processed cheese and processed cheese preparations consist of a wide variety of products in which cheese is melted and emulsified, usually with the addition of other milk components or foodstuffs. The products range from those which consist

© Woodhead Publishing Limited, 2011

mainly of cheese to products where the cheese content is important in contributing to the flavour of the product, but is present in relatively small amounts.

The ingredients in addition to cheese are cream, butter and butteroil, and for processed cheese preparations other dairy ingredients such as milk powder.

The range of processed cheese products is extensive, with some products being hard and sliceable, others soft and spreadable, and others intended for dipping. A further complication is the characterisation of some processed cheese by variety name, such as 'Processed Emmental cheese' or 'Spreadable Processed Emmental Cheese'.

Although Codex Standards for these various product types exist (CODEX, 1978a, 1978b, 1978c), in practice trade both nationally and internationally has developed independently of these standards to meet consumers' needs and at the time of writing (2010) it is likely that these standards will be withdrawn.

These products contain sodium from two sources: the sodium chloride present in the natural cheese used in the formulation, and the emulsifying salts such as sodium citrate or polyphosphates which are needed to produce a uniform stable product. Reduced saturated fat versions of these products can be made by using a lower fat natural cheese as starting point, and by reducing the quantities of cream, butter and butteroil, and increasing the quantities of milk powder and water. The use of lower fat natural cheese produced by the addition of buttermilk has been reported as improving the quality of the resultant processed cheese (Raval and Mistry, 1999). A study by Lee et al (2003) has shown that in the manufacture of processed cheese the creaming reaction which occurs is primarily a protein-based interaction, which takes place with or without the presence of fat, indicating that reduced fat formulations are capable of development.

9.4   Butter and spreadable fats

Butter is the traditional spreadable fat used on bread in many countries. As a relatively stable product it is important in national and international trade, and as a consequence is defined in both international (Codex Alimentarius), European Union and often national legislation.

In Codex Alimentarius (CODEX, 1971) butter is described as a fatty product derived exclusively from milk and/or products obtained from milk, principally in the form of an emulsion of the type water-in-oil. Its composition is also defined as having a minimum milkfat content of 80% m/m, a maximum water content of 16% m/m, and a maximum milk solids-not-fat content of two per cent m/m. In the European Union the compositional requirements for butter are identical to those of Codex Alimentarius and given in Annex XV of Regulation 1234/2007.

With such tight constraints the opportunities for reducing the saturated fat content of butter are limited and Wilbey (2009) describes the main methods. In practice two are the most important: reducing the saturated fat content of the milk from the cow (see section 9.5 and Chapter 12), or by fractionating the butterfat and using a fraction relatively rich in unsaturates to produce the butter.

© Woodhead Publishing Limited, 2011

For the former, use can be made of the seasonal variability in the saturated fat content of milk, which results from feed modification. Milk from cows fed on grass is relatively lower in saturates, with the consequence that summer milk has a lower saturates content than winter milk. For example, Soyeurt et al (2008) found that milkfat produced in spring and summer had a saturated fat content of 63%, compared to winter milkfat with a saturated fat content of 69%. The advantage of feed modification, or choice of summer milkfat, is that there is no additional processing involved, and all of the milkfat is used in the butter. The disadvantage is that the reduction in saturates is relatively modest, although useful in producing a butter which is more easily spread at refrigerated temperatures.

Fractionation can produce more important reductions in saturates, but this requires processing modifications, although fat fractionation is usually achieved purely by physical processes involving heating the butterfat to liquefy it, followed by cooling to allow different fractions to be separated. An important commercial requirement is to find viable commercial applications for each butterfat fraction. The process of fractionating anhydrous milk fat followed by recombining desired fractions to produce speciality butters has been described by Kaylegian (1999). First the anhydrous milk fat is placed in a stainless steel-jacketed tank with an agitator and heated to 60°C to remove all prior crystals, then cooled slowly and allowed to crystallise in a serious of steps. At the end of any step there are two fractions, one solid and one liquid, and it is most common to refractionate the liquid fraction by reheating then recooling to a temperature lower than the first step. The desired fat fraction is then combined with an aqueous phase of skim milk, reconstituted skim milk or buttermilk (the aqueous liquid obtained when cream is churned to produce butter), stirred and homogenised. The resultant emulsion is then texturised by passing the emulsion through a scraped-surface heat exchanger which induces rapid fat crystallisation.

A further possibility is to whip butter, thereby incorporating air in the product and increasing its volume with the result that the fat content is present in a larger volume, which can lead to a smaller amount per serving (Illingworth et al., 2009).

In many countries an easier route to producing spreadable butter-like products has been to blend the butterfat with vegetable oils low in saturates. These products are not of course 'butter', though in the marketing of these products considerable emphasis is often given to the butter content, or to the fact that the product contains buttermilk, or to the buttermaking process (e.g. reference to churning). Whether such references are legal in that they are trading on the image of dairy products, and may be in breach of the Regulations (in the European Union, Regulation 1234/2007), is an issue for the enforcement authorities and law courts.

Consumers have readily accepted these products, and Codex standards and regulations have been developed which cover them, as well as products of lower fat than butter, including dairy, non-dairy and blends. CODEX STAN 253–2006 (CODEX, 2006) defines dairy fat products from 10% to less than 80% m/m while CODEX STAN 256–2007 (CODEX, 2007) covers fat products from 10% to not more than 90% fat intended as spreads, but excluding products derived exclusively

© Woodhead Publishing Limited, 2011

from milk or dairy products. Consequently CODEX STAN 253–2006 covers reduced fat dairy spreads and CODEX STAN 256–2007 covers blends of dairy fats with other fats. In the European Union, Annex XV of Regulation 1234/2007 defines the marketing standards applying to spreadable fats, and this Regulation includes butter, dairy spreads at fat levels less than 80%, and blends of milkfat and vegetable fats.

As a consequence of this flexibility a wide range of fat spreads of different types and saturated fat contents exist. These reduced fat spreads can either be made using dairy technology involving churning (Frede and Buchheim, 1994) or scraped-surface heat exchangers akin to margarine technology (Lane, 1998).

9.5   Reducing the saturated content of milk fat through feed

A very active area of current research is into the possibilities of reducing the saturated fatty acid content of milk as produced by the cow by feed modifications. The aim is to achieve this using natural feedstuffs and without significantly increasing the *trans* unsaturated fatty acid content, and without affecting the milk yield or milkfat yield. A major advantage of this approach is that saturated fatty acids are tackled at source, removing the criticism that reducing the saturates in dairy products may merely result in the saturates from milk being incorporated in other food products without a net dietary benefit to consumers.

Numerous feed trials have been carried out using various oilseeds including linseed, rapeseed, soybeans and sunflower. A meta-analysis of 145 supplementation experiments has confirmed that significant modification of the fatty acid profile of milkfat is possible (Glasser *et al.*, 2008). In addition to reductions in saturates, significant reductions in the methane emissions from cows fed modified diets have also been reported (Martin *et al.*, 2008).

While this is encouraging there are many practical issues to be considered. These include quantifying the actual reduction in saturates, measuring this on an ongoing basis, and considering any animal health or welfare issues. Also important is the extent to which the reduction in saturates is accompanied by increases in undesirable *trans* fatty acids.

The cost of producing the milk is also important, and whether there are any practical issues which would dissuade milk producers from pursuing this, and how milk producers can be persuaded to move to new feeds. It is also important to establish if this milk requires modified processing to produce the required dairy products, and whether the resultant products are acceptable to consumers.

The final and perhaps the most important issue is whether these products will in fact result in consumers obtaining health benefits from moving from dairy products obtained from conventional milk to these products obtained from milk naturally lower in saturates. This is by no means certain since the evidence that conventional products can be harmful to health is not robust. Detailed trials will be necessary to evaluate the effects on various markers for coronary disease using the new products and appropriate controls.

© Woodhead Publishing Limited, 2011

9.6   Future trends

It is always difficult to predict the future but there are three areas which are currently the subjects of intense research. These are the role of dairy fat in cardiovascular disease, the development of reduced and low fat cheeses, and the ability to modify the composition of dairy fat through feed changes.

On the role of dairy fat in cardiovascular disease, the hypotheses that reducing both the total fat in the diet and the amount of saturated fat in the diet will improve people's health are increasingly being re-examined. The FAO and WHO have recently concluded (FAO/WHO, 2010) an Expert Consultation on Fats and Fatty Acids in Human Nutrition and decided against any further advice to reduce the energy contribution from saturates from the previously recommended 10% level. This review also finds no benefit in replacing saturated fat by refined carbohydrates. This Consultation is clear that energy balance is the critical factor in maintaining a healthy body weight, regardless of the percentage of energy from total fat.

It will be many years before nutritionists agree on the dietary benefits or otherwise of continuing to reduce saturated fats in the diet, and in the meantime the dairy industry will continue to develop reduced and low-fat cheeses to satisfy consumer demand. Fat reductions in other dairy products are much easier to achieve, with milks, yogurts and spreads already offering consumers a wide choice of products and fat contents. Cheeses such as Cheddar are the real challenge, although already the eating qualities of some reduced fat cheeses are comparable to the standard product. We can expect the quality to continue to improve. The requirement for making a reduced fat claim in the Codex is a 25% reduction, which is a significant hurdle, but the requirement for making a low-fat claim is a fat content of below 3%, which is very much more difficult. Nevertheless, I expect to see increased marketing of low-fat cheddar type cheeses, which at the very least are used as pizza toppings and in situations which are less critical than on the cheeseboard.

The third area is that of modified feed for dairy cattle. In principle this would appear to offer the advantages of reduced saturated fat in the milk together with reduced methane emissions from the cow, which would appear to be a winning combination. Time will tell if the resultant products do improve the health of the population, and if reduced methane emissions are part of sustainable agricultural developments.

9.7   Sources of further information and advice

9.7.1   The Society of Dairy Technology

The Society of Dairy Technology (SDT), founded in 1943, is the professional organisation dedicated to the advancement of Dairy Science and Technology in the British and Irish dairy industries. The Society organises conferences, symposia and residential courses on relevant technical topics, and it publishes the renowned

© Woodhead Publishing Limited, 2011

International Journal of Dairy Technology and a range of technical publications/ manuals. A 'Technical Forum' section on its website provides answers to technical questions, based on the Society possessing, through its members, a specialist and unique knowledge base in Dairy Technology. Its website is http://www.sdt.org.

9.7.2   Dairy UK Information Hub
The Dairy UK Information Hub provides advice and solutions to anyone who wishes to develop new products or working practices, or refine existing ones, but is unaware of where to source the funding, advice, equipment or raw materials to achieve this. The information includes help from the start (funding sources, suppliers, consultancies, factsheets), development (training courses), complying with legal requirements (labelling, health and safety, accreditation, copyrights, certification, health claims, environmental issues), nearing completion (transport, wholesalers, multiples) and then (once the process is complete) how to compare the product / process with those of your competitors (benchmarking). Its website is http://www.dairyuk.org/dairyukhubmicrosite0/about.html

9.7.3   UK-IDF
UK-IDF is the UK National Committee of the International Dairy Federation (IDF). Membership of UK-IDF is open to any organisation, company or individual in the UK who has a connection with or interest in the dairy sector, and currently includes representatives from dairy trade and producer organisations as well as academic and research establishments. Its website is http://www.ukidf.org.

9.7.4   International Dairy Federation (IDF)
IDF is an international source of scientific and technical expertise for all stakeholders of the dairy chain. Membership covers 56 countries and is growing. IDF accounts for about 86% of current total milk production worldwide. The mission of IDF is to represent the dairy sector worldwide by providing the best global source of scientific expertise and knowledge in support of the development and promotion of quality milk and dairy products to deliver nutrition, health and well-being to consumers. Its website is http://www.fil-idf.org.

9.8   References

Abbasi H, Mousavi ME, Ehsani MR, Jomea ZE, Vaziri M, Rahimi J, and Aziznia S (2009) 'Influence of starter culture type and incubation temperatures on rheology and microstructure of low fat set yoghurt' Int. J. of Dairy Technol. 62 (4) 549–55.
Annex XII of Council Regulation (EC) No 1234/2007 of 22 October 2007 establishing a common organisation of agricultural products and on specific provisions for certain agricultural products. Official Journal L299, 16.11.2007, p 1.

Annex XV of Council Regulation (EC) No 1234/2007 of 22 October 2007 establishing a common organisation of agricultural products and on specific provisions for certain agricultural products. Official Journal L299, 16.11.2007, p 1.

Ares G, Goncalvez D, Perez C, Reolon G, Segura N, Lema P and Gambaro A (2007) 'Influence of gelatin and starch on the instrumental and sensory texture of stirred yogurt' Int. J. of Dairy Technol. 60 (4) 263–9.

Banks, JM Brechany EY, and Christie WW. 1989. 'The production of low fat Cheddar cheese'. Int. J. Soc. Dairy Technol. 42 (1): 6–9.

CODEX (1966) Codex Standard for Cheddar (CODEX STAN 263–1966). Amended 2008. Available from http://www.codexalimentarius.net/ [Accessed 26 May 2010].

CODEX (1971) Codex Standard for Butter (CODEX STAN 279–1971). Amended 2006. Available from http://www.codexalimentarius.net/ [Accessed 26 May 2010].

CODEX (1978) Codex General Standard for Cheese (CODEX STAN 283–1978). Revised 2008. Available from http://www.codexalimentarius.net/ [Accessed 26 May 2010].

CODEX (1978a) Codex General Standard for Process(ed) Cheese and Spreadable process(ed) Cheese (CODEX STAN 286–1978). Available from http://www.codexalimentarius.net/ [Accessed 26 May 2010].

CODEX (1978b) Codex General Standard for Process(ed) Cheese Preparations, Process(ed) Cheese Food, and Process(ed) Cheese (CODEX STAN 287–1978). Available from http://www.codexalimentarius.net/ [Accessed 26 May 2010].

CODEX (1978c) Codex General Standard for Named Variety Process(ed) Cheese and Spreadable Process(ed) Cheese (CODEX STAN 285–1978). Available from http://www.codexalimentarius.net/ [Accessed 26 May 2010].

CODEX (1999) Codex General Standard for the Use of Dairy Terms (CODEX STAN 206–1999). Available from http://www.codexalimentarius.net/ [Accessed 26 May 2010].

CODEX (1999a) Codex Group Standard for Cheeses in Brine (CODEX STAN 208–1999). Amended 2001. Available from http://www.codexalimentarius.net/ [Accessed 26 May 2010].

CODEX (2001) Codex Group Standard for Unripened Cheese including Fresh Cheese (CODEX STAN 221–2001). Amended 2008. Available from http://www.codexalimentarius.net/ [Accessed 26 May 2010].

CODEX (2003) Codex Standard for Fermented Milks (CODEX STAN 243–2003). Revised 2008. Available from http://www.codexalimentarius.net/ [Accessed 26 May 2010].

CODEX (2006) Codex Standard for Dairy Fat Spreads (CODEX STAN 253–2006). Amended 2008. Available from http://www.codexalimentarius.net/ [Accessed 26 May 2010].

CODEX (2007) Codex Standard for Fat Spreads and Blended Spreads (CODEX STAN 256–2007. Amended 2009. Available from http://www.codexalimentarius.net/ [Accessed 26 May 2010]

Council Regulation (EC) No 361/2008 of 14 April 2008 amending Regulation (EC) No 1234/2007 establishing a common organisation of agricultural markets and on specific provisions for certain agricultural products. Official Journal of the European Union L 121 page 1of 7.5.2008.

DairyUK (2009) Code of Practice for Yogurt. Available from http://www.dairyuk.org [Accessed 26 May 2010].

Eatwell Plate (2010) Food Standards Agency. Available from http://www.eatwell.gov.uk/healthydiet/eatwellplate/ [Accessed 26 May 2010].

Earley R (1998) 'Liquid milk and cream' in The Technology of Dairy Products, edited by Earley R, Second Edition, Blackie Academic and Professional.

Elwood PC, Strain JJ, Robson PJ, Fehily AM, Hughes J, Pickering J and Ness A (2005) 'Milk consumption, stroke, and heart attack risk: evidence from the Caerphilly cohort of older men' J Epidemiol Community Health 59: 505.

Elwood PC, Givens DI, Beswick AD, Fehily AM, Pickering JE, and Gallacher (2008) 'The survival advantage of milk and dairy consumption: an overview of evidence from cohort

© Woodhead Publishing Limited, 2011

studies of vascular diseases, diabetes and cancer' J. American College of Nutrition 27(6) 723S–734S.

Elwood PC, Pickering JE, Givens DI, and Gallacher JE (2010) 'The consumption of milk and dairy foods and the incidence of vascular disease and diabetes: an overview of the evidence' Lipids, published online 16 April 2010.

FAO (2010) Food and Agriculture Organization of the United Nations, Food-based Dietary Guidelines. Available from http://www.fao.org/ag/humannutrition/nutritioneducation/fbdg/en/ [Accessed 26 May 2010].

FAO/WHO (2010). Expert Consultation on Fats and Fatty Acids in Human Nutrition. Interim summary available from http://www.who.int/nutrition/topics/FFA_human_nutrition/en/index.html [Accessed 26 May 2010].

Fenelon MA, Beresford TP, and Guinee TP (2002) 'Comparison of different bacterial culture systems for the production of reduced-fat Cheddar cheese' Int. J. of Dairy Technol. 55 (4): 194–203.

Food Standards Agency (2002) McCance and Widdowson's 'The Composition of Foods', Sixth summary edition, Cambridge: Royal Society of Chemistry.

Frede E and Buchheim W (1994), 'Buttermaking and the churning of blended fat emulsions', J. Soc. Dairy Techn. 47 (1): 17–27.

FSA (2010) Guidance on the Legislation on the Protection of Dairy Designations. Available from Food Standards Agency, London.

German JB, Gibson RA, Krauss RM, Nestel P, Lamarche B, van Staveren, WA, Steijns JM, de Groot LC, Lock AL, Destaillats F, (2009) 'A reappraisal of the impact of dairy foods and milk fat on cardiovascular disease risk', Eur J Nutr 48(4): 191–203.

Glasser F, Ferlay A and Chilliard Y (2008) 'Oilseed Lipid Supplements and Fatty Acid Composition of Cow Milk: A Meta-Analysis', J. Dairy Sci. 91: 4687–703.

Guinee TP, Fenelon MA, Mulholland EO, O'Kennedy BT, O'Brien N, and Reville WJ. 1998 'The influence of milk pasteurization temperature and pH at curd milling on the composition, texture and maturation of reduced fat Cheddar cheese', Int. J. of Dairy Technol., 51: 1–10.

Guinee TP and Fox PP (2004) 'Salt in cheese: physical, chemical and biological aspects' in Cheese: Chemistry, Physics and Microbiology, Volume 1 General Aspects, 3rd Edition 2004, Edited by Patrick F Fox, Paul L H McSweeney, Timothy M Cogan, Timothy P Guinee, Elsevier Academic Press.

Guven, M, Yasar K, Karaca, OB, and Hayaloglu (2005) 'The effect of inulin as a fat replacer on the quality of set-type low-fat yogurt manufacture' Int. J. of Dairy Technol. 58 (3): 180–4.

Illingworth D, Patil GR, and Tamime AY (2009) 'Anhydrous milk fat manufacture and fractionation', in Dairy Fats and Related Products, edited by Tamine AY, Society of Dairy Technology, Wiley-Blackwell.

Kaylegian KE (1999), 'The production of speciality milk fat ingredients', J Dairy Sci 82: 1433–9.

Komorowski ES (1987) 'Additive milks', J. Soc. of Dairy Technol. 40: 94–5.

Lane R (1998) 'Butter and mixed fat spreads' in The Technology of Dairy Products, edited by Earley R, Second Edition, Blackie Academic and Professional.

Lawrence, R. C. and J. Gilles. 1980. 'The assessment of potential quality of young Cheddar cheese'. New Zealand J. Dairy Sci. Technol. 15: 1.

Lee SK, Buwalda RJ, Euston SA, Foegeding EA and McKenna AB (2003) 'Changes in the rheology and microstructure of processed cheese during cooking' Lebensmittel-Wissenschaft und-Technologie, 36(3): 339–45

Martin C, Rouel J, Jouany JP, Doreau M, and Chilliard Y, (2008) 'Methane output and diet digestibility in response to feeding dairy cows crude linseed, extruded linseed, or linseed oil', J. Anim Sci. 86: 2642–50.

NDNS (2002) A survey carried out in Great Britain on behalf of the Food Standards Agency and the Departments of Health. Available from http://www.food.gov.uk/multimedia/pdfs/ndnsprintedreport.pdf [Accessed 26 May 2010].

© Woodhead Publishing Limited, 2011

NDNS (2004) A survey carried out in Great Britain on behalf of the Food Standards Agency and the Departments of Health. Available from http://www.food.gov.uk/multimedia/pdfs/ndns5full.pdf [Accessed 26 May 2010].

Punidadas P, Tung MA, and Fiertag J (2000) 'Potential use of homogenized whey protein dispersions and process modification for the manufacture of low fat and reduced fat cheddar type cheeses' Int. J. of Dairy Technol. 53(2): 45–50.

Raval DM and Mistry VV (1999) 'Application of ultrafiltered sweet buttermilk in the manufacture of reduced fat process cheese' J Dairy Sci 82: 2334–43.

Soyeurt, H, Dardenne, P. Dehareng, F. Bastin, C and Gengler, N (2008) 'Genetic parameters of saturated and monounsaturated fatty acid content and the ratio of saturated to unsaturated fatty acids in bovine Milk' J. Dairy Sci. 91: 3611–26.

Shakeel-Ur-Rehman, Frakye NY, and Drake M (2003) 'Reduced-fat Cheddar cheese from a mixture of cream and liquid milk protein concentrate' Int. J. of Dairy Technol. 56(2): 94–8.

Siri-Tarino PW, Sun Q, Hu FB and Krauss RM (2010) 'Meta-analysis of prospective cohort studies evaluating the association of saturated fat with cardiovascular disease' Am J Clin Nutr. 91: 535–46.

Tamime AY and Robinson RK (2004) 'Yoghurt Science and Technology', Second Edition, Woodhead Publishing Ltd.

Wilbey RA (2009) 'Butter', in Dairy Fats and Related Products, edited by Tamime AY, Society of Dairy Technology, Wiley-Blackwell.

© Woodhead Publishing Limited, 2011

10

Saturated fat reduction in butchered meat

K. R. Matthews, Agriculture and Horticulture Development Board, UK

Abstract: This chapter describes the measurement of fat in carcases and the change in fat in red meat cuts over time. The fat in the carcases and red meat cuts of cattle, sheep and pigs has been reduced dramatically over recent decades. This has been achieved through a combination of animal breeding, management and selection for slaughter. The fat content of meat cuts has been further reduced by refined butchery techniques responding to consumer demands. Even the mince consumed has, on average, a reduced fat content as the range of mince available has increased and 'leaner' options have increased in sales.

Key words: saturated fat, carcase, beef, pork, lamb.

10.1   Introduction

The aim of rearing cattle, sheep and pigs is to produce muscle (lean tissue) with the amount of fat required by the market. Indeed, in European Union law, for use as a product ingredient, meat is defined as 'Skeletal muscles of mammalian and bird species recognised as fit for human consumption with naturally included or adherent tissue where the total fat and connective tissue content does not exceed [certain values]' (Commission Directive 2001/101/EC, 2001). For example, meat from mammals (other than rabbits and porcines) has a maximum fat content of 25% and a maximum connective tissue content also of 25%.

Over time, particularly in the UK, the quantity of fat that is considered desirable has generally declined. Historically, large quantities of fat were required. Indeed, getting animals ready for slaughter was traditionally referred to as 'fattening' and this was seen as necessary for quality. For example, Bull (1916) stated: 'The main object in fattening is to improve the flavour, tenderness and quality of the lean meat by the deposition of fat between the fibres.' The fact that the preferred term is now 'finishing' indicates the change in perception. The importance of pigs for the production of fat was emphasised in the *Book of the Pig* in 1886, which states: '. . . wherever the pig is dealt with as an article of commerce, the lard which it

© Woodhead Publishing Limited, 2011

furnishes is sufficient to create a great trade in itself' (Long, 1886). The production of clean, edible fat from feedstuffs not suitable for human consumption was a vital part of animal production. Fat carcases were also desirable because, as well as providing an energy-rich food, the fat had other important uses. Animal fat was used to make candles, for example, for centuries.

This history has led to the farmed red meats being considered 'fatty' foods. Today's policy makers and health professionals all too often subscribe to this dated view and doctors all too often prescribe a reduction in meat in the diet for those with high cholesterol. This chapter will show how this is no longer necessarily the case, describing how changes in animal production, carcase dressing, butchery and meal preparation have all contributed to a reduction in the fat consumed with red meat. It is also a misunderstanding to consider that the fat associated with red meat is saturated fat. It is true that a proportion of the fatty acids are saturated, but that is not the whole picture. In fact, leaner animals not only have less fat but the fat they contain is also less saturated. This will be explored further in section 10.2. Inevitably, however, the easiest way to reduce the saturated fatty acid intake from red meat is the reduction in total fat intake rather than changing the fatty acid composition. In the main then, this chapter will focus on the overall reduction in fat in red meat with the assumption that this is directly related to the reduction in the saturated fat content. Finally, the role that fat plays in meat eating quality will be considered.

10.2   Animal production

10.2.1   Animal growth and selection for slaughter

The objective of rearing animals for meat is to maximise the production of those parts that command the highest price in the market. In Western countries this is lean muscle. That does not mean that other parts of the animal have no value but that the largest returns to the supply chain can be obtained by maximising the highest-value parts. The main components of the carcase are bone, muscle and fat. In growing animals these tissues mature in that order. This means that in a newborn animal bone is a relatively high proportion of the body weight and, as the animal matures, bone growth slows and muscle growth increases, followed by fat tissue. The fat content of the carcase of an animal of a particular genotype is largely determined, therefore, by the stage of maturity at which it is slaughtered.

Different tissues also have different nutrient requirements for growth. Of particular interest is the energy requirement for muscle and fat tissue. On a weight-for-weight basis fat requires about six times the energy needed to deposit lean meat. Fat contains 56.35 kJ/g whereas protein contains 46.2 kJ/g (Orskov and Ryle, 1990), but lean tissue is some 75% water. This means that producing an animal fatter than is required for the market not only results in a greater degree of trimming required, but also incurs unnecessary cost in growing that fat.

It follows from the above description that producing meat with the required ratio of fat to lean, without the need for excessive trimming, depends on sending

© Woodhead Publishing Limited, 2011

animals for slaughter at the right stage in their growth. In pig production this is often achieved by selecting on finished weight. A known genotype, on a ration of known formulation, will generally produce animals of a similar fat level at a similar weight. The producer who knows his pigs will learn the right weight to target the fat level to optimise the price received. In cattle and sheep, where forage of variable composition often makes up much of the diet, selection of animals for slaughter at the right degree of finish is a highly skilled task. Programmes such as the EBLEX Better Returns Programme aim to increase the producer's awareness of market requirements and develop the skills needed to meet them.

10.2.2   Assessing carcase composition

The payment that producers receive for slaughter animals is largely determined by the value of the carcases to the slaughterer, whether they are purchased liveweight (through an auction market) or deadweight (purchased direct with the price being determined by the carcase weight). Over time the proportion of animals being sold deadweight has increased markedly. The basis for assessing the value of the animal is essentially an estimate of the saleable product that can be derived from the carcase, whether the transaction is on a liveweight or deadweight basis. Various methods are used as indicators of the yield of saleable meat from the carcase. These vary by species and are described separately below.

Measuring the composition of pig carcases
The vast majority of pigs are sold deadweight and the price paid is based on the classification of the carcase. The European Union rules for the classification of pig carcases require that the lean meat percentage of the carcase is estimated (Council Regulation (EC) 1234/2007, 2007). The main determinant of the lean percentage in a carcase at a given weight is the fat content of the carcase. Some 70% of the fat in a pig carcase is just beneath the skin (Kempster *et al.*, 1986), known as subcutaneous fat, which means that in most cases the determination of the lean meat percentage is based on some measure of the fat depth of the carcase coupled with either a measure of muscle depth and/or the weight of the carcase. In the UK, trade in pig carcases has historically been based on weight and the P_2 fat depth (the depth of subcutaneous fat at the head of the last rib and 6 cm from the midline of the carcase). Most classification methods are based on these assessments. The instruments approved for use for the classification of pigs in Great Britain are summarised in Table 10.1.

From the measurements taken, the lean meat percentage of the carcase is estimated according to equations determined by dissection of a representative set of carcases and set down in European Commission Decisions. The Decision currently applicable in the UK is Commission Decision 2004/370/EC as amended (Commission Decision 2004/370/EC, 2004, Commission Decision 2006/374/EC, 2006).

© Woodhead Publishing Limited, 2011

Table 10.1   Instruments approved for pig carcase classification in Great Britain

Device	Type	Parameters used for prediction of lean meat percentage
Intrascope (optical probe)	Manual insertion probe	Thickness of back fat measured at 6 cm off the midline at the last rib ('P_2') Weight of the cold carcase in kg
Fat-O-Meater	Semi-automatic insertion probe	P_2 Thickness of back fat measured at 6 cm off the midline between the third and fourth last ribs ('rib-fat') Thickness of muscle measured at the same time and in the same place as rib-fat ('rib-muscle')
Hennessy Grading Probe (HGP 4)	Semi-automatic insertion probe	P_2 rib-fat rib-muscle
CSB Ultra-Meater	Hand held ultrasonic scanner	rib-fat rib-muscle
Autofom	Fully automatic ultrasonic apparatus	108 measurements across the carcase

Source: Commission Decision 2004/370/EC

Assessing the quality of beef and lamb carcases
There are two main reasons why a simple measurement of fat depth and weight of the carcases of ruminant animals is not as effective as in pigs as criteria for assessment of carcase composition:

- Removal of the hide during dressing can result in damage to the subcutaneous fat so that the depth at a single point may no longer represent the degree of fat cover across the carcase.
- The proportion of carcase fat that is subcutaneous fat is, in any case, lower than in pigs.

In the absence of an objective measurement that relates to the yield of meat from a beef or lamb carcase, a visual scale is used to describe the shape and fatness of carcases.

The European Community Scale for beef carcase is mandatory for beef abattoirs slaughtering more than 75 adult bovine animals per week. A licensed classifier assesses the carcase for conformation (shape) on the scale EUROP, where E is excellent conformation and P is poor. An additional S (or 'superior') grade can also be used. Fatness is assessed on a scale of 1 (extremely lean) to 5 (very fat). Some classes are subdivided. In Britain, traditionally the beef fat classes 4 and 5 are subdivided into L (low) and H (high) and the conformation classes U, O and (optionally) P are subdivided into plus and minus.

A Community Scale exists for sheep classification and is broadly similar to the beef system. In Great Britain the scale developed by the Meat and Livestock

© Woodhead Publishing Limited, 2011

Commission, and now owned by Meat and Livestock Commercial Services Limited, is widely used. This is basically the same as the Community Scale. Conformation class P is not given fat classes, and the fat classes 3 and 4 are subdivided into L and H.

10.2.3   Changes in carcase fatness over time

The modern meat market no longer requires animals to carry excessive amounts of fat. Meat cuts presented for sale are usually required to have a small amount of associated fat. There is often a cost to the disposal of fat that has to be trimmed off to present steaks and joints acceptably. In any case, fat is of much lower value than lean and there is therefore strong commercial pressure to reduce the fat content of meat animals. This has resulted in significant changes in the composition of the carcases of animals reared for meat production.

Reduction in fat content of pig carcases
The back fat depth of pig carcases has been reducing 'since records began'. Table 10.2 gives the fat depth at the P_2 position, carcase weight and an approximate lean meat percentage every five years since 1983. This clearly shows a reduction in the fat content of the carcases. This can be contrasted even more dramatically with the fat content of pig carcases in the late nineteenth century, with the carcase of a 'fat pig' (i.e. one ready for slaughter) being in the region of 40% fat (Long, 1886).

In more recent years the fat depth has remained fairly constant while carcase weight has increased. While less obvious, this represents a continuing increase in the leanness of animals, as can be seen by the estimated lean meat percentage comparing 2003 and 2008.

A number of factors have contributed to this dramatic decline in the fat content of pig carcases. The very strong market signals mean that producers have sought leaner breeding stock, and pig breeding companies responded by selecting animals with increased genetic potential for lean growth and lower fat deposition. Coupled with this, nutritional management on the farm is now clearly aimed at achieving

Table 10.2   Changes in the average carcase characteristics of pigs

Year	P2 fat depth (mm)	Carcase weight (kg)	Estimated lean meat percentage
1983	13.8	61.0	57.5
1988	11.9	62.9	59.5
1993	10.8	66.7	60.8
1998	11.2	70.1	60.6
2003	10.9	73.5	61.1
2008	10.8	75.8	61.4

Source: BPEX, a Division of the Agriculture and Horticulture Development Board

Lean meat percentage estimated using the currently approved equation for Great Britain: Lean meat % = 66.5 − 0.95 × P2 + 0.068 × carcase weight

© Woodhead Publishing Limited, 2011

lean growth and not simply weight gain. Initially restricting the intake of pigs ('restrict feeding') was used to minimise fat deposition. Modern genotypes, however, can produce lean carcases on properly formulated ad-libitum diets.

Until the late 1970s most male pigs in Britain would have been castrated. Primarily this practice developed as a means of managing male animals for meat production without the risk of unwanted pregnancy in their female contemporaries. Castrates are also more placid and easy to manage. Unfortunately, however, they have a tendency to deposit more fat. Better management and more rapid growth to slaughter weights means that the main problems perceived with entire male pigs no longer apply. The vast majority of male pigs in Britain are now left entire. This results in more efficient growth and leaner carcases (Lundström *et al.*, 2009). At the same weight an entire male has anything from four to forty per cent less fat.

Despite the changes in breeding, management and nutrition, it remains important for producers to ensure that the animals they produce are sent for slaughter at the right point in their development. The market clearly no longer requires large, fat pigs where the lean is used for processed products and any surplus fat is used for other products such as pastry. The modern British slaughter weight pig averages 75.8 kg with a P_2 fat depth of 10.8 mm (BPEX, 2009).

Changes in the carcase quality of cattle and sheep
The ruminant sector has a very different structure to the pig industry. There is a wide range of production systems utilising a large range of breeds and types. Genetic improvement, instead of being in the hands of a few professional breeding companies, is the result of individual pedigree breeders who come together in breed societies. This means that breeding has to be managed differently. Estimated breeding values (EBVs) can be derived for animals across a breed by collection of data (such as weights and ultrasound back fat depths) from individual herds and flocks centrally and analysis using methods which separate the environmental (farm) effect from the genetic effect. In this way the merit of an animal for breeding can be compared with others of the same breed on other farms. This approach has certainly resulted in breed improvement within the pedigree breeds. To deliver significant benefits in the population of slaughter animals, however, requires widespread use of high genetic merit breeding animals across the commercial production. Inevitably, uptake is not uniform across the industry!

A further challenge to the progress towards leaner animals in the ruminant sector has been the lack of strong market signals. The main reasons for this are twofold. The Common Agricultural Policy, historically, meant that producers were rewarded with subsidies simply for producing animals. Secondly, the shortage of animals for slaughter relative to the capacity of the abattoir sector means that slaughterers are reluctant to penalise less desirable animals too heavily for fear they cannot maintain their throughput. The former is beginning to change. Reform of the Common Agricultural Policy and the introduction of the Single Farm Payment means that individual farm enterprises no longer attract subsidy payments and therefore can, and indeed should, stand or fall on their profitability. The price received for a slaughtered animal becomes much more critical and

© Woodhead Publishing Limited, 2011

Table 10.3 Fat class distribution for lamb carcases in Great Britain over ten years

Fat class	1	2	3L	3H	4L	4H	5	P
1999	1.0	19.0	47.5	20.7	4.9	1.9	0.7	4.3
2000	0.6	19.0	49.2	21.0	5.3	1.9	0.6	2.4
2001	0.8	18.7	51.9	19.8	5.2	1.8	0.7	1.2
2002	0.7	20.1	50.9	19.2	4.8	1.6	0.5	2.1
2003	0.5	20.5	49.9	19.8	5.3	1.7	0.5	1.7
2004	0.6	19.2	49.4	20.9	5.8	2.1	0.8	1.3
2005	0.8	21.3	51.5	18.1	4.5	1.3	0.6	1.9
2006	1.2	24.0	51.8	16.0	4.1	1.1	0.5	1.3
2007	0.9	21.3	49.9	19.0	5.0	1.7	0.7	1.4
2008	1.0	21.9	53.3	17.0	4.0	1.1	0.5	1.1
2009	1.6	21.6	51.5	20.4	3.7	0.8	0.3	0.6

Source: EBLEX, a Division of the Agriculture and Horticulture Development Board

Table 10.4 Fat class distribution for prime beef carcases in Great Britain over ten years

Fat class	1 and 2	3	4L	4H	5L	5H
1999	5.4	24.0	49.5	19.3	1.5	0.2
2000	6.1	24.1	49.5	18.6	1.5	0.2
2001	8.1	25.7	48.6	15.9	1.5	0.2
2002	8.1	25.5	48.7	16.0	1.4	0.2
2003	8.2	27.6	47.1	15.5	1.3	0.2
2004	8.3	28.2	46.4	15.8	1.0	0.1
2005	8.8	27.1	46.1	16.6	1.3	0.2
2006	10.3	27.7	45.8	15.0	1.0	0.1
2007	11.3	28.7	44.5	14.4	1.0	0.1
2008	13.4	31.1	43.8	11.0	0.6	0.1
2009	12.1	30.8	44.0	12.1	0.9	0.1

Source: EBLEX, a Division of the Agriculture and Horticulture Development Board

therefore a greater focus is placed on meeting the market requirement for lean and well-conformed animals.

The change in the distribution of carcase fat classes over the last ten years are shown in Tables 10.3 and 10.4. In both cases the distribution has shifted towards the leaner carcases. The proportion in what is generally considered the target range of fat classes has risen for lambs (fat class 1 to 3L) from 67.5% to 74.7%; and for beef (1 to 4L) from 78.9% to 86.9%.

Changes in fat available for consumption
In 1996 we published an assessment of the fat available for consumption from cattle, sheep and pigs in Great Britain in 1982 and 1992 (Matthews and Warkup, 1996). This showed that there had been a substantial decline (around 26%) in the carcase fat available for consumption between the two years as a result of a

© Woodhead Publishing Limited, 2011

reduction in fat produced in animal production and a reduction in imported fat. In 1992 it was clear, however, that there were still substantial imports of fat in order to make food products that required fat as an ingredient. We simply were not producing enough fat to meet our appetites! This is still the case, but the imported fat is declining. Net imports of rendered pig and poultry fat, for example, have fallen from 40 603 tonnes in 1997 to 5096 tonnes in 2009 (Her Majesty's Revenue and Customs import statistics), indicating a huge reduction in demand for animal fats. Consumer demand clearly determines to a large extent the population intake of animal fats. Further changes in animal production to reduce fat production will only be made in response to this. A change in the demand for high-fat products, or reformulation of products to contain less fat (where this is possible) is necessary to change the overall dietary intake.

10.2.4   Current carcase composition

Overall carcase composition
In 1993 the Meat and Livestock Commission undertook assessment of the chemical composition of beef. This involved the full dissection of carcases into their component parts (mainly lean, fat and bone) and chemical analysis of the resulting tissues. Regression equations were derived that enable the estimation of the composition of animals from their classification. Table 10.5 gives the estimated physical composition for the average carcase in 2009 for prime cattle based on current classification results and predictions from the chemical composition study.

In comparison with the composition of carcases in the first half of the twentieth century, there have been dramatic changes. Hammett and Nevell (1929) gave figures for the percentage of the carcase that was 'lean flesh' of 33% for lean sheep and 36% for lean cattle. In Table 10.5 it can be seen that the most common carcase currently for prime beef gives figures for lean ranging from 63.4% to 68.1%. Similar changes will have been seen in pigs and sheep over the same time period.

Table 10.5   Estimated physical composition of beef carcases in 2009

	Steers	Heifers	Young Bulls
Classification	R4L	R4L	R3
Mean side weight	172.5	151.5	164.5
As % of side:			
Lean	63.4	65.9	68.1
Intermuscular fat	12.5	11.2	9.8
Subcutaneous fat	7.7	7.1	5.3
Bone and waste	16.5	15.7	18.1

Source of classification data: EBLEX, a Division of the Agriculture and Horticulture Development Board

© Woodhead Publishing Limited, 2011

Fatty acid composition

In 1996, Enser and colleagues examined the fatty acid content of English beef, lamb and pork at retail (Enser *et al.*, 1996). The data show that only 41, 44 and 37% of the fatty acids in the muscle of beef sirloin steaks, lamb chops and pork loin chops/steaks respectively were saturated fatty acids. Even in the adipose tissue, the corresponding percentage saturated fatty acids are 42, 39, and 38%. The authors demonstrated that the red meats make an important contribution to the total polyunsaturated fatty acids in the diet.

The regressions derived from chemical composition studies described above show that the leaner the carcase, the lower the proportion of saturated fatty acids. This is logical, as the fatty acids deposited in storage fats are generally more saturated and fatter animals have more of these storage fats. On the other hand, the fatty acids are contained in all tissues in cell membranes. To maintain membrane flexibility and function these are required to be primarily unsaturated fatty acids. The quantity of these membrane lipids changes little over time, whereas the deposited fats accumulate as an animal matures, thus the proportion shifts towards more saturated fatty acids in fatter animals. Thus the requirement for leaner animals *per se* has meant that the fatty acid composition has become less saturated.

In their review of red meat in the diet, Williamson *et al.* (2005) discussed the fatty acid composition of red meat. They also pointed out that the level of saturated fatty acids was similar to that of monounsaturated fatty acids, with relatively low levels of polyunsaturated fatty acids. Nevertheless, in a diet low in oily fish, they highlighted the importance of red meat for the provision of the long chain n-3 polyunsaturated fatty acids. The authors also discussed the main saturated fatty acids found in red meat. It is not the place of this chapter to discuss the nutritional importance of different fatty acids, but it is worth noting that one of the main saturated fatty acids in red meat is stearic acid, which is considered to have no effect on cholesterol levels, perhaps the most important negative impact of saturated fatty acids in the diet.

10.3   Preparation of cuts

10.3.1   Changes to butchery

Any interested observer walking alongside the retail shelves will see that there is a great deal less fat associated with whole-muscle cuts than there would have been a generation ago. In part this is the result of the changes in animal production and selection for slaughter already described, but even where a carcase still carries too much fat for the modern consumer, leaner cuts can often be presented by changes to butchery practice.

In broad terms, the larger the carcase, the easier it is to present lean cuts from an overfat animal. Thus beef cuts contain less muscles and the fat around the muscles can relatively easily be removed by knife, whereas lamb cuts present a more difficult challenge because they are often composed of several muscles and

© Woodhead Publishing Limited, 2011

the intermuscular fat (that between the muscles) is not possible to remove without destroying the cut.

Nevertheless, alternative methods of preparing cuts present opportunities for trimming more fat. So-called 'seam butchery', where muscles are removed along the natural lines between them rather than cutting to the bone structure, allows for intermuscular fat to be almost entirely removed if the market requires it. Higgs (2000) described how the fat content of pork loin can be reduced from 19.5% to 7.9% by simply removing the backfat, and further reduced to 3.9% by seam cutting.

10.3.2 Mince

Mince now accounts for close to 50% of beef sales. The fat sold with mince is therefore an important component of the contribution of animal fat to the intake of saturated fat. It is noteworthy, therefore, that lean beef mince now makes up some 42% of beef mince sales.

10.4   In the kitchen and on the plate

It is clear that the fat sold with meat cuts is not necessarily consumed. There are three main aspects of the reduction of fat intake from red meat once in the home (or indeed catering premises). Firstly, there may be further trimming of the raw meat before cooking. This will not be considered further here because the effect is essentially the same as trimming by the butcher and this has been considered above. Cooking itself results in changes to the weight and composition of the meat and this will be considered. Finally, the person eating the meat often trims fat from the cut during the meal. This 'plate waste' is rarely quantified or taken into account in considering the dietary impact of red meat but can be important.

10.4.1   Effect of cooking on fat content

When cooked, meat cuts lose weight. This weight loss is primarily made up of water and fat. The cooking loss, for example, from a beef sirloin roast is around 29% (Lawrie, 1998). In leaner meat the loss of water is generally higher than the loss of fat so that the final steak may have a percentage fat content that is unchanged or even higher, but in fattier cuts a higher proportion of the weight loss is fat. In either case, the weight of fat consumed from the steak will have been reduced by the weight of fat that has been lost during cooking. Thus, if we took a notional steak of 200 g with a fat content of 10% (including the band of subcutaneous fat), the raw steak would contain 20 g of fat. A cooking loss of 30% would reduce the weight to 140 g. Assuming this weight loss was water and fat in the ratio of 3:1 the loss of fat would be 15 g, leaving 5 g (or 3.6%) in the final product. Thus the fat intake, compared with the raw product, has been reduced by 75%. It is important, therefore, when comparing the fat content of raw meat with other foods, particularly ready-to-eat foods, that the likely cooking loss is taken into account.

© Woodhead Publishing Limited, 2011

10.4.2   Trimming on the plate ('plate waste')

It is a natural assumption that many people trim fat from meat cuts during consumption and do not eat it. The degree to which this influences fat intake has not been widely studied. In 1997 we published a preliminary study and evaluation of methods of assessing trimming at the table (Leeds *et al.*, 1997). In a relatively small group of subjects (51) trimming behaviour was quantified using pork loin steaks with an average total fat content of 29.1 g/100 g. Trimming reduced, on average across the whole group, the fat content to 12.9 g/100 g. For the 36 subjects who trimmed the steaks the fat content was reduced, on average, to 6.1 g/100 g. The study also validated a method for assessing trimming habits using shading of photographs. The advantage of this approach would be that large study groups could be accommodated by postal survey.

10.5   Effect on meat quality

There is concern, particularly among the more traditional parts of the meat industry, that reducing the fat content of meat will have a negative impact on meat eating quality. It is worth noting that a broader definition of meat quality would include visual appeal and nutritional quality, both of which are improved by reducing fat content. Nevertheless, eating quality is of critical importance to the enjoyment of meat eating. Indeed, if meat is consistently of poor eating quality it can be assumed that people will cease to purchase it.

It is suggested that the fat in meat can influence each of the three main eating quality attributes that determine consumer acceptability: tenderness, juiciness (or succulence) and flavour. Each of these is considered in turn. There is a large body of published evidence on the effect of fatness on the eating quality of meat. It is not always easy to interpret the results, however, because the differences in fat content are inevitably confounded with other differences.

10.5.1   Role of fat in the tenderness of meat

It is mainly the intramuscular fat that is considered important for the tenderness of meat. This is the fat within the muscle itself, which at low levels is invisible and at higher levels becomes visible as 'marbling'. This might be thought to have an effect on tenderness in a number of ways. Fat tissue within the muscle might substitute for muscle that, within a given piece, is diluted with softer tissue, thus reducing the overall force required to bite through the meat. This might be considered to be a likely effect at higher levels of intramuscular fat. Alternatively, or in combination, the fat might weaken the structural integrity of muscle, perhaps preventing cross links forming between connective tissue of muscle fibre proteins, thus enabling the muscle to be broken up more readily in the mouth. A further possible effect in the mouth is the potential for fat to lubricate during chewing, reducing resistance to the teeth through reduced friction. Studies to evaluate these effects in the mouth are very difficult to conduct and generally sufficient useful

© Woodhead Publishing Limited, 2011

information is obtained by the use of trained sensory panels assessing the overall tenderness (or toughness) of the meat. The complex nature of chewing, however, means that care should be taken in the interpretation of results from instrumental measures of toughness. These should only be relied upon as a guide to the sensory perception of quality.

Where an effect of fatness on the tenderness of meat has been observed it is usually positive. Across the range of fat contents seen normally in British red meat, however, the effect is generally small, such that even a doubling of the fat content would have only a very small impact on the sensory perception of tenderness. Having said that, the literature is consistent, with a decline in tenderness for meat from those animals at the very leanest end of the scale, suggesting that a minimum level of intramuscular fat is required to prevent damaging tenderness. Below about 2.5% intramuscular fat beef tenderness has been seen to decline sharply, but above that there is very little effect of intramuscular fat (Buchter, 1986). Similarly, research at the Meat and Livestock Commission's Stotfold Pig Development Unit found that P_2 fat depths below 8 mm were associated with tougher meat (MLC, unpublished data).

A further benefit of fat in meat tenderness is the insulating effect it has on the carcase immediately post slaughter. The muscle in fatter carcases cools more slowly post slaughter. When muscle chilling is too rapid a toughening effect, called cold shortening, can occur. The slower cooling of fatter carcases can reduce this effect, resulting in apparently more tender meat. If chilling is considerate, however, this advantage to fatter carcases disappears. This effect is particularly apparent in smaller lamb carcases, which cool more rapidly.

10.5.2   Fatness and flavour

Those who advocate increased fatness often claim that fat imparts stronger flavour to meat. Indeed fat does play a part in meat flavour development during cooking. The main reaction developing flavour of meat is the Maillard reaction between amino acids and sugars. Following this, the Maillard reaction products interact with fatty acids to generate a range of compounds involved in flavour. Generally speaking, however, the 'species flavour' – that is, the unique flavour of beef, lamb or pork – is imparted with the minimal amount of fat present in every muscle. Additional fat can impart additional species flavour but generally only adds fatty flavour, which is liked by some people and not by others.

10.5.3   Fat in meat and juiciness

It is very difficult in sensory studies to separate the perception of juiciness (or succulence) from that of other textural traits, particularly tenderness. The traits are highly correlated, meaning that a tender piece of meat is usually also perceived as juicy. Increased fatness may impart a greater perception of juiciness where the meat is cooked to well done, but in medium or rare cooked meat there is little difference. Fatness can thus be seen as an insurance against overcooking!

© Woodhead Publishing Limited, 2011

10.6   Future trends

The meat industry already has the tools at its disposal necessary to deliver lean meat cuts to the consumer and lean raw materials for further processing. Further reductions in the fat consumed that has been derived from the carcases of cattle, sheep and pigs is likely to be driven by market forces. If the rewards for producing leaner meat are sufficient then this will ensure that the industry responds.

In the area of animal breeding, selection for more efficient lean growth is likely to continue. This both improves the financial efficiency of animal production and, by happy coincidence, reduces the environmental impact of producing meat animals. Selection against overfat animals also remains a part of ruminant breeding programmes.

A key to delivering against the consumer demand for lean meat remains the selection of animals for slaughter at the appropriate stage of growth. Knowledge transfer programmes with farmers, to improve understanding of market requirements and develop the skills to select for slaughter, will be important in ensuring the meat industry has the right raw materials with which to work.

The presentation of lean cuts is already possible. It is likely that butchery will further adapt to provide a greater choice of lean, tender and easy-to-cook products that meet the needs of today's consumer. The area in which the greatest further advances are likely to be seen is the adoption of new tools for carcase classification, providing better market signals and therefore a stronger motivation to produce the carcases that are required. Video image analysis systems have already been developed that can assess the conformation and fat class of cattle and sheep carcases using a picture captured by camera and predictive software. They have not yet been adopted for classification or payment purposes in the UK. These are likely to improve with time, and prediction of meat yield is likely to be used for payment in the future. In pigs, objective measures of fatness are already employed, but these may, again, be further developed to increase the ability to predict composition.

In lean red meat further reductions in saturated fatty acid intakes can be achieved by shifting the fatty acid composition of the meat, making it less saturated. Much research is currently under way in this area and this is discussed in Chapter 12.

10.7   Conclusions

The fat in the carcases of cattle, sheep and pigs red meat cuts has been reduced dramatically over recent decades. This has been achieved through a combination of animal breeding, management and selection for slaughter. The fat content of meat cuts has been further reduced by refined butchery techniques responding to consumer demands. Even the mince consumed has, on average, a reduced fat content as the range of mince available has increased and 'leaner' options have increased in sales.

© Woodhead Publishing Limited, 2011

10.8   Sources of further information and advice

EBLEX and BPEX (Divisions of the Agriculture and Horticulture Development Board) collect data on the current carcase classification of cattle, sheep and pigs in Great Britain. Their websites (http://www.eblex.org.uk and http://www.bpex.org. uk) also contain a great deal of information on butchery and presentation of meat. The EBLEX Better Returns Programme provides producers with materials and training to facilitate the selection of cattle and sheep to meet market requirements.

Two recent reviews (Williamson *et al.*, 2005 and McAfee *et al.*, 2010) provide useful overviews of meat consumption and of the role of red meat in the diet. Indeed, the British Nutrition Foundation is a good source of balanced information about human nutrition and diet and health.

10.9   References

BPEX (2009). *Pig Yearbook*, Kenilworth, Warwickshire, BPEX, A Division of the Agriculture and Horticulture Development Board.

Buchter, L. (1986). Eating quality in low fat beef. *In:* Staff colloquium of Merck Sharp and Dohme Reasearch Laboratories, 1986, Heathrow, London.

Bull, S. (1916). *The principles of feeding farm animals*, New York, The Macmillan Company.

Commission Decision 2004/370/EC of 15 April 2004 authorising methods for grading pig carcases in the United Kingdom OJ L116, 22.4.2004, p 32.

Commission Decision 2006/374/EC of 22 May 2006 amending Decision 2004/370/EC authorising methods for grading pig carcases in the United Kingdom OJ L142, 30.5.2006, p 34.

Commission Directive 2001/101/EC of 26 November 2001 amending Directive 2000/13/EC of the European Parliament and of the Council on the approximation of the laws of the Member States relating to the labelling, presentation and advertising of foodstuffs. OJ L310, 28.11.2001, p 19.

Council Regulation (EC) 1234/2007 of 22 October 2007 establishing a common organisation of agricultural markets and on specific provisions for certain agricultural products (Single CMO Regulation) OJ L299, 16.11.2007, p 1.

Enser, M., Hallett, K., Hewett, B., Fursey, G. A. J. and Wood, J. D. (1996). Fatty acid content and composition of English beef, lamb and pork at retail. *Meat Science*, 42, 443–56.

Hammett, R. C. and Nevell, W. H. (1929). *A Handbook on Meat and Text Book for Butchers*, London, Meat Trades Journal.

Higgs, J. D. (2000). Leaner meat: an overview of the compositional changes in red meat over the last 20 years and how these have been achieved. *Food Science and Technology Today*, 14, 22–6.

Kempster, A. J., Cook, G. L. and Grantley-Smith, M. (1986). National estimates of the body composition of British cattle, sheep and pigs with special reference to trends in fatness. A review. *Meat Science*, 17, 107–38.

Lawrie, R. A. (1998). *Meat Science*, Cambridge, Woodhead.

Leeds, A. R., Randall, A. and Matthews, K. R. (1997). A study into the practice of trimming fat from meat at the table, and the development of new study methods. *Journal of Human Nutrition and Dietetics*, 10, 245–51.

Long, J. (1886). *The Book of the Pig*, London, L Upcott Gill.

Lundström, K., Matthews, K. R. and Haugen, J.-E. (2009). Pig meat quality from entire males. *Animal*, 3, 1480–7.

© Woodhead Publishing Limited, 2011

Matthews, K. R. and Warkup, C. C. (1996). The production and utilisation of fat from cattle, sheep and pigs in the United Kingdom in 1982 and 1992. *Meat Focus International*, 5, 410–14.

Mcafee, A. J., Mcsorley, E. M., Cuskelly, G. J., Moss, B. W., Wallace, J. M. W., Bonham, M. P. and Fearon, A. M. (2010). Red meat consumption: An overview of the risks and benefits. *Meat Science*, 84, 1–13.

Orskov, E. R. and Ryle, M. (1990). *Energy Nutrition in Ruminants*, London and New York, Elsevier Science.

Williamson, C. S., Foster, R. K., Stanner, S. A. and Buttriss, J. L. (2005). Red meat in the diet. *Nutrition Bulletin*, 30, 323–55.

© Woodhead Publishing Limited, 2011

11

Saturated fat reduction in processed meat products

S. Barbut, University of Guelph, Canada

Abstract: Animal fats vary in their saturation level depending on species, diet and climate. The degree of saturation affects the fats' melting point, plasticity and behavior in a food product. Early work on fat reduction resulted in lower cook yield, mushy interior, skin formation and sensory changes after reheating. Later work focused on finding fat replacers that could mimic the mouthfeel and textural characteristics of animal fat. Ingredients such as hydrocolloid gums, starches and dietary fiber helped improve the quality of the products. Flavor issues could be resolved by using extracts. A better understanding of the mechanisms involved in fat perception will help bring the industry to the next level.

Key words: beef, meat, hydrocolloid gum, lard, meat, pork, poultry, oil, saturated and unsaturated fats, sensory, tallow, texture, vegetable oil.

11.1 Introduction

Animal fats play important functional, sensory and nutritional roles in many food products including processed meats. Animal fats have been used for centuries in the manufacturing of meat products (sausages, hams, pies) and other foods (baked goods, dairy products). The fat, which can be part of the meat cuts or added into a meat product, is important in providing a unique texture and creating a unique taste profile (Giese, 1996; Hughes *et al.*, 1998; Jiménez-Colmenero, 2007; Dransfield, 2008; Youssef and Barbut, 2009). Animal fats can vary in their composition (Wood *et al.*, 2008) but are relatively high in saturated fatty acids compared to vegetable oils such as canola, and animal fats contain cholesterol; both factors have been implicated in increasing plasma low-density lipoprotein (see Chapter 4). Overall, fats from animal sources can be ranked based on their degree of saturation (beef>pork>chicken>fish), which affects their melting point, plasticity at a given temperature and behavior in a food product (e.g. liver paté can be made more or less spreadable at room temperature.)

© Woodhead Publishing Limited, 2011

Studies on fat reduction in meat products started to appear in the scientific literature in the 1970s but intensified in the early 1990s. Today fat substitution/ reduction is a hot topic as some common products such as frankfurters and breakfast sausages often contain 25% to 30% fat. Early work on reducing fat in ground-meat products, (e.g. from 25% to 10% and below) often resulted in cooked hamburger patties that were bland and dry with a hard, rubbery or mealy texture (Berry and Leddy, 1984; USDA, 1986). However, reformulation with certain fat substitutes could improve some of the poor binding, lack of beef flavor (mainly coming from fat), reduced browning reactions and shorter microbiological shelf-life (Keeton, 1994). Sausages (e.g. salami, bologna) produced with low fat ($\leq$10%) showed lower cook yield, soft mushy interior, rubbery skin formation, excessive purge in vacuum packages, shorter shelf-life and changes in sensory qualities after cooking or reheating. Later work has been focusing on finding fat replacers that could mimic the mouthfeel and textural characteristics of fat, for the development of low-fat meat products.

It is important to note that in fresh and processed meat products the characteristic meat flavor is produced during cooking by a complex series of reactions that occur between non-volatile components of lean and fatty tissues (see reviews by Mottram, 1998; Dransfield, 2008). Currently, over a thousand volatile compounds have been identified. Early work suggested that the species differences in flavor are largely explained by differences in lipid-derived volatile components in cooked meat. There are also several hundred volatile compounds, derived from lipid degradation, that have been identified. They include aliphatic hydrocarbons, aldehydes, ketones, alcohols, carboxylic acids and esters. Some aromatic compounds, especially hydrocarbons, have been described, as well as oxygenated heterocyclic compounds such as lactones and alkylfurans. In general, these compounds result from oxidation of the fatty acid components of lipids. The fact that a lot of the texture and especially flavors are derived from a specific animal fat (e.g. cooking lean chicken meat with beef fat will provide typical beef flavor and aroma) represents a big challenge when animal fat is reduced/substituted.

In general, studies that have been published on strategies to reduce animal fat in meat products include: formulating with leaner meats (fat-reduced, partially defatted); substituting some of the fat with water; utilizing protein-based ingredients such as proteins from blood plasma, egg, milk and soy; carbohydrate-based substitutes such as cellulose, starches, hydrocolloid gums; and using synthetic compounds such as Polydextrose® and Olestra®. As will be discussed in this chapter, the most common approach today is to employ a combination of several of the strategies mentioned above. Overall, the meat industry has gained a lot of knowledge over the past two decades regarding the use of fat replacements; however, more insight and better understanding are needed to elucidate the interactions among the meat ingredients, processing conditions and consumer preferences.

Since there are so many types of meat products, the chapter is divided into the following sections: ground-meat products (burgers), sausages (coarse-ground, emulsion-type, dry fermented), and prepared and/or coated meat products (nuggets, pies).

© Woodhead Publishing Limited, 2011

11.2   Ground-meat products (burgers)

As indicated in the introduction, a straight fat reduction in ground beef type patties to 10% or below results in an inferior product. This can also be seen in the data provided in Table 11.1. Reitmeier and Prusa (1987) also reported that as fat level was reduced in pork patties from 23 to 4%, the product became less tender and juicy and had a lower oily mouth coating. Pork flavor was much less pronounced in the 4% fat patties. As observed with the beef patties, fat reduction by itself will not likely produce palatable low-fat pork patties. The authors suggested that additional ingredients be tried/used to enhance the eating quality of reduced fat products.

Huffman and Egbert (1990) reported that beef patties produced with approximately 20% fat were highest in overall acceptability compared to fat content ranging from 5 to 25%. When changing the particle size they noted that overall palatability of low-fat ground beef was slightly improved by a final grind through a 0.48 cm (3/16 inch) plate rather than the more common 0.32 cm (1/8 inch) plate.

Table 11.1   Effects of fat level on composition, sensory, texture and yield parameters of ground-beef patties

| Characteristic | Effect | Fat level % | | | | | | SE |
		0	4	8	12	16	20	
Fat content, raw, %	ab	1.3	5.2	9.5	12.5	16.6	21.3	0.12
Fat content, cooked, %	ab	1.8	7.2	11.6	15.2	17.2	20.0	0.10
Moisture content, raw, %	ab	79.0	76.0	72.0	70.0	66.0	62.0	0.09
Moisture cont, cooked, %	ab	67.0	64.0	62.0	59.0	58.0	55.0	0.11
Initial tenderness[x]	ab	3.8	4.0	4.8	5.0	5.1	5.2	0.04
Juiciness[x]	ab	3.8	4.5	4.9	5.1	5.8	5.6	0.04
Beef flavor intensity[x]	ab	4.0	4.6	5.1	5.4	5.8	5.7	0.04
Peak load, kg	ab	8.1	7.0	6.3	6.3	5.9	5.3	0.05
Cooking yield, %		69.6	69.7	69.9	70.9	69.4	69.6	0.26
Reduction in patty thickness, %	a	13.5	18.7	19.8	23.7	25.4	25.9	0.32
Reduction in patty diameter, %		18.3	16.0	15.8	15.4	15.9	15.1	0.27

[a] Linear effect (P < 0.01)
[b] Quadratic effect (P < 0.01)

Tenderness, juiciness and flavor: [x] Scores are based on 8-point system where 8 = extremely tender, juicy, intense in flavor.

Source: data from Berry, 1992

© Woodhead Publishing Limited, 2011

Huffman and Egbert (1990) and Egbert *et al.* (1991) have evaluated the use of a carrageenan gum in a large-scale study targeted to bring a new low-fat product to the market. They compared beef patties containing 20% fat to those with 8% fat with or without 0.5% iota carrageenan, 10% water, 0.4% encapsulated salt and 0.2% hydrolyzed vegetable proteins. Broiled carrageenan patties with 8% fat were rated more tender by a sensory panel and contained 16% more moisture, 58% less fat, 16% less cholesterol (14 mg/100 g) and 37% fewer calories (100 kcal/100 g) than the 20% fat control. Reducing the fat content to 8% without any additives resulted in patties that were less juicy, had lower flavor intensity, and greater shear force values than either the 20% control or 8% fat/carrageenan patties. Patties with 20% fat had the highest cooking losses but lowest shear force. Serving temperature also appeared to be more critical for low-fat patties than regular fat patties. The McDonald's Corporation adapted a low fat/carrageenan formulation pretty similar to the one described by Huffman and Egbert (1990) and introduced the McLean Delux™ hamburger in 1991. The product was on the market for several years but then removed (in around 1996), probably due to low sale volumes. It is interesting to note that in consumer surveys, most people indicate that they would like to buy low-fat hamburgers (e.g. when asked in focus groups), but when they enter a fast food restaurant they would actually like to have a juicy/full flavor hamburger. Since the 1991 introduction, there has been quite a lot of development done in this area by various meat and/or ingredient companies and quality has dramatically improved, but the McLean has not been re-introduced. Overall, the application of any water:gum substitution combination (e.g. water:carrageenan) must be carefully done, otherwise unexpected product changes can negatively affect acceptability. For example, when using carrageenan one must remember that it has a low melting point and it forms a so-called reversible gel (melts at about 50°C). This can cause premature moisture loss and/ or loss of water-soluble flavors; fewer browning reaction products may develop during grilling/broiling, thus reducing meaty flavor (both just after cooking and more so during warming under a fast food service situation). This is on top of natural variations in carrageenan performance (e.g. the gum is extracted from seaweeds at different locations around the world, refined by different processes, and is affected by the presence of mono and divalent salts).

Another approach has been the replacement of some fat with water. Pork sausage patties containing 25% fat and 13% added water showed higher cooking losses than 15% or 35% fat patties prepared with 13% added water (Ahmed *et al.*, 1990). However, 15% and 25% fat patties with 3% added water had less cooking losses than their 35% fat counterparts. Generally speaking, it appears that for low-fat patties, the addition of excess water alone may be detrimental to cook yield, juiciness, and tenderness as well as causing higher springiness and cohesiveness. As with ground beef, added water must be well bound to produce a desirable low-fat pork product.

The use of starches and maltodextrins, which are glucose polymers typically derived from corn, oats, potatoes, rice, tapioca and waxy maize, represent another strategy. Upon hydration and heating of the native starch, two polymeric forms (i.e. amylose and amylopectin) create a three-dimensional gel network that can entrap water. Most fat replacement starches are pregelatinized to enable cold water swelling, which is an important feature in binding water prior to the denaturation of meat proteins by heat. Berry and Wergin (1993) incorporated 8% modified pregelatinized potato starch gel (3% starch, 5% water) in beef patties with 4% or 20% fat. Starch-treated patties had lower sensory flavor and juiciness scores, higher tenderness ratings, improved cook yields (4–6%) and a cost advantage due to the price of the starch. In a slightly different study, Minerich *et al.* (1991) formulated ground-beef patties (10, 15 and 30% fat) with and without 0, 15 or 30% Minnesota wild rice. As the rice level increased, proportional decreases in cholesterol, fat, protein and ash content were observed. Patties with rice, regardless of fat level, had higher cook yields, lower oxidation and were preferred by consumer panelists over regular ground beef. Troutt *et al.* (1992) concluded that a three-way combination of polydextrose, potato starch, and either sugar beet, oat or pea fiber reduced firmness and cohesiveness of 5% and 10% fat beef patties when compared to a 20% fat control. The ingredient combination lightened raw patty color and reduced cooking losses (by 20–40%), beef flavor intensity, juiciness and oily mouth coating scores. The authors recommended further research to optimize the use of these ingredients in beef patties because high-level use can result in reduced firmness and cohesiveness, lightened color, as well as reductions in beef flavor intensity and juiciness.

Oat bran and oat fiber have also been evaluated by themselves or in combination with other ingredients. Overall, they appear suited as a fat replacer, up to a certain point, in ground beef and pork products due to their ability to retain water and emulate some of the texture and particle definition in ground meat in terms of both color and texture. Some of the new fiber preparations such as citrus fibers (e.g. Citri-fi®) are advertised to be able to hold 1:7 water. The use of fiber is also becoming attractive to certain manufacturers as they can add a nutritional claim to their meat products. Such labels in products containing soy fibers are already on the market. However, it should be mentioned that overuse or misuse of oat bran or other fiber can result in poor binding of the raw product, causing difficulties with patty formation (reduced particle binding), reduced raw color appearance and stability, as well as a crumbly or mealy texture after cooking. Also, careful formulation and selection of flavor extracts and/or enhancers are required to retain the meat flavor and texture equal to that of regular fat ground beef. Revised cooking procedures are also needed to avoid overcooking and loss of juices, or creating palatability problems resulting in rejection of low-fat ground beef.

Piñero *et al.* (2008) reported on the beneficial effect of using an oat fiber source of β-glucan (13% homogenate) in low-fat (<10%) beef patties as compared to 20% fat control patties. Significant improvements in cooking yield (74%), retentions of fat (79%), and moisture (48%) seen in the low-fat patties were attributed to the water binding ability of β-glucan. Low-fat patties received a lower degree of likeness in the taste panel, but were reported juicer than control. Appearance, tenderness and color were not affected by the addition of oat's soluble fiber. The author suggested that oat fiber could be used successfully as a

© Woodhead Publishing Limited, 2011

fat substitute in low-fat beef patties and today a number of burger-type products are produced with added fibers. In a more recent example, Sánchez-Zapata *et al.* (2010) used tiger nut fiber to successfully improve the quality characteristics of pork burgers and showed higher cook yield, fat and moisture retention as well as higher nutritional value.

The development of a bacon product with a more attractive fatty acid profile is a nice example of a concept that now represents a popular product on the market. Walters *et al.* (1992) reported on the development of a turkey bacon where some of the appearance of the white pork fat is mimicked by ground/minced white turkey breast meat. Overall, thigh and breast meat are included to give the alternating colors of white and red characteristic of pork bacon, respectively. The turkey thigh meat was ground (9.5 mm) or cut in 1 × 5 cm pieces. It was then mixed with curing brine to prepare the darker portion of the bacon. Breast meat was ground (6.35 mm) or chopped, and mixed with the other non-meat ingredients except nitrite. A skin paste (10 to 20%) was also blended with the meat materials, or added to the breast meat section. The dark and white portions were alternately layered in aluminum foil pans. The fabricated loaves were fully smoked and cooked to 60°C. After chilling, the bacons were removed from the pans and sliced. Turkey bacon was analyzed before reheating for serving and found to contain 70.1% water, 8.7% fat, 17.8% protein, and 3.6% ash. Microwave heating of the product decreased the amount of water more than heating by pan frying. A consumer taste panel found the turkey bacon to have acceptable sensory qualities when compared with other products. Today this product is successfully manufactured by various leading brands and can be found in most stores in North America.

The use of minced meat from fish, poultry or red meat with or without prior washing is an interesting alternative. Bonifer *et al.* (1996) reported on the potential use of washed poultry skin (sometimes called Surimi) in bologna product. The skin was washed with a sodium bicarbonate (0.5%) solution in a pilot plant facility to remove fat and pigments from skin and used at 0, 10, and 20%. Washing followed by draining the wash water or centrifugation reduced fat, and increased total protein and moisture in skin. With reference to emulsion stability, skin content did not affect fat or gelwater losses and lowered solids loss when compared to bologna with 0% skin (P < 0.05). Kramer shear peak force was not significantly different for bologna at each treatment level. Total energy was higher for bologna with 0% skin. Skin addition did not affect compression measurements of hardness, springiness, cohesiveness and chewiness when compared to bologna with 0% skin. Consumer panelists rated bologna with 10% skin highest in texture, flavor, and texture and appearance acceptability.

11.3   Sausages – coarse-ground (e.g. cooked salami, breakfast sausage)

The sausage area has seen fairly similar approaches for fat reduction/substitution to those discussed for the ground-meat products; however, the technological

© Woodhead Publishing Limited, 2011

requirements from the additives used can vary quite a bit from hamburger-type products. In practice, most reduced fat products on the market today contain a combination/mixture of a few ingredients to compensate for the reduced/substituted fat in the original product. Ingredients such as simple and complex carbohydrates include starches, hydrocolloid gums, maltodextrins and dextrins, which are used to modify the product's texture, improve cooking yield, increase moisture retention and reduce formulation cost as well as improve freeze-thaw stability. As there are so many types of sausages, this topic is divided into three sections: coarse-ground sausages, finely comminuted sausages, and prepared/coated products.

Barbut and Mittal (1992) investigated the effects of kappa and iota carrageenans as well as xanthan gum on the quality of reduced-fat pork sausage (17 to 8%; water added to keep the protein level constant in all products). Iota carrageenan and xanthan gum retained more moisture compared to kappa carrageenan or products with no gum. Fat reduction resulted in higher cohesiveness, gumminess and chewiness values, which were not overcome by the gums. In any case, kappa carrageenan formulation provided a more tender product than the other low-fat products. Xanthan gum (0.5%) resulted in good fat and moisture retention during cooking; however, it was detrimental to textural parameters and sensory acceptability.

Xiong et al. (1999) studied the production of low-fat (4%) beef sausages with 23% added water, and compared them to a regular-fat control (25%) as well as comparing the use of 1.0% or 2.5% salt, different polysaccharide gums (0.5%), and pH adjusted meats (5.2, 5.6 or 6.2). The iota and kappa carrageenans increased ($P < 0.05$) cooking yield, hardness, and bind strength in the 1.0% salt sausage, but had little effect on the 2.5% salt sausage. Sausages containing alginate, locust bean gum and xanthan gum were softer, more deformable, crumbly and slippery, when compared to non-gum controls. It appears that in this study the fat level was too low for this kind of product, and most gums could not compensate for it. As has already been discussed, certain ingredients/gums have been found beneficial when used as texture-modifying compounds in sausage products; however, some do not work, or actually interfere with meat matrix structure formation. Among possible factors which could hinder the application of certain gums in commercial meat processing is the incompatibility between salt-soluble muscle proteins and certain polysaccharides, especially under high-salt conditions (Tolstoguzov, 1991; Xiong et al., 1999).

Konjac flour is another hydrocolloid gum which forms a strong hydrophilic elastic gel, claimed to have some of the sensory properties of fat, and can provide a substantial reduction in calorie content. Osburn (1992) incorporated rehydrated konjac gel into a 10% fat prerigor pork sausage at levels of 0%, 10% or 20% (0.00%, 0.25% and 0.50% konjac on a dry weight basis) and compared it to sausages with 40% fat. Konjac-containing sausage patties were redder in color, similar to controls in overall appearance and slightly detectable at the 20% level. In comparison to the 40% fat control, patties with 10% konjac had 3% greater cook yield, were rated only slightly higher for shear force, springiness, cohesiveness, chewiness, hardness, denseness and fracturability and slightly lower for juiciness. Some konjac gels are translucent and should be colored to

© Woodhead Publishing Limited, 2011

avoid pigment absorption from the muscle tissues resulting in a 'blood splash' appearance. In addition, seasonings and ingredients can be included in the gel to avoid flavor voids. It was also noted that during pan frying, surface browning did not occur without caramel coloring in the seasoning mix. It is interesting to note that industry sources indicate that the use of konjac gel has gained more popularity in Europe than in North America.

Another approach is the utilization of preformed gels prepared by polysaccharides and/or non-meat proteins, which are later incorporated into meat products as a fat replacer system. Lyons *et al.* (1999) evaluated various combinations of such preformed gels. They reported that mixed gels containing high-gelling whey protein concentrate (8%) and carrageenan (1.5%) with dry addition of tapioca starch (3%) produced low-fat (<3% fat) pork sausages with similar characteristics to those of full-fat (20% fat) controls. On the other hand, addition of preformed gel and tapioca starch had a significant negative interactive effect on cook loss, and showed a significant positive linear effect for mechanical textural values. Increasing levels of preformed gel blends with tapioca starch resulted in a general decrease in flavor intensity and overall flavor scores. It should also be mentioned that there are several patents describing such a technology and in some the use of flavor extracts is included.

The evaluations of barley β-glucan (0.3 and 0.8%) and carboxymethyl cellulose (CMC; 0.3%) in reduced-fat breakfast sausage (22 to 12% fat) was reported by Morin *et al.* (2004). Barley β-glucan is a non-starch polysaccharide that shows potential to be used as a fat replacer in low-fat sausages. It is a water-soluble hydrocolloid that functions to provide water control by thickening and/or gelling. As a soluble fibre component, β-glucan has the health benefits of reducing blood serum cholesterol. Cook loss results showed that β-glucan held more water in the sausages compared to the control, mainly due to its ability to form a tighter network (physical entrapment of water) within the meat protein matrix (investigated using scanning electron microscopy). Overall, the water-holding capacity is largely dependent on the reactive groups available to form the gel (e.g. as indicated before some are said to hold 1:7 water). Based on Morin *et al.*'s (2004) results, it appears that CMC was not as effective, as it interfered with protein network formation, by partially remaining in the spaces between the muscle fibre cells. Cheftal *et al.* (1985) suggested that due to CMCs negatively charged polyelectrolytic features, it prevents a strong protein network from forming, resulting in a lower cook yield, as water is easily able to move out. On the other hand, the β-glucan treatments demonstrated a higher cook yield since they did not inhibit protein cross-linking. Instead, they formed dense matrices, which had the ability to hold large amounts of water within the protein and fat network. This agrees with Bernal *et al.* (1987) and DeFreitas *et al.* (1997), who found that carrageenans increased water-holding capacity and gel strength of meat protein networks due to physical entrapment of water, not because of molecular interactions with meat proteins.

The use of pork skin or rind has also been evaluated as a fat replacer in reduced fat products. Abiola and Adegbaju (2001) reported that replacing pork back-fat with rind decreased refrigeration and cook weight losses. Overall, values obtained for sensory properties decreased with increase rind levels in the sausage. However,

© Woodhead Publishing Limited, 2011

up to 66% pork back-fat could be replaced with rind in pork sausage without any adverse effect on processing yield. Osburn *et al.* (1997) indicated that pre-heating (70°C) pork skin connective tissue (PCT) increased water binding. Gels (with 100–600% added water) were formed by heating PCT (70°C) for 30 minutes. Higher added water levels increased gel moisture content, while decreasing fat, melting points, collagen content, and hardness. Addition of PCT gels in bologna decreased hardness and increased juiciness, indicating the potential of PCT gels as water binders and texture-modifying agents.

11.4   Sausages – emulsion-type products (e.g. bologna, frankfurters)

Emulsion-type meat products represent a significant part of the market where a unique process is employed to incorporate and retain the fat/oil within the product. The process requires the use of a single pass through an emulsion mill or the continuous use (4–10 minutes) of the so-called silent cutter to reduce the fat particle to the micron size. The formation of this unique microstructure represents a big challenge in terms of keeping the fat/oil within the product during the cooking process (i.e. prior to the meat protein gelation). It should also be mentioned that the reference to emulsion-type meat products is due to the fact that these products do not conform to the true emulsion definition where fat/oil particles size is $< 20\mu m$ (Barbut, 2002).

The strategy of replacing some of the fat with water has been reported in bologna-type meat product by Claus *et al.* (1989). Formulations ranging from 30% fat (plus 10% added water) to 5% fat (plus 35% added water), all with similar protein content, were produced. The authors observed low-fat, high-added-water bologna to be generally softer, juicier, more cohesive, and darker in color with greater cooking and vacuum package purge loss than a control. Regression analysis indicated that bologna with 10% fat would require 24.3% added water to approximate the sensory firmness of the control. The results indicate that water retention and duplication of the textural characteristics of fat become major problems when formulating low-fat emulsion products simply by fat substitution with water only. When fat was kept at 14–16%, Park *et al.* (1989) indicated that processing yields, aroma, flavor, juiciness and overall desirability of frankfurters containing 14–16% added water with 14–16% fat (~75% as high-oleic sunflower oil) were equal to or greater than control frankfurters with 29% fat.

Bishop *et al.* (1993) reported that replacing fat (half of the 30%) with added water prevented the increase in firmness normally associated with low-fat bologna. However, during storage, accumulated purge in vacuum packages increased with water content in the products, and also with the use of pre-emulsified oil. In terms of modifying processing methods, the authors also tried pre-emulsifying the fat or oil. They indicated that it helped to decrease the firmness of low-fat bologna. The color was darker for all the reduced-fat bologna except the one pre-emulsified with corn oil. Flavor and overall acceptability scores, from a consumer sensory

© Woodhead Publishing Limited, 2011

panel, did not differ among bologna samples, but juiciness scores were higher in bologna containing additional water.

The effect of heating rate was studied by Cofrades *et al.* (1997). They compared regular fat level (23%) and low fat (9%; produced with high added water level) in frankfurters heated at 0.55, 1.10 and 1.90°C min^{-1}. They evaluated moisture binding properties (cooking and purge losses) and texture (compression test). Low-fat frankfurters exhibited poorer (P < 0.05) binding properties; they were less hard and chewy but more cohesive and springy than high-fat frankfurters. Heating rate had little effect on binding properties. Hardness, cohesiveness, springiness and chewiness were greater (P < 0.05) at the slowest heating rate than at the other rates.

Various researcher groups have investigated the option of using different vegetable oils in emulsion-type meat products as animal fat substitutes (Bloukas *et al.*, 1997; Pappa *et al.*, 2000; Tan *et al.*, 2001; Severini *et al.*, 2003; Youssef and Barbut, 2009) as the liquid oil is emulsified into small droplets that can be held within the product. Some vegetable oils contain large amounts of monounsaturated fatty acids (MUFA), and are obviously free of cholesterol. MUFA and PUFA can help decrease plasma low-density lipoprotein (LDL). Moreover, a higher level of PUFA can increase high-density lipoprotein (HDL) and thus reduce incidences of coronary heart disease (see Chapter 4). Canola oil has one of the lowest levels of saturated fatty acids and linolenic acid of any other conventional vegetable oils and is a good source of the antioxidant tocopherol (Giese, 1992, 1996).

Vegetable oils differ considerably in their color, flavor and fatty acid content, which may affect the quality characteristics of meat products. Marquez *et al.* (1989) reported that low-fat frankfurters made with a 60% substitution of the traditional beef fat with peanut oil had lower emulsion stability, firmer texture and darker color. Hammer (1992) produced frankfurter-type sausages using olive oil and sunflower oil (25% fat level). The products were lighter in color and no processing problems occurred, even without the use of non-meat additives such as blood plasma, phosphate or an emulsifier. Bloukas and Paneras (1993) produced low-fat frankfurters using olive oil, but the product had a lower processing yield and overall palatability. Paneras and Bloukas (1994) reported that low-fat frankfurters (10% fat, 12.5% protein) made with olive, corn, sunflower or soybean oils showed lower processing yields, darker color, firmer texture, lower juiciness, as well as lower levels of saturated fatty acids, calories and cholesterol compared to a control (29.1% pork fat, 10.4% protein). Ambrosiadis *et al.* (1996) reported that replacing the pork back-fat with soybean, sunflower, cottonseed, corn, or palmine oil (19.5% level) resulted in good emulsion stability in beef meat frankfurters, but firmness and lightness (internal color) were lower compared to the control. However, Park *et al.* (1989) reported that replacing animal fat with high-oleic-acid sunflower oil and fish oil had little effect on emulsion stability of low-fat frankfurters. Hsu and Yu (2002) looked at reducing fat in kung-wans, which are emulsified meatballs. They had three controls (25% pork back-fat, 10% fat and 10% water) and 11 plant oils, including coconut, sunflower, palm, corn, peanut, soybean, tea seed and olive, and hydrogenated oils from coconut, palm and soybean were compared. Results indicated that replacing 25% pork back-fat

© Woodhead Publishing Limited, 2011

with 10% water did not change the textural properties. In general, all plant-oil products had similar textural properties to the control kung-wans except for tea seed oil and peanut oil, which showed higher textural profile analysis data. Tea and peanut oils were inferior due to bitter taste and strong odor. Overall, coconut, palm, soybean, olive and hydrogenated soybean oils indicated as fat substitutes.

Understanding the mechanism(s) of different fats/oils stabilization in meat emulsion is of great importance to the industry. When substituting animal fat with vegetable oil, care should be given to potential problems with higher cooking loss and reduced emulsion stability. Youssef and Barbut (2010) reported that replacing beef fat with 25% canola oil, palm oil, hydrogenated palm oil or rendered beef fat in high-protein meat batters caused instability with some of the fats/oils (Fig. 11.1). As indicated earlier, canola oil resulted in significantly higher cooking losses as protein level was raised. The fact that no differences were found between the regular and rendered beef fat treatments may suggest that the collagenous network around the fat cells does not contribute to fat holding; however, fat hardness plays an important role in the emulsion stability (i.e. difference between liquid canola oil and beef fat/palm oil). When protein content was reduced to 8%, small fat losses started to appear in the beef fat, rendered beef fat and palm oil treatments. However, it should be mentioned that 8% is a very low level and is not used for practical

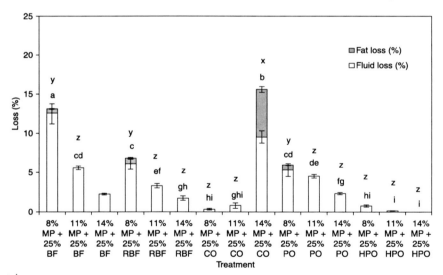

[a–i] Means related to fluid loss with no common superscript are significantly different (P < 0.05); error bars indicate the standard error.

[x–z] Means related to fat loss with no common superscript are significantly different (P < 0.05); error bars indicate the standard error.

From Youssef and Barbut (2010); with permission.

Fig. 11.1   Fat and fluid losses from meat batters prepared with 8, 11 and 14% meat protein. (MP – meat protein; BF – beef fat; RBF – rendered beef fat; CO – canola oil; PO – palm oil; HPO – hydrogenated palm oil).

© Woodhead Publishing Limited, 2011

reasons, as well as because of legal requirements in countries such as Canada (e.g. a minimum of 11% protein is required). Raising the amount of meat proteins reduced fat and fluid losses in the beef fat, rendered beef fat and palm oil containing batters. It is assumed that a high protein level formed a denser protein network within the batter, and helped restrict fat and fluid migration out of these products (microstructure results provided in the paper support this assumption). It could also be that an increase in protein content resulted in more side chains capable of interacting with water molecules during heating, and thus improved yield.

The use of hydrocolloid gums to partially replace animal fat and/or tie the extra water added has also been investigated. In some of the earliest studies Wallingford and Labuza (1983) reported xanthan gum to be more effective than carrageenan, locust bean gum and low methoxy pectin in preventing water loss from a low-fat meat emulsion model system. Whiting (1984) noted that alginate or xanthan gums (0.1–0.3%) improved water binding in low-fat frankfurters but were detrimental to gel strength. Foegeding and Ramsey (1986), however, concluded that kappa and iota carrageenan at levels of <1% were the most beneficial for holding moisture and increasing hardness of 11.5% fat frankfurters. Hedonic scores indicated that low-fat frankfurters with iota/kappa carrageenan were as acceptable as the 27% fat control frankfurter.

The production of low fat kung-wan, an emulsified meatball (1% vs. 20% fat), with 13 different gums was reported by Hsu and Chung (1999). Replacing fat with water resulted in lower cooking yield, smaller diameter, inferior sensory qualities and lower texture profile analysis indices. Eight gum-hydrates produced kung-wans with higher cooking yields than the 20% fat control. Seven gum-hydrates produced low fat kung-wans with similar texture profile analysis indices as the control. Six gum-hydrates produced products with similar sensory qualities as the control. Overall, kappa carrageenan, sodium alginate with $CaCO_3$, curdlan gum and locust bean gum, appeared to be good fat substitutes for making low fat emulsified kung-wan meatballs.

Using a mixture of ingredients to develop an ultra low-fat bologna (<2% fat) was reported by Chin et al. (2000). They evaluated two levels (0.5% or 1.0%) of konjac blends (KB; KSS = konjac flour/starch; KNC = konjac flour/carrageenan/starch) and the replacement of meat proteins with 2% soy protein isolate (SPI). Increased levels of KB decreased (P < 0.05) most texture profile analysis values as well as lightness and yellowness. Bologna containing 1.0% KB with 2% SPI showed texture profile analysis values and sensory flavor/taste attributes similar to the control (30% fat). However, based on sensory evaluation, low-fat bologna formulated with KSS had textural characteristics more similar to the control than those with KNC.

The use of carbohydrate derivatives such as maltodextrin to replace fat in reduced-fat (30% to 12% and 5%) frankfurters was reported by Crehan et al. (2000). Reducing the fat from 30% to 5% increased cook loss and decreased emulsion stability. Panelists detected a decrease in overall texture and overall acceptability as well as an increase in juiciness, when the fat level was reduced from 30% to 5%. Texture profile analysis showed a decrease in hardness, chewiness and gumminess and an increase in springiness with decreasing fat

© Woodhead Publishing Limited, 2011

level. Maltodextrin addition caused a significant decrease in cook loss but also decreased the emulsion stability. An interactive effect was seen between fat level and maltodextrin, resulting in no significant difference in hardness, gumminess and chewiness values when maltodextrin was present in the reduced-fat frankfurters. The authors concluded that maltodextrin can be used as a suitable fat replacer since it offset some of the changes brought about by fat reduction (i.e. decreasing cook loss and maintaining a number of the textural and sensory characteristics of the frankfurters).

Enzyme-modified potato starch (MPS) was evaluated at 2% and 4% as a fat replacer in reduced-fat (30% to 15% and 10%) emulsion-type sausage (Liu *et al.*, 2008). The 15% and 5% fat sausages containing 2% MPS had a similar hardness to the 30% fat control. Sensory evaluation indicated that the presence of MPS in reduced-fat sausages increased the product's tenderness. Overall, the 15% fat sausage with 2% MPS was comparable to the 30% fat control in color, texture profile and sensory properties, but was lower in energy, suggesting that the MPS can be used as a potential fat replacer in emulsified sausages. Roller and Swinton (1990) also conducted specific enzymatic modifications (at 65°C) of potato starch for the production of fat mimetics. The hydrolyzed potato starch with dextrose equivalent (DE) of 6.0 was used in laboratory formulated full-fat and low-fat sausages, which compared favorably with commercial samples when assessed by a trained panel.

Overall, some starches can help provide the mouthfeel of high-fat emulsions in low-fat or fat-free products and lend a glossy, fat-like appearance (Tharanathan, 2005). The advantages of enzyme-modified starches are that they can have specific functional and sensory properties compared to other carbohydrate-based products on the market (e.g. unmodified starches, fiber-based materials). Certain enzyme-modified potato starches can perform well in high-moisture foods, such as meat emulsion-type sausages. Some new commercial starch preparations, recently introduced on to the market, claim that they are miscible with fat/oil and can form a thermo-stable gel with a smooth, fat-like texture and natural taste.

In developing a low-fat fish sausage Cardoso *et al.* (2008) evaluated the use of 4% of dietary fiber obtained from inner pea (DF-P), different levels of pork meat replacement (0%, 50% and 100%) by hake fish mince and the combination of varying amounts of dietary fiber obtained from chicory root (DF-CR) and hake minces (DF-CR: to hake mince ratio, 2.6:5.2, 5.2:2.6 and 7.8:0.0, % w/w) as a substitute for pork fat. They indicated that adding DF-P to pork sausage favored greater gel strength and hardness. On the contrary, increasing levels of pork meat replacement by hake fish mince reduced the sausages' gel strength and hardness. Sausages without pork fat showed promising textural and color parameters. High-DF-CR sausages were less cohesive and chewable than pork fat sausages (control) but also exhibited a greater gel strength. Low-DF-CR sausages presented almost all textural properties similar to the control, with the exception of hardness and gumminess. Their conclusion was that it is possible to produce low-fat fish sausages similar to ordinary pork sausages.

The use of fiber derived from lemon (lemon albedo, a high-fiber part of the citrus fruit peel) as a source of fiber and potentially as a fat replacer was reported by

Fernández-Ginés *et al.* (2004). They used raw and cooked albedo at 0%, 2.5%, 5.0%, 7.5% and 10% level. The formulations that provided sensory qualities similar to the conventional sausages were produced with 2.5% and 5.0% raw albedo and 2.5%, 5.0% and 7.5% cooked albedo (Fig. 11.2). Other authors have also worked on

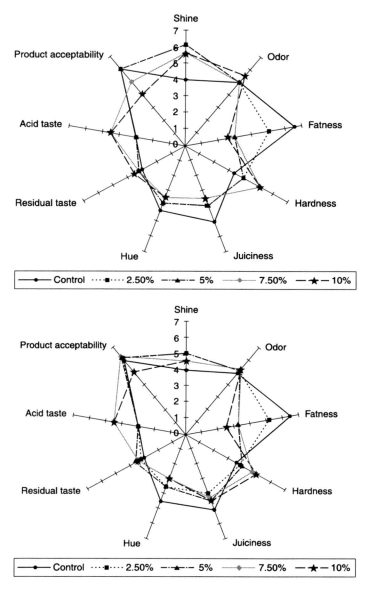

Fig. 11.2 Sensory evaluation results of quantitative descriptive analysis carried out in bologna sausages formulated with different raw (top) and cooked (bottom) lemon-albedo concentrations. From Fernández-Ginés *et al.*, 2004 (with permission).

© Woodhead Publishing Limited, 2011

incorporating this ingredient to sausages and, as mentioned before, some of the citrus fiber products can bind up to four to seven times the weight in water.

The combined effects of carbohydrate and protein-based ingredients has also been studied in ground-meat products (see previous section) and in emulsion products as this approach can usually better mimic the mouthfeel and textural characteristics of a regular fat product. Protein-based fat replacements appear to offer several advantages to low-fat products; however, improvements to textural characteristics (reduced cohesiveness, hardness and springiness) are still required. Carballo *et al.* (1995) examined the combined effects of fat reduction (7 to 22%), starch (0 to 10%) and egg white (0.6 to 3.0%) addition into a bologna-type sausage while employing a surface response methodology approach to study those combined effects. Of the three variables studied, starch most influenced binding and textural properties. Starch reduced cooking loss and purge loss during storage, as well as increasing hardness, chewiness and penetration force. Egg white helped to increase hardness, chewiness and penetration force but did not affect binding properties. Each individual variable was generally not influenced by the other two. Using this kind of surface response approach allows evaluation of the cumulative effect of different additives, which is helpful when using several ingredients at the same time. Claus and Hunt (1991) reported on using isolated soy protein, oat fiber, pea fiber, commercial dietary fiber, wheat starch and modified starch to enhance the textural and sensory characteristics of low-fat (10%), high-water-added (30%) bologna. Test products were less firm than the high-fat control but more firm than the low-fat control. Fiber-containing bolognas were more grainy and less juicy than the high-fat control. Commercial dietary fiber and oat fiber had greater cooking losses than the low-fat control, but purge was reduced by all test ingredients, particularly modified starch. Lower vacuum level in packages also resulted in less purge. The authors concluded that 'test ingredients had beneficial effects on properties of low-fat, high-added-water bologna, thus providing a way to alter product characteristics'.

The effects of CMC and two types of microcrystalline cellulose (MCC-I and II) were investigated in low-fat (13% vs. 26%) frankfurters (Barbut and Mittal, 1996). Fat was replaced with water in the low-fat products. Moisture loss during cooking was reduced in low-fat products from 10% to 6% due to CMC addition; however, both MCCs increased overall moisture loss by 12 to 15%. Product hardness, brittleness, gumminess and chewiness increased with the decrease in fat level. MCC-II improved the textural properties of the low-fat product over those of the high-fat product. Sensory panel results indicated a decrease in tenderness with low fat and this was not improved by MCC-II. The viscoelastic properties (relaxation time, elastic moduli) were not found to be affected by the level of fat reduction used here.

Lin *et al.* (1988) examined the use of four types of CMC with varying degrees of substitution (DS) and molecular weights (250,000 to 700,000) in low-fat, high-moisture and high-protein frankfurters. Generally speaking, as the CMC molecular weight decreased, the emulsion stability also decreased;

© Woodhead Publishing Limited, 2011

however, processing yield and proximate composition of the products were not significantly affected by the treatments. With the exception of springiness and cohesiveness, addition of the CMC significantly decreased the textural parameters, but there were no textural differences in frankfurters due to molecular weights or degree of substitution of the CMC. The ability to soften low-fat frankfurters demonstrated the potential for inclusion of CMC in low-fat meat emulsion products.

Cofrades *et al.* (2000) reported on the effects of fat level reduction (30% to 12% and 5%), carrageenan, and oat fiber combination in frankfurters. Overall textural acceptability decreased as fat level was reduced. Carrageenan and oat fiber improved the acceptability of the 12% fat frankfurters, but neither ingredient offset the detrimental effects on texture acceptability when fat was reduced to 5%. Carrageenan and oat fiber differed in their effects on texture profile analysis values but the latter was more effective at improving texture. The results demonstrate that carrageenan and oat fiber can partially offset some of the textural changes which occur in low-fat frankfurters when added water replaces fat and the protein level remains constant. The results also emphasize the point that there is a limit to fat reduction. An 8 to 10% limit is currently used by quite a few meat companies in their production of reduced-fat meat products. That should also withstand the tough cost constraints in this highly competitive market of emulsified meat products (e.g. bologna, hotdogs).

Nowak *et al.* (2007) replaced fat with inulin and also studied the effects of substituting citrate for phosphate in a traditional German-type mortadella. Fat was replaced with increasing amounts of inulin (used as a frozen gel) to yield 3%, 6%, 9% and 12% inulin in the final product. Replacing fat with inulin led to significant calorie reductions of up to 47.5% (with 12% inulin). However, the sensory properties were also different from those of the control; fracturability fell, hardness and adhesiveness rose, and the product became darker. In any case, the substitution of citrate for phosphate significantly reduced the negative effects of inulin. The sensory attributes (texture, color) of the 6% inulin-citrate sausages were comparable to the control sausages, and the sausages were microbiologically stable for three weeks of storage. The study illustrates the overall point that certain dietary fibers, such as inulin, can be useful in maintaining the organoleptic qualities of fat and also contribute other health benefits (Beylot, 2005). It is also interesting to mention that inulin has been used to improve the stability of foams and emulsions, and in a gel form it also displays exceptional fat-like characteristics.

11.5   Sausages – dry fermented (e.g. summer sausage, dry salami)

In dry fermented meat products there are different requirements from the fat/oil used, especially as the products go through acidification (fermentation by lactic acid bacteria), subsequent slow drying and expected long shelf-life, often at room

© Woodhead Publishing Limited, 2011

temperature. Muguerza *et al.* (2001) produced six Chorizo de Pamplona, a traditional Spanish fermented sausage, by replacing 0%, 10%, 15%, 20%, 25% and 30% of pork back-fat with pre-emulsified olive oil, using soy protein isolates for pre-emulsification. Sausages with 10–25% substitution were acceptable from a sensory point of view. It was concluded that up to 25% of pork back-fat could be replaced with pre-emulsified olive oil. Higher replacing levels were unacceptable due to considerable dripping of fat during the ripening process. Cholesterol content showed a reduction of about 12% in sausages with 20–25% replacement level as well as a significantly lower saturated fatty acid level.

Fat reduction in dry fermented sausages is usually more difficult because replacement of fat by lean meat further increases the hardness of the product due to the high water loss during ripening and drying. Mendoza *et al.* (2001) used inulin in low-fat, dry fermented sausages prepared with a 50% and 75% fat reduction. The 75% reduced fat batch was supplemented with different amounts of the soluble dietary fiber as both a powder and in an aqueous solution. Ripening was followed by physico-chemical and microbiological analysis. Sensory analysis indicated an overall improvement in the sensory properties due to a softer texture provided by inulin. Texture profile analysis results for tenderness, springiness and adhesiveness were similar to the conventional high-fat sausage. Thus, with the addition of inulin a low-calorie product (30% of the original), enriched with soluble dietetic fibre (~10%), could be produced.

In a later study, acceptable dry meat products were developed, reaching a 25% substitution of pork back-fat with pre-emulsified soy oil (Muguerza *et al.*, 2003). However, the maximum effective substitution level (with olive oil) proposed in the literature is around 40–50% of the total fat. Higher levels of oil provoked a dripping effect, perspiration through the casings, inhibition of molds, separation of the casing from the meat batter and breaking up of the cured products. For this reason, the next approach was to capture/trap some of the oil using a separate protein or carbohydrate base matrix.

Del Nobile *et al.* (2009) used that approach to retain olive oil and replace pork back-fat in dry Italian salami. They used whey protein-based crumb or white bread crumb to absorb the oil. Five types of salamis were manufactured, under commercial conditions, by replacing 0% (control), 60% and 100% of pork back-fat with whey protein-based crumb (WP60, WP100) and white pan bread (PB60, PB100). Results indicated that pH, weight loss, color and microbial counts did not significantly change between the control and the modified salamis. Modified salamis resulted in a better fatty acid profile (lower saturated and higher monounsaturated fatty acids) than control (Table 11.2). The control showed the highest values for Warner-Bratzler shear, hardness, cohesiveness, gumminess and chewiness. Textural evaluations of the WP60 did not reveal significant differences compared to the control, whereas PB100 and WP100 were unacceptable for taste. This is an important step as some dry fermented products show high fat content per serving and fat reduction is attractive to the customer.

© Woodhead Publishing Limited, 2011

Table 11.2   Effect of fat replacement on chemical composition (%) fatty acids, texture and sensory parameters of dry Italian salami manufactured with traditional formulation and with substitution of pork back-fat with whey protein-based crumb (WP60–WP100) and pan bread (PB60–PB100) respectively, soaked in oil (60% and 100%) (means ± SEM)

	Control	PB100	PB60	WP100	WP60	SEM	Effect-*P*
Moisture	26.01 d	37.40 a	31.11 b	28.39 c	27.50 cd	0.52	**
Fat	27.98 b	25.99 c	23.64 d	29.84 a	28.26 b	0.48	***
Protein	38.52 a	30.88 c	38.48 a	34.92 b	37.42 a	0.38	**
Ash	7.49 a	5.73 b	6.77 a	6.85 a	6.73 a	0.26	*
SFA	40.37 a	26.81 c	30.39 b	25.26 c	29.33 b	0.54	***
MUFA	46.54 c	63.07 a	57.87 b	64.84 a	58.62 b	0.72	**
PUFA	13.09 a	10.12 c	11.74 b	9.90 c	12.03 b	0.25	**
			Sensory				
Hardness	97.85 a	55.98 c	82.26 b	40.69 d	73.93 b	0.32	**
Cohesiveness	0.25 a	0.17 c	0.15 c	0.20 b	0.16 c	0.01	*
Gumminess	24.46 a	9.55 c	11.95 b	8.28 c	11.83 b	0.06	**
Color[a]	7.18 a	6.31 b	7.31 a	5.93 b	6.89 ab	0.19	***
Odor[a]	7.03 a	6.00 b	6.65 a	5.84 b	6.67 a	0.20	***
Taste[a]	7.07 a	5.61 c	6.38 b	5.68 c	6.57 ab	0.22	***

* $P < 0.05$, ** $P < 0.01$, *** $P < 0.001$. SFA = saturated fatty acids; MUFA = mono unsaturated fatty acids; PUFA = polyunsaturated fatty acids.
[a] Score: 1, extremely dislike

Source: Del Nobile *et al.*, 2009.

11.6   Prepared and coated meat products (e.g. nuggets, pies)

In the area of prepared and coated products there has been an emphasis on reducing the fat added or absorbed during processing. Since fried foods such as chicken nuggets can absorb quite a lot of oil during their preparation, various attempts have been made to reduce oil uptake during frying. This is no small challenge because, as the product is fried, water rapidly evaporates from the surface and the voids are usually filled with oil. Sahin *et al.* (2005) studied the effects of various gums (guar gum, methylcellulose, xanthan gum, gum arabic) on the quality of deep-fat-fried chicken nuggets. Chicken breast portions were coated with batters composed of a 3:5 solid to water ratio by immersion. The solid content of batter formulations contained equal amounts of corn and wheat flours, 1.0% gum, 1.0% salt and 0.5% leavening agent. As a control, batter without gum addition was used. Samples were fried at 180°C for 3, 6, 9 and 12 minutes. The hardness and oil content of the chicken nuggets increased whereas the moisture content decreased during frying. Methylcellulose and xanthan gums significantly reduced oil absorption compared with other gums and the control. When gum arabic was added to the batter formulation, a product with the highest oil content and porosity was obtained.

© Woodhead Publishing Limited, 2011

Later, Mah *et al.* (2008) examined the effectiveness of a whey protein isolate (WPI) solution as a post-breading dip to reduce oil absorption in deep-fried, battered and breaded chicken patties. Chicken patties were battered, breaded with either crackermeal or Japanese breadcrumbs, and dipped in WPI solutions prepared at four different protein concentrations (0%, 2.5%, 5% and 10%, w/w WPI) that were adjusted to pHs 2, 3 and 8 before being deep fried. Undipped chicken patties served as the control. Overall, the most effective treatment was observed for WPI solutions made at high concentrations (5% and 10% WPI) at low pH levels (pHs 2 and 3). The highest lipid reduction observed for crackermeal patties (CMP) was 31.2%, seen in patties treated with 5% protein solutions at pH 2, while the highest lipid reduction for Japanese breadcrumb patties (JBP) was 37.5%, seen in patties treated with 10% protein solutions at pH 2. Oil degradation and batter, breading and whey pickup did not significantly affect final lipid and moisture content. Moisture content was generally lower in patties treated at low pH levels (pHs 2 and 3). The results indicate that the usage of WPI as a post-breading dip is a promising alternative in reducing fat content in fried foods. In a subsequent publication the authors also reported on the sensory characteristics of these treatments and showed that the only perceivable changes in treated patties were related to color, some hardness, and crunchiness properties (Mah and Brannan, 2009). Increasing WPI concentration caused darkening of JBP but made CMP lighter. Patties treated at pH 8 were significantly darker across all WPI concentrations. The presence of WPI increased hardness and crust fracture for CMP but not JBP. The former could probably be corrected by reducing crumb use.

In another study the use of whey protein, as an additional coating, in combination with basic, well-described pre-dust, batter and breading ingredients, for fat uptake reduction in fried chicken was investigated (Dragich and Krochta, 2010). Chicken breasts were cut into strips and coated with wheat flour (WF) as a pre-dust, dipped in batter, coated with WF as a breading, then dipped in 10% denatured whey protein isolate (DWPI) aqueous solution. Coated chicken strips were deep fried at 160°C for five minutes. Fat content of the meat fraction of fried samples, the coating fraction of fried samples, raw chicken and raw coating ingredients were determined. The WF-batter-WF-10% DWPI solution had significantly lower fat uptake than the WF-batter-WF control, by 31% on a dry basis. Overall, it was demonstrated that it is possible to achieve fat reduction while maintaining a simple procedure applicable to actual food processing lines. It should be mentioned that the food industry is currently using and evaluating various ingredients (e.g. modified starches, gums) to reduce oil absorption in fried foods (e.g. nuggets and French fries).

In the area of meat pies and similar products where meat is used as a filler, the idea is also to reduce total fat and/or form a more favorable fatty acid profile. The same approaches mentioned above for ground-meat products and sausages have been employed. Since other ingredients such as vegetables and gravy are included it is sometimes easier to incorporate gums, fiber and starches to create a creamy texture that will mimic some of the fat characteristics. Overall, as in sausages, not all the animal fat is usually replaced as it contributes to some of the unique flavor and textural properties. In any case, there are not many scientific papers published

© Woodhead Publishing Limited, 2011

in the area of meat pies. This might be because of the overlap of meat, vegetables and pastry. However, most ingredient suppliers have quite a lot of practical proprietary information regarding formulations. As indicated before, an increasingly popular ingredient used today for fat reduction is fiber (e.g. inulin, citrus fiber, pea fiber) which can have the ability to bind four to seven times its weight in water, enhance mouthfeel (e.g. provide a smooth, creamy texture) and is used as an ingredient to boost nutritional claims.

In conclusion, various combinations of carbohydrates (e.g. starches, hydrocolloid gums, fiber) have been demonstrated to offer some solutions for fat reduction in meat products either alone or in combination with non-meat proteins and/or modification in processing conditions. As can be seen in this chapter, the industry continues to look at optimizing ingredient combinations in order to maximize water-binding, textural characteristics, flavor perception, cook yield and shelf-life.

11.7   Future trends

Over the past two to three decades, scientists and product developers have been working on finding ways to reduce fat content and/or improve the fatty acid profile of a variety of meat products. During the last ten years there has been more pressure on the food industry to come up with improved low-/no-fat food products (e.g. dairy, baked goods, meat). The formation of an acceptable texture and flavor are essential in gaining market acceptability and sustainability for low-fat products. As described in this chapter, various carbohydrates (starches, gums, fiber) and proteins as well as non-digestive fats have been tried and some combinations have been successful in the marketplace. Work on better understanding the contribution of fat to the rheological and flavor characteristics of meat products will continue along with the search for new ingredients/combinations. Substitution with vegetable oils is gaining more acceptance in the marketplace as a way to get a more attractive nutritional profile. Olive oil, for example, is one of the most monounsaturated vegetable oils. It contains 55–85% monounsaturated fatty acids, 8–25% saturated and 3–21% polyunsaturated fatty acids and is rich in tocopherols and phenolic substances (antioxidants). It also has a high biological value attributed to its high ratio of vitamin E to polyunsaturated fatty acids content and shows beneficial effects on postprandial lipid metabolism and thrombosis. Whatever the approach is, the positive effects for consumer health should be the main driver. Improving meat products with a simultaneous reduction in fat level, partial replacement of some animal fat with vegetable oils, and the inclusion of beneficial dietary components (e.g. fiber) seem to be the main approaches currently employed.

11.8   Sources of further information

Material cited in the chapter ranges from studies concerning the understanding of fat flavor perception (receptor level) to practical experiments involving the use of

© Woodhead Publishing Limited, 2011

various formulations and trying to explain the role of individual ingredients. Ingredient suppliers also have information that is usually kept confidential, but can be accessed by clients from the meat industry (some is available on the web). Future developments will be dictated by the marketplace and the ability of the meat industry to deliver products that are perceived to be of high value in terms of texture, flavor, cost and improved nutrition profile.

11.9   References

Abiola S S, and Adegbaju S W (2001), Effect of substituting pork backfat with rind-on quality characteristics of pork sausage. *Meat Sci*, 58, 409–12.

Ahmed P O, Miller M F, Lyon C E, Vaughters H M and Reagan J O (1990), Physical and sensory characteristics of low-fat fresh pork sausage processed with various levels of added water, *J Food Sci*, 55, 625–8.

Ambrosiadis J, Vareltzis K P and Georgakis S A (1996), Physical, chemical and sensory characteristics of cooked meat emulsion style products containing vegetable oils, *Int J Food Sci Technol*, 31, 189–94.

Barbut S (2002), *Poultry Products Processing*, New York, CRC Press, 256–72.

Barbut S and Mittal G S (1992), Use of carrageenans and xanthan gums in reduced fat breakfast sausage, *Food Sci Technol*, 25, 509–13.

Barbut S and Mittal G S (1996), Effects of three cellulose gums on the texture profile and sensory properties of low fat frankfurters, *Int J Food Sci Technol*, 31, 241–7. doi: 10.1046/j.1365+2621.1996.00337.x.

Bernal V M, Smajda C H, Smith J L and Stanley D W (1987), Interactions in protein/ polysaccharide/calcium gels, *J Food Sci*, 52, 1121–5, 1136.

Berry B W (1992), Low fat level effects on sensory, shear, cooking, and chemical properties of ground beef patties, *J Food Sci*, 57, 537–40, 574.

Berry B W and Leddy K F (1984), Effects of fat level and cooking method on sensory and textural properties of ground-beef patties, *J Food Sci*, 49, 870–5.

Berry B W and Wergin W P (1993), Modified pregelatinized potato starch in low-fat ground beef patties, *J Muscle Foods*, 4, 305–20. doi: 10.1111/j.1745-4573.1993.tb00511.x

Beylot M (2005), Effects of inulin-type fructans on lipid metabolism in man and in animal models, *Brit J Nutr*, 93(Suppl 1), S163–8.

Bishop D J, Olson D G and Knipe C L (1993), Pre-emulsified corn oil, pork fat, or added moisture affect quality of reduced fat bologna quality, *J Food Sci*, 58(3), 484–7. doi: 10.1111/j.1365-2621.1993.tb04306.x

Bloukas J G, and Paneras E D (1993), Substituting olive oil for pork for pork backfat affects quality of low-fat frankfurters, *J Food Sci*, 58, 705–9.

Bloukas J G, Paneras E D and Fournitzis G C (1997), Effect of replacing pork backfat with olive oil on processing and quality characteristics of fermented sausages, *Meat Sci*, 45, 133–44.

Bonifer L J, Froning G W, Mandigo R W, Cuppett S L and Meagher M M (1996), Textural, color, and sensory properties of bologna containing various levels of washed chicken skin, *Poult Sci*, 75(8), 1047–51.

Carballo J, Barreto G and Jiménez-Colmenero F (1995), Starch and egg white influence on properties of bologna sausage as related to fat content, *J Food Sci*, 60(4), 673–7. doi:10.1111/j.1365-2621.1995.tb06204.x

Cardoso C, Mendes R and Nunes M L (2008), Development of a healthy low-fat fish sausage containing dietary fibre, *Int J Food Sci Technol*, 43, 276–83. doi:10.1111/j.1365-2621.2006.01430.x

© Woodhead Publishing Limited, 2011

Cheftal J C, Cug J L and Lorient D (1985), Amino acids, peptides and proteins, in Fennema O R (Ed.), *Food Chemistry – 2nd ed.*, New York, Marcel Dekker Inc., 245–369.

Chin K B, Keeton J T, Miller R K, Longnecker M T and Lamkey J W (2000), Evaluation of konjac blends and soy protein isolate as fat replacements in low-fat bologna, *J Food Sci*, 65(5), 756–63.

Claus J R and Hunt M C (1991), Low-fat, high added-water bologna formulated with texture-modifying ingredients, *J Food Sci*, 56(3), 643–52.

Claus J R, Hunt M C and Kastner C L (1989), Effects of substituting added water for fat on the textural, sensory and processing characteristics of bologna, *J Musc Food*, 1, 1–21.

Crehan C M, Hughes E, Troy D J and Buckley D J (2000), Effects of fat level and maltodextrin on the functional properties of frankfurters formulated with 5, 12 and 30% fat, *Meat Sci*, 55(4), 463–69.

Cofrades S, Carballo J and Jiménez-Colmenero F (1997), Heating rate effects on high-fat and low-fat frankfurters with a high content of added water, *Meat Sci*, 47(1–2), 105–14.

Cofrades S, Hughes E and Troy D J (2000), Effects of oat fibre and carrageenan on the texture of frankfurters formulated with low and high fat, *Eur Food Res Technol*, 211(1), 19–26.

DeFreitas Z, Sebranek J G, Olson D G and Carr J M (1997), Carrageenan effects on salt-soluble meat proteins in model systems, *J Food Sci*, 62, 539–43.

Del Nobile M A, Conte A, Incoronato A L, Panza O, Sevi A and Marino R (2009), New strategies for reducing the pork back-fat content in typical Italian salami, *Meat Sci*, 81(1), 263–9. doi: 10.1016/j.meatsci.2008.07.026

Dragich A M, Krochta J M (2010), Whey protein solution coating for fat-uptake reduction in deep-fried chicken breast strips, *J Food Sci*, 75(1), 43–50. doi: 10.1111/j.1750-3841.2009.01408.x

Dransfield E (2008), The taste of fat, *Meat Sci*, 80(1), 37–42. doi: 10.1016/j.meatsci.2008.05.030

Egbert W R, Huffman D L, Chen C-M and Dylewski D P (1991), Development of low fat ground beef, *Food Technol*, 45, 64–71.

Fernández-Ginés J M, Fernández-López J, Sayas-Barberá E, Sendra E and Pérez-Álvarez J A (2004), Lemon albedo as a new source of dietary fiber: Application to bologna sausages, *Meat Sci*, 67(1), 7–13. doi: 10.1016/j.meatsci.2003.08.017

Foegeding E A and Ramsey S R (1986), Effect of gums on low-fat meat batters, *J Food Sci*, 51, 33–6, 46.

Giese J (1992), Developing low-fat meat products, *Food Technol*, 46, 100–8.

Giese J (1996), Fats and fat replacers: balancing the health benefits, *Food Technol*, 50(9), 76–8.

Hammer G F (1992), Processing vegetable oils into frankfurter-type sausages, *Fleischwirtschaft*, 72, 1258–65.

Hsu S Y and Chung H-Y (1999), Comparisons of 13 edible gum-hydrate fat substitutes for low fat kung-wan (an emulsified meatball), *J Food Eng*, 40(4), 279–85.

Hsu S Y, Yu S H (2002), Comparisons on 11 plant oil fat substitutes for low-fat kung-wans, *J Food Eng*, 51(3), 215–20.

Huffman D L and Egbert W R (1990), Chemical analysis and sensory evaluation of the developed lean ground beef products, in *Advances in Lean Ground Beef Production*. Alabama Agric Exp Sta Bull No. 606, Auburn University, Alabama, USA.

Hughes E, Mullen A M and Troy D J (1998), Effects of fat level, tapioca starch and whey protein on frankfurters formulated with 5% and 12% fat, *Meat Sci*, 48, 169–80.

Jiménez-Colmenero F (2007), Healthier lipid formulation approaches in meat-based functional foods. Technological options for replacement of meat fats by non-meat fats, *Trends Food Sci Technol*, 18, 567–78.

Keeton J T (1994), Low-fat meat products – technological problems with processing, *Meat Sci*, 36, 261–76.

Lin K C, Keeton J T, Gilchrist C L and Cross H R (1988), Comparisons of carboxymethyl cellulose with differing molecular features in low-fat frankfurters, *J Food Sci*, 53(6), 1592–5. doi: 10.1111/j.1365-2621.1988.tb07792.x

Liu H, Xiong Y L, Jiang L and Kong B (2008), Fat reduction in emulsion sausage using an enzyme-modified potato starch, *J Sci Food Agric*, 88, 1632–7. doi: 10.1002/jsfa

Lyons P H, Kerry J F, Morrissey P A and Buckley DJ (1999), The influence of added whey protein/carrageenan gels and tapioca starch on the textural properties of low fat pork sausages. *Meat Sci*, 51(1), 43–53.

Mah E, Price J and Brannan, R.G (2008), Reduction of oil absorption in deep-fried, battered, and breaded chicken patties using whey protein isolate as a postbreading dip: effect on lipid and moisture content, *J Food Sci*, 73(8), S412–8.

Mah E and Brannan, R.G (2009), Reduction of oil absorption in deep-fried, battered, and breaded chicken patties using whey protein isolate as a postbreading dip: effect on flavor, color and texture, *J Food Sci*, 74(1), S9–16. doi: 10.1111/j.1750-3841.2008.00973.x

Marquez E J, Ahmed E M, West R L and Johnson D D (1989), Emulsion stability and sensory quality of beef frankfurters produced at different fat or peanut oil levels, *J Food Sci*, 54, 867–70, 873.

Mendoza E, García M L, Casas C and Selgas M D (2001), Inulin as fat substitute in low fat, dry fermented sausages, *Meat Sci*, 57(4), 387–93.

Minerich P L, Addis P B, Epley R J and Bingham C (1991), *J Food Sci*, 56, 1154–7.

Morin L A, Temelli F and McMullen L (2004), Interactions between meat proteins and barley (Hordeum spp.) β-glucan within a reduced-fat breakfast sausage system, *Meat Sci*, 68(3), 419–30.

Mottram D S (1998), Flavor formation in meat and meat products: a review, *Food Chem*, 62, 415–24.

Muguerza E, Gimeno O, Ansorena D, Bloukas J G and Astiasaran I (2001), Effect of replacing pork backfat with pre-emulsified olive oil on lipid fraction and sensory quality of Chorizo de Pamplona – a traditional Spanish fermented sausage, *Meat Sci*, 59(3), 251–8.

Muguerza E, Ansorena, D and Astiasaran I (2003), Improvement of nutritional properties of Chorizo de Pamplona by replacement of pork backfat with soy oil, *Meat Sci*, 65, 1361–7.

Nowak B, von Mueffling T, Grotheer J, Klein G and Watkinson B –M (2007), Energy content, sensory properties, and microbiological shelf life of German bologna-type sausages produced with citrate or phosphate and with inulin as fat replacer, *J Food Sci*, 72(9). doi: 10.1111/j.1750-3841.2007.00566.x.

Osburn W N (1992), Evaluation of physical, chemical, sensory and microbial characteristics of low-fat precooked lamb and fresh pork sausages made with konjac flour, MS thesis, Texas A&M University, College Station, Texas, USA.

Osburn W N, Mandigo R W, and Eskridge K M (1997), Pork skin connective tissue gel utilization in reduced-fat bologna. *J Food Sci*, 62, 1176–82.

Paneras E D and Bloukas J G (1994), Vegetable oils replace pork backfat for low-fat frankfurter, *J Food Sci*, 59, 725–8, 733.

Park J, Rhee K S, Keeton J T, and Rhee K C (1989), Properties of low-fat frankfurters containing monounsatured and omega-3 polyunsaturated oils, *J Food Sci*, 54, 500–4.

Pappa I C, Bloukas J G and Arvanitoyannis I S (2000), Optimization of salt, olive oil and pectin level for low-fat frankfurters produced by replacing pork backfat with olive oil, *Meat Sci*, 56, 81–8.

Piñero M P, Parra K, Huerta-Leidenz N, Arenas de Moreno L, Ferrer M, Araujo S and Barboza Y (2008), Effect of oat's soluble fibre (β-glucan) as a fat replacer on physical, chemical, microbiological and sensory properties of low-fat beef patties, *Meat Sci*, 80, 675–80. doi: 10.1016/j.meatsci.2008.03.006

Reitmeier C A and Prusa K J (1987), Cholesterol content and sensory analysis of ground pork as influenced by fat level and heating, *J Food Sci*, 52, 916–18.

© Woodhead Publishing Limited, 2011

Roller S and Swinton S (1990), Enzymes and the food industry: the role of the Leatherhead Food Research Association, *Food Sci Tech Today*, 4, 111–14.

Sánchez-Zapata E, Muñoz C M, Fuentes E, Fernández-López J, Sendra E, Sayas E, Navarro J A and Pérez-Alvarez J A (2010), Effect of tiger nut fibre on quality characteristics of pork burger, *Meat Sci*, 85, 70–6.

Sahin S, Sumnu G and Altunakar B (2005), Effects of batters containing different gum types on the quality of deep-fat fried chicken nuggets, *J Sci Food Agric*, 85, 2375–9.

Severini C, Pilli T D and Baiano A (2003), Partial substitution of pork backfat with extra-virgin olive oil in 'salami' products: effects on chemical, physical and sensorial quality, *Meat Sci*, 64, 323–33.

Tan S S, Aminah A, Affandi Y M S, Atil O and Babji A S (2001), Chemical, physical and sensory properties of chicken frankfurters substituted with palm fats, *Int J Food Sci Nutr*, 52, 91–8.

Tharanathan R N (2005), Starch – value addition by modification, *Crit Rev Food Sci Nutr*, 45, 371–84.

Troutt E S, Hunt M C, Johnson D E, Claus J R, Kastner C L and Kropf D H (1992), Characteristics of low-fat ground beef containing texture-modifying ingredients, *J Food Sci*, 57(1), 19–35.

Tolstoguzov V B (1991), Functional properties of food proteins and role of protein-polysaccharide interaction, *Food Hydrocoll*, 4, 429–68.

USDA (1986), Composition of food: beef products, *Agriculture Handbook Number 8–13*, United States Department of Agriculture, Human Nutrition Service, Hyattsville, Maryland.

Wallingford L and Labuza T P (1983), Evaluation of the water binding properties of food hydrocolloids by physical/chemical methods and in a low fat meat emulsion, *J Food Sci*, 48, 1–5.

Walters B S, Lourigan M M, Racek S R, Schwartz J A and Maurer A J (1992), The fabrication of turkey bacon, *Poult Sci*, 71(2), 383–7.

Whiting R C (1984), Addition of phosphate and gums to reduced salt frankfurter batters, *J Food Sci*, 49, 1355–9.

Wood J D, Enser M, Fisher A V, Nute G R, Sheard P R, Richardson R I, Hughes S I and Whittington F M (2008), Fat deposition, fatty acid composition and meat quality: A review, *Meat Sci*, 78(4), 343–58. doi: 10.1016/j.meatsci.2007.07.019

Xiong Y L, Noel D C and Moody W G (1999), Textural and sensory properties of low-fat beef sausages with added water and polysaccharides as affected by pH and salt, *J Food Sci*, 64(3), 550–4. doi: 10.1111/j.1365-2621.1999.tb15083.x

Youssef M and Barbut S (2009), Effects of protein level and fat/oil on emulsion stability, texture, microstructure and color of meat batters, *Meat Sci*, 82, 228–33.

Youssef M and Barbut S (2010), Physicochemical effects of the lipid phase and protein level on meat emulsion stability, texture, and microstructure, *J. Food Sci.* 75(2), 108–14.

© Woodhead Publishing Limited, 2011

12

Altering animal diet to reduce saturated fat in meat and milk

A. P. Moloney, Teagasc, Ireland

Abstract: The range in saturated fatty acids (SFA) content of beef, pigmeat, chicken meat and bovine milk will be illustrated and the contribution of these foods to consumer SFA consumption summarised. Strategies to decrease the SFA content in meat and milk include inclusion of forage in the ration of ruminants and supplementation of ruminants and monogastrics with polyunsaturated fatty acid (PUFA)-rich oilseeds, fish oil or marine algae. The influences of these manipulations will be illustrated. The chapter will end with a commentary on likely future trends in the SFA content of meat and milk.

Key words: saturated fatty acids, cows, beef, poultry, chicken, milk.

12.1 Introduction

Based on the relationships between dietary fat and the incidence of human disease, particularly coronary heart disease, medical authorities have developed guidelines in relation to fat in the diet. Thus it is recommended that energy intake from total fat should not exceed 30–35%, that energy intake from saturated fatty acids (SFA) should not exceed 10% of total energy intake and that energy intake from monounsaturated fatty acids (MUFA) and polyunsaturated fatty acids (PUFA) should be approximately 16% and 7%, respectively, of energy intake. Furthermore, an increase in omega-3 PUFA consumption such that the ratio of omega-6: omega-3 PUFA is < 4:1 has also been recommended (WHO, 2003). Currently, PUFA and MUFA are generally regarded as beneficial for human health while reducing the intake of SFA and increasing the intake of omega-3 PUFA are particularly encouraged.

Meat is considered to be a good source of protein and micronutrients (including vitamins A, B_6, B_{12}, D, E, and the minerals iron, zinc and selenium). In addition, fat in meat supplies fatty acids that cannot be synthesised by humans and can act as a carrier of lipid-soluble vitamins and antioxidants while it is also an essential

© Woodhead Publishing Limited, 2011

component of the sensory perception of juiciness, flavour and texture. Similarly, milk has long been recognised as a source of fatty acids, amino acids and other nutrients such as calcium. Historically, animal products were considered to be wholesome, versatile foods for humans and important for human health, and consequently meat and milk make a major contribution to population energy consumption, e.g. 23% and 14% (excluding butter), respectively, of total energy consumption by United Kingdom consumers in 2003 (Henderson *et al.*, 2003). Moreover, the consumption of meat and milk is projected to increase at 0.8% and 0.6% per annum, respectively, up to 2010 in the developed world with corresponding projections for the developing world of 3.0 and 2.9% (Delgado, 2005). However, as shown in Table 12.1, meat and milk also contain considerable amounts of SFA. Lean beef, lamb, pork meats and chicken provide similar proportions of MUFA, making meat an important source of these fatty acids. Within the meats, the proportion of SFA can be ranked lamb > beef > pork > chicken. Lean pork has a higher proportion of PUFA than ruminant meat but a lower one than chicken. Cow and goat milk, in contrast, contain up to 70% SFA. However, of the SFA, only lauric acid (C12:0), myristic acid (C14:0) and palmitic acid (C16:0) raise total and low-density lipoprotein cholesterol which are risk factors for coronary heart disease, with C14:0 the most potent, while stearic acid (C18:0) has been shown to be neutral in humans (Bonanome and Grundy, 1988).

Table 12.1   Saturated fatty acid composition of milk and meat (g/100g)

Fatty acid	Cow's milk		Goat's milk	Lean beef	Lean lamb	Lean pork	Chicken	
	Whole	Skimmed					Dark	Light
C4:0	4.0	5.0	2.1	–	–	–	–	–
C6:0	2.6	–	2.4	–	–	–	–	–
C8:0	1.4	–	2.7	–	–	–	–	–
C10:0	3.1	5.0	8.7	–	0.3	–	–	–
C12:0	4.3	5.0	4.8	–	0.6	–	–	–
C14:0	11.7	10.0	10.5	2.7	5.9	1.1	0.8	1.0
C15:0	1.1	–	1.5	0.5	0.8	–	–	–
C16:0	30.2	30.0	27.9	26.2	24.8	23.4	21.0	21.8
C17:0	0.6	–	0.6	1.1	1.3	0.3	0.4	–
C18:0	11.7	15.0	9.3	15.9	20.2	12.7	6.2	6.9
C20:0	–	–	0.3	–	0.2	0.3	–	–
C22:0	–	–	0.3	–	–	–	–	–
SFA	70.7	65.0	71.2	47.0	54.1	38.3	28.8	30.7
MUFA	26.5	30.0	24.9	47.6	40.3	42.3	49.8	47.5
PUFA	2.8	5.0	3.9	5.4	5.6	19.4	21.4	21.8
Fat (%)	4.0	0.3	3.7	4.3	8.0	4.0	2.8	1.1

Source: adapted from MAFF, 1998

© Woodhead Publishing Limited, 2011

For shorter SFA, Steijns (2008) concluded that more research is needed but 'a tentative conclusion would be that saturated dairy fatty acids with a chain length below 10 C-atoms will not significantly contribute to blood lipid levels at actual intakes of dairy products'. Cholesterol-raising SFA represent 46.5%, 28.9%, 24.5% and 22% for cow's milk, lean beef, lean pork and chicken, respectively.

Nevertheless, the SFA content of milk and meat combined with their level of consumption results in them making a large contribution to population SFA consumption. This is illustrated in Table 12.2, which is an extract of data from the EU TRANSFAIR study (Hulshof et al., 1999). While there was considerable variation between EU countries examined, on average, meat and milk contributed 20 and 40% of total SFA consumption. Total energy consumption from SFA exceeded on average the 10% target advised by medical authorities. Animal products are obvious targets therefore for strategies to decrease population SFA consumption. The options appear to be either a decrease in the contribution of animal products to the diet of the population or maintenance of the position of animal products in the diet but a decrease in their SFA concentration. The latter option has provided impetus for an enormous research effort on modifying the fatty acid composition of meat and milk over the past 30 years. Food animal production systems represent the combined and interacting effects of genotype, gender (meat animals), age and nutrition, all of which can contribute to differences in the amount and composition of the fat in animal-derived food. In

Table 12.2 Contribution of milk and meat products to saturated fatty acid consumption by European consumers

Country	SFA intake (g/d)	SFA intake (% energy)	SFA (% from milk)	SFA (% from meat)
Belgium	40.5	15.4	30.2	25.1
Finland	29.0	12.7	44.9	19.5
France	30.1	15.4	56.7	20.2
Germany	44.1	18.1	57.1	18.2
Greece	23.4	11.7	27.4	13.9
Iceland	46.2	17.7	39.8	18.9
Ireland[1]	37.8	14.0	28.1	21.1
Italy	30.9	10.6	47.3	15.3
Netherlands	35.4	14.1	33.9	20.1
Norway	31.7	12.5	41.3	18.6
Portugal	28.1	11.2	32.5	28.1
Spain	33.5	11.7	27.5	29.0
Sweden	32.8	14.8	48.5	17.6
United Kingdom	27.1	13.2	38.8	17.1
Unweighted mean	33.6	13.8	39.6	20.2

[1] Adapted from Joyce et al., 2008

Source: adapted from Hulshof et al., 1999

© Woodhead Publishing Limited, 2011

this chapter, the impact of alterations to the diet of cattle, pigs and chickens on the SFA composition of the resulting meat and milk will be discussed. Where appropriate, examples from the more recent literature will be given with reference to more comprehensive reviews of specific aspects of the discussion made as required.

12.2   The fat content of meat and milk

12.2.1   Meat

The fat content of meat varies with the choice of cut or meat product, the species of animal and the production system through which that animal has come. Fat is present in meat as structural components of the muscle membranes, as storage droplets of triacylglycerol between the muscles (intermuscular fat), as adipose tissue within the muscles (intramuscular fat or marbling) and as subcutaneous fat (under the skin). Most of the fat in adipose tissue is present as glycerol esters but the fat in muscle also contains considerable quantities of phospholipids. The different lipid fractions in muscle are characterised by different fatty acid profiles and the relative proportions of these fractions can confound comparison of dietary treatments. Within a carcass there is considerable variation among muscles in total fat content and in fatty acid composition. In general, the *longissimus dorsi* (striploin) is intermediate in fat content between the semitendinosus (outside round) and the supraspinatus muscle (chuck) (Lawrie, 2006).

12.2.2   Milk

Lipids occur as globules emulsified in the aqueous phase of milk. The globules contain nonpolar or core lipids such as triacylglycerol, cholesterol esters and retinol esters. They are coated with bipolar materials, phospholipids, proteins, cholesterol, enzymes, etc., into a loose layer called the milk lipid globule membrane. This membrane prevents the globules from coalescing and acts as an emulsion stabiliser. Ruminant milk fat contains an array of individual fatty acids that differ primarily in chain length and number and orientation of unsaturated bonds. Over 95% by mass of the fatty acids are esterified in triacylglycerol while the remainder are found in phospholipid, cholesterol ester, diacylglycerol, monoacylglycerol and free fatty acids. Short- and medium-chain fatty acids (4 to 14 carbons) and a portion of the 16-carbon fatty acids are derived from *de novo* synthesis from acetate and to a lesser extent β-hydroxybutyrate. On a molar basis, about half of milk fatty acids are synthesised *de novo*. Preformed fatty acids account for the remaining 16-carbon and all the longer-chain fatty acids (>16 carbons), and are taken up from the circulating plasma pool. These originate from absorption from the digestive tract or mobilisation from body reserves (Givens and Shingfield, 2006).

© Woodhead Publishing Limited, 2011

12.3   Dietary effects on the fat content and fatty acid composition of meat

12.3.1   Fat content

Within a species, the degree of fat deposition in the animal is determined by genotype, the weight of the carcass and how close the animal is to its ultimate mature size when slaughtered. In animal production systems which evolve to optimise economic efficiency, several of these factors may vary and interactions between these factors and nutrition are likely and should also be considered. When examining the effects of diet on the fat content of meat it is important to separate the direct effects of dietary ingredients from indirect effects of possible differences in energy and/or protein intake on carcass weight and fatness. Carcass fatness in ruminants and monogastrics can be influenced by the energy and protein concentration in the diet. In pigs, restricting the energy intake by feeding a low-energy (low fat and/or high fibre) diet while supplying adequate protein will reduce carcass fat deposition. Feeding excess protein, i.e. excess essential amino acids, to pigs will result in a higher proportion of lean to fat in the carcass but the effect is primarily a result of energy restriction relative to protein. The converse, restricting protein supply while supplying adequate energy, will increase fat deposition (Teye *et al.*, 2006).

Knowledge of energy and amino acid nutrition of ruminants is not as advanced as for monogastrics mainly due to pre-fermentation and transformation of dietary ingredients in the rumen of ruminants. Nevertheless, there is a body of evidence that unwilted, extensively fermented grass silage can increase fatness relative to wilted silage/hay or non-silage-based diets and that high-starch ingredients promote greater fatness than digestible fibre-based ingredients. In a grass silage-based ration, protein supplied in excess of requirement increased carcass fatness (Steen and Robson, 1995). Increasing propionate supply from the rumen by addition of sodium propionate to the diet decreased fat deposition (Moloney, 1998; 2002). In general for any particular ration, an increase in intake by a meat-producing animal will promote a higher growth rate and a fatter carcass (at a similar carcass weight), i.e. growth rate *per se* will increase fat deposition relative to protein deposition (Owens *et al.*, 1995). However, there is some opportunity to decrease fatness by manipulating the growth path relatively close to slaughter. Thus Moloney *et al.* (2008) reported that, compared to cattle finished on a grass silage and concentrate ration, feeding unsupplemented silage for 56 days followed by the same amount of concentrates offered *ad libitum* decreased internal fat weight and *longissimus dorsi* lipid concentration. This also illustrates the close association between whole-body fat deposition and intramuscular fat concentration. Clearly, one strategy to decrease the SFA content in meat is to produce leaner meat!

12.3.2   Saturated fatty acids in beef

In general, increasing fat deposition in a meat animal results in greater unsaturation of lipids, with the MUFA proportion increasing and SFA proportion decreasing.

© Woodhead Publishing Limited, 2011

This is illustrated by the data in Table 12.3. In this study, dairy steers from medium maturing breed sires (Holstein/Friesian) and late-maturing breed sires (Belgian Blue) were slaughtered at two weights and the fatty acid composition of the *longissimus* muscle examined. On average, the total fatty acid concentration was higher for the earlier maturing breed. For both breeds, increasing slaughter weight increased the concentration of fatty acids but the increase was considerably less for the later maturing breed. The increase in intramuscular fat was accompanied by a decrease in the SFA and PUFA proportions and an increase in the MUFA proportion in both breeds. Comparisons between dietary treatments are often confounded by such differences in fatty acid composition resulting from differences in intramuscular fat. Breed differences and effects of maturity or growth stage on the subcutaneous or intramuscular fatty acid composition of beef have been reviewed by de Smet *et al.* (2004), who concluded that much of the difference in fatty acid composition apparently due to genotype could be explained by variation in intramuscular fat concentration and that effects of genotype were in general much smaller than effects due to diet. One strategy to decrease the SFA content in meat animals, particularly cattle and pigs, is to use late-maturing breeds and slaughter them at lighter weights. This may not be economically attractive in many production environments.

In ruminants, dietary MUFA and PUFA are hydrogenated to SFA but a proportion of dietary unsaturated fatty acids bypasses the rumen intact and is absorbed and deposited in body fat (e.g. Noci *et al.*, 2005a). Increasing the dietary supply of unsaturated fatty acids is one strategy to increase MUFA and PUFA concentrations in ruminant meat, which may be accompanied by a decrease in SFA concentration.

Table 12.3   Saturated fatty acid composition of intramuscular lipids from *M. longissimus dorsi* from Holstein/Friesian (HF) or Belgian Blue (BB) × Holstein steers slaughtered at two target bodyweights (mg/100g muscle, proportions in parentheses)

Fatty acid	HF: Slaughter weight (kg)		BB: Slaughter weight (kg)	
	578	631	550	630
C10:0	6.6 (0.17)	6.6 (0.10)	9.7 (0.36)	4.1 (0.16)
C12:0	1.0 (0.03)	1.7 (0.03)	0.7 (0.02)	0.5 (0.03)
C14:0	231.1 (5.89)	284.2 (4.22)	380.1 (10.76)	188.0 (6.86)
C15:0	41.2 (1.17)	54.9 (0.83)	52.0 (1.82)	36.7 (1.17)
C16:0	948.1 (24.10)	1659.0 (25.21)	680.5 (22.69)	727.0 (24.93)
C17:0	66.5 (1.73)	100.9 (1.54)	60.9 (2.09)	53.1 (1.77)
C18:0	631.7 (15.62)	933.0 (14.30)	424.6 (14.13)	435.0 (13.81)
C20:0	2.3 (0.06)	2.7 (0.04)	2.3 (0.07)	1.2 (0.04)
C22:0	2.0 (0.05)	2.3 (0.04)	2.3 (0.07)	1.2 (0.04)
SFA	1931.4 (48.8)	3045.0 (46.3)	1541.2 (52.1)	1447.2 (48.8)
MUFA	1738.0 (43.6)	2975.0 (45.0)	1152.1 (38.7)	1263.0 (43.2)
PUFA	151.2 (4.1)	212.2 (3.3)	171.0 (5.9)	128.6 (4.2)
PUFA:SFA	0.08	0.07	0.11	0.09
Total Fatty acids	3954	6578	2962	3084

Source: adapted from Moreno *et al.*, 2008

© Woodhead Publishing Limited, 2011

Rapeseed/oil is the main source of MUFA; sunflower seed/oil, safflower seed/oil and soyabean/oil are rich in PUFA, particularly the omega-6 linoleic acid; while linseed/oil and flaxseed/oil are also rich in PUFA, particularly the omega-3 linolenic acid. Fish oil and marine algae are the main sources of long-chain omega-3 fatty acids (Woods and Fearon, 2009). All of these sources of unsaturated fatty acids have been examined in beef, pigmeat and poultry meat production (see below).

The process of ruminal biohydrogenation of dietary PUFA also results in the production of unsaturated fatty acids that may contain one or several *trans* double bonds. In contrast, monogastric-derived foods are practically devoid of *trans* fatty acids. Epidemiological associations between the risk of coronary heart disease and the consumption of *trans* PUFA has focused attention on their concentration in food products and it is now mandatory in many countries to declare the *trans* fatty acid content on food labels. The most common source of *trans* fatty acids in the human diet is industrially produced partially hydrogenated vegetable oils used as food ingredients. Measurement of *trans* fatty acids is complex and consequently their concentration is not always reported. Advances in analytical procedures have facilitated the measurement of individual *trans* fatty acids and it has become clear that the profile of *trans* fatty acids differs between that of ruminant products and hydrogenated vegetable oils (see Scollan *et al.*, 2006b). Recent studies have concluded that consumption of ruminant *trans* fatty acids does not pose a risk to human health, most likely due to the high proportion of *trans* 11 C18:1 in ruminant-derived foods (Stender *et al.*, 2008; Jakobsen *et al.*, 2008). In the fatty acid data relating to ruminants in this chapter, where *trans* C18:1 is reported, it is included in MUFA. Similarly, where isomers of C18:2 such as conjugated linoleic acid (below) are reported they are included in PUFA.

Pasture or forage
Grass has higher PUFA and particularly higher omega-3 PUFA, primarily as linolenic acid, than grain-based ruminant feeds. In temperate climates grass, either grazed or conserved, is usually the cheapest form of cattle feed. The impact of pasture in the ration of beef cattle on the fatty acid composition of muscle has been widely studied (see reviews by Scollan *et al.*, 2006a and Daley *et al.*, 2010) and selected examples are given in Table 12.4. As far as possible, studies were chosen where there was no significant difference between treatments in intramuscular fat content so the possible confounding discussed earlier could be avoided. In general, at constant intramuscular fat content, grass-fed beef has a lower proportion of SFA and a higher proportion of PUFA in intramuscular lipids. An increase in the proportion of grass in the diet of finishing steers and an increase in the duration of grazing decreased the SFA concentration (and increased the PUFA) concentration (French *et al.*, 2000; Noci *et al.*, 2005a). Where reported, this reduction seemed to be particularly evident in C16:0, one of the 'dangerous' SFA from a human health perspective. The apparent inconsistency in the study of Leheska *et al.* (2008), which was a survey of commercially available beef in the United States, is explained by the difference in intramuscular fat as outlined in Table 12.3. There is increasing interest in cattle production from botanically

© Woodhead Publishing Limited, 2011

Table 12.4 Influence of pasture on the fatty acid composition of bovine muscle

Source	Fat %	C12:0	C14:0	C16:0	C18:0	SFA	MUFA	PUFA	PUFA:SFA	Reference
				Fatty acid (g/100 g total fatty acids)						
Control	3.41	0.09	2.74	27.40	15.95	48.1	41.5	4.9	0.09	French et al. (2000)
Grass 510	4.49	0.08	2.52	24.72	16.13	45.7	40.9	4.5	0.10	
Grass 770	4.02	0.08	2.61	24.07	15.51	44.9	42.3	4.7	0.11	
Grass 1000	4.36	0.09	2.71	22.84[L]	14.72	42.8[L]	43.1	5.4[L]	0.13[L]	
Control	2.92	0.05	2.08	24.13	16.94	45.4	41.6	5.6	0.12	Noci et al. (2005a)
40 days	2.76	0.06	2.53	23.44	17.51	45.8	39.6	6.3	0.14	
99 days	3.25	0.06	2.31	24.07	16.92	45.5	41.2	5.6	0.12	
158 days	2.99	0.06	2.09[Q]	21.71[C]	17.12	43.1[Q]	41.1	6.6[L]	0.15	
Control	4.40	0.07	3.45[a]	26.3	13.2[a]	45.1[a]	46.2[a]	2.8[a]	0.06	Leheska et al. (2008)
Grass–fed	2.80	0.05	2.85[b]	26.9	17.0[b]	48.8[b]	42.5[b]	3.4[b]	0.07	
Control	3.7	NR	NR	NR	NR	44.9	47.2	8.0[a]	0.18	Steen et al. (2003)
Grass	3.9	NR	NR	NR	NR	47.3	42.9	9.9[b]	0.21	
Experiment 1										
Control	2.7	NR	NR	NR	NR	43.0[a]	43.2	13.8	0.32	Steen et al. (2003)
Grass	2.7	NR	NR	NR	NR	41.7[b]	43.4	14.8	0.34	
Experiment 2										
Control	S	0.05	2.81	28.8[a]	13.2	47.0	46.3	4.5[a]	0.10	Engle and Spears (2004)
Grass	S	0.07	2.62	25.7[b]	13.0	44.2	47.7	5.8[b]	0.13	

S = Stated by authors to be similar; NR = not reported; L, Q, C = linear, quadratic or cubic effect of treatment; Within an experiment, means with different superscripts (a, b) differ (P < 0.05)

© Woodhead Publishing Limited, 2011

diverse pastures but there is a paucity of information on the fatty acid composition of such beef. This topic was comprehensively reviewed by Lourenco *et al.* (2008) and, for lamb at least, there was a general tendency for an increase in total PUFA proportions in intramuscular fat due to modest reductions in SFA and MUFA.

In general, conserving grass as silage or hay decreases the concentration of fatty acids and this tends to dilute the positive effect of fresh pasture in meat from cattle subsequently consuming the conserved forages. In most conserved forage-based beef production systems, concentrate supplements are used which, unless they are enriched in PUFA (see below), will also add to this dilution. With regard to forage type, mixtures of grass and red clover silage relative to grass silage alone increased the deposition of PUFA in muscle of finishing beef steers, resulting in increases in the PUFA:SFA ratio, but did not affect the proportion of SFA (Scollan *et al.*, 2006b). Similarly, feeding cattle whole-crop wheat silage rather than grass silage (Noci *et al.*, 2005b) or wilting grass prior to ensiling (Noci *et al.*, 2007) did not affect the SFA proportion in muscle for cattle fed these silages.

Supplementation with unprotected lipids
Since dietary inclusion of fatty acids must be restricted (to 60 g/kg dry matter consumed, approx.) to avoid impairment of rumen function, the capacity to manipulate the fatty acid composition by use of ruminally available fatty acids is limited. Typical supplementation strategies examined are illustrated in Table 12.5. The objective generally has been to enhance the PUFA, and in particular the omega-3 PUFA, rather than decrease the proportion of SFA *per se*. Of note is that supplementation with SFA increased the SFA proportion in lipids, mainly at the expense of MUFA (Hutchison *et al.*, 2006; Jordan *et al.*, 2006). The rationale for the latter study was to decrease methane production. Supplementation with PUFA generally causes a modest but statistically significant decrease in SFA proportion and in particular the C16:0 proportion of intramuscular lipids. Consequently, while the supplementation strategies described above can cause sizeable changes in the omega-6:omega-3 PUFA ratio they generally do not increase the PUFA:SFA ratio in the meat above that observed for the control rations.

Supplementation with protected lipids
Abomasal infusion, thereby bypassing the rumen, demonstrated the potential to markedly increase the concentration of PUFA in beef muscle if ruminal saturation could be avoided. For practical exploitation of the capacity of muscle to deposit PUFA, and in particular omega-3 PUFA, methods to protect dietary lipids from ruminal degradation are under ongoing investigation. A variety of procedures have been explored including the use of intact oilseeds, heat/chemical treatment of intact or processed oilseeds, chemical treatment of oils to form calcium soaps or amides, and emulsification/encapsulation of oils with protein and subsequent chemical protection. Of these, the most effective seems to be the last. Some studies using this technology are summarised in Table 12.6. The objective of one of the earlier studies by Ashes *et al.* (1993) was to increase the MUFA proportion of beef adipose tissue and resulted in a 45% increase accompanied by a decrease in the proportion of

© Woodhead Publishing Limited, 2011

Table 12.5 Influence of lipid sources on the fatty acid composition of bovine muscle: oils and oilseeds

Source	Fat%	C12:0	C14:0	C16:0	C18:0	SFA	MUFA	PUFA	PUFA:SFA	Reference
				Fatty acid (g/100 g total fatty acids)						
Control	3.5	0.11	3.45	28.37	14.68	46.6	40.5	4.8	0.07	
Linseeds	4.2	0.11	3.67	25.32	13.74	42.8	42.7	4.8	0.07	Recalculated from
Fish oil	4.3	0.11	4.16	30.36	12.95	47.6	37.9	4.3	0.05	Scollan et al. (2001)
Linseeds/fish oil	4.0	0.11	3.98	27.36	12.39	43.9	41.1	4.8	0.05	
Control	3.4	0.07	2.63	27.45	14.01	45.6	43.3	7.1	0.16	
Sunflower oil–1	3.3	0.08	2.69	26.86	13.91	44.9	43.2	7.8	0.18	Noci et al. (2005b)
Sunflower oil–2	3.3	0.08	2.71	25.98[L]	14.42	44.6	42.7	8.9[L]	0.20[L]	
Control	3.9	0.07	2.85	26.94[a]	16.90	46.4[a]	43.4	4.7	0.10	Andrae et al. (2001)
High oil corn	3.6	0.07	2.75	25.78[b]	15.93	44.3[b]	43.6	5.9	0.13	
Control	S	NR	2.07	28.7[a]	12.05	42.8[a]	45.0	8.5[a]	0.20	
Soyabean oil	S	NR	1.87	25.9[b]	13.49	41.2[a]	45.8	10.1[a]	0.25	Ahroni et al. (2005)
Full fat soya	S	NR	1.87	26.1[b]	12.30	40.3[b]	44.6	12.0[b]	0.30	
Control	1	0.08[a]	2.48[a]	29.46	13.33	45.2[a]	47.5	7.3	0.16	
Coconut oil	1	0.17[b]	3.45[b]	25.10	15.12	44.3[a]	48.1	7.6	0.17	Jordan et al. (2006)
Copra meal	1	0.16[b]	3.24[b]	29.11	14.95	49.0[b]	45.2	5.9	0.12	
Control	M	NR	2.93	26.75	12.90[a]	44.3[a]	49.4[a]	5.6	0.13	
Tallow	M	NR	3.19	28.13	13.72[ab]	46.8[b]	47.4[b]	5.5	0.12	
Poultry fat	M	NR	3.26	28.04	14.28[b]	47.0[b]	46.7[b]	5.9	0.13	Hutchison et al. (2006)

S = stated by the authors to be similar; I = indices of fatness similar; M = marbling score similar; NR = not reported; L = linear effect of treatment; Within a study, means with different superscripts (a, b) differ (P < 0.05)

© Woodhead Publishing Limited, 2011

Table 12.6 Influence of lipid sources on the fatty acid composition of bovine muscle: protected lipids

Source	Fat%									Reference
		C12:0	C14:0	C16:0	C18:0	SFA	MUFA	PUFA	PUFA:SFA	
Control	3.6[a]	NR	3.00	27.92	14.36	45.3	40.9	6.3	0.06[a]	Recalculated from
PLS–500g/d	3.4[a]	NR	2.60	25.83	12.79	41.2	41.4	10.2	0.19[b]	Scollan et al. (2003)
PLS–1000g/d	2.6[b]	NR	2.67	24.65	13.52	40.9	36.9	14.3	0.28[c]	
Control	4.7	NR	3.05	28.12	13.78	45.0	39.2	4.2	0.11	Recalculated from
PFO–50g/d	4.1	NR	3.16	28.52	13.42	45.1	38.0	4.6	0.12	Richardson et al. (2004)
PFO–100g/d	3.9	NR	2.99	28.41	13.47	44.9	37.8	5.2	0.13	
PFO–200g/d	4.3	NR	3.08	27.75	13.30	44.1	38.5	5.0	0.13	
Control*	–	NR	2.90	26.1[a]	13.80	42.8	51.1	1.8	0.04	Ashes et al. (1993)
PCS–10%	–	NR	2.80	22.6[b]	12.70	38.1	53.3	5.9	0.16	
PCS–15%	–	NR	2.60	20.3[c]	14.20	37.1	53.3	7.2	0.19	
Control	NR	NR	3.32	26.6[a]	16.8	46.7	46.2	2.9	0.05[a]	Gilbert et al. (2003)
Canola lipid	NR	NR	2.65	24.0[b]	17.6	44.4	45.7	6.7	0.13[b]	

Fatty acid (g/100 g total fatty acids)

* Subcutaneous adipose tissue; NR = not reported; PLS = protected lipid supplement; PFO = protected fish oil; PCS = protected rapeseed oil; Within an experiment, means with different superscripts (a, b, c) differ (P < 0.05)

© Woodhead Publishing Limited, 2011

C16:0 and SFA of 23% and 14% respectively. Using this technology, Scollan *et al.* (2003) showed that a protected plant oil supplement markedly improved the PUFA:SFA ratio (from 0.08 to 0.27) and decreased the proportion of SFA in muscle by 10%. It is interesting that in this study the increase in PUFA:SFA was associated with an increase in PUFA content but also a reduction in intramuscular fat content. Based on the earlier discussion this would be expected to increase the proportion of SFA so underestimates the treatment effect. Supplementation with ruminally protected fish oil did not affect the SFA proportion of intramuscular lipids. Since the most effective protection strategies to date have been on a non-commercial scale and involved formaldehyde, the use of which may not be permitted by some regulatory authorities, development of alternative protection technologies is needed. Progress in this area is reflected in the studies presented in Table 12.11, below. Many of the strategies examined above for beef have also been examined for sheep meat. These studies were recently reviewed by Sinclair (2007).

12.3.3   Saturated fatty acids in other meats

Pigmeat
Across the world, pig production systems can differ in the breed and gender used, whether males are used as boars or castrates and the target slaughter weight. Ration formulation for pigs is more refined than that for ruminants with frequently different formulations being used at different phases of the production cycle. In addition, the formulation of the control ration can also confound the apparent effect of the test ration, i.e. whether it is low in fat or both rations have similar oil content and the nature of the oil. All these factors can influence the response to a particular treatment, so comparison of responses across experiments should be made with caution. Earlier studies focused on adipose tissue because it is more amenable to manipulation than intramuscular lipid and contains the bulk of the body's fatty acids. The motivation was mainly from a processing perspective with a focus on increasing the MUFA fraction at the expense of the SFA fraction. More recent studies have sought to manipulate pig muscle fatty acid composition from a human health perspective with a focus on increasing the PUFA fraction and within that the omega-3 PUFA in particular. The array of lipid sources examined is illustrated in Table 12.7. As before, the intramuscular lipid concentration is shown to assist interpretation of the data. Fatty acid deposition in pigmeat largely reflects dietary fatty acid composition. This is illustrated in Apple *et al.* (2009), where inclusion of beef tallow, poultry fat and soyabean oil, which are characterised by decreasing proportion of SFA, results in a corresponding decrease (albeit small) in muscle SFA proportion. Similarly, in the study of Rentfrow *et al.* (2003), relative to a control ration, high oil corn characterised by high PUFA, decreased SFA and increased PUFA without affecting MUFA. In contrast, high oleic corn, characterised by high MUFA, similarly decreased SFA but increased MUFA and decreased PUFA. Teye *et al.* (2006) compared rations containing palm kernel oil high in C12:0, C14:0 and C18:0; palm oil high in

© Woodhead Publishing Limited, 2011

Table 12.7 Influence of lipid sources on the fatty acid composition of pig muscle

Source	Fat %	Fatty acid (g/100 g total fatty acids)								Reference
		C12:0	C14:0	C16:0	C18:0	SFA	MUFA	PUFA	PUFA:SFA	
Control	H	0.06	1.18	23.5	11.5	36.8[a]	47.8[a]	13.1	0.30	
Beef tallow	L	0.04	1.17	23.0	11.6	36.4[ab]	47.1[a]	14.7	0.34	
Poultry fat	L	0.05	1.14	23.0	11.3	36.0[b]	46.5[a]	15.8	0.37	
Soyabean oil	H	0.07	1.18	22.7	11.2	35.7[b]	44.6[b]	18.2	0.45	Apple et al. (2009)
Palm kernel oil	2.5	0.2[a]	1.41[a]	22.9	11.1[a]	35.6[a]	45.2	14.4[a]	0.30[a]	
Palm oil	2.2	0.09[b]	0.99[b]	22.1	10.3[b]	33.4[b]	44.1	16.0[ab]	0.36[ab]	
Soyabean oil	2.3	0.13[b]	1.09[b]	22.7	11.0[a]	34.9[a]	42.9	17.7[b]	0.41[b]	Teye et al. (2006)
Control	8.7	NR	1.28	25.4	13.7	40.7	45.7[a]	13.6[a]	0.33	
Extruded linseed	9.6	NR	1.24	24.4	14.0	40.0	42.8[b]	17.3[b]	0.43	Guillevic et al. (2009)
Control	1.0*	NR	0.95	21.3	12.5	35.0	37.0	27.0	0.80	
Rapeseed/fishoil	1.0	NR	1.04	21.9	12.3	36.0	40.0	24.0	0.70	Leskanich et al. (1997)
Control	4.5[a]*	NR	1.7	23.8[a]	11.7[a]	38.6[a]	52.0[b]	9.3[d]	0.24	
Animal fat	3.9[ab]	NR	1.7	22.5[b]	11.1[a]	36.7[b]	48.9[c]	14.4[b]	0.39	
Safflower oil	3.7[ab]	NR	1.6	21.7[bc]	10.0[b]	34.3[c]	52.5[b]	13.2[b]	0.39	
Sunflower oil	3.4[a]	NR	1.5	21.0[bc]	9.4[b]	33.3[c]	55.6[a]	11.1[c]	0.33	
Rapeseed oil	2.8[bc]	NR	1.6	20.6[c]	9.8[b]	33.6[c]	49.5[c]	16.6[a]	0.49	Miller et al. (1990)
Low fat	15.5	0.16[a]	1.49[a]	24.2[a]	12.7	38.8[ab]	52.0[b]	7.35[a]	0.28	
Low fat/fish oil	16.0	0.14[a]	1.43[a]	23.0[a]	13.8	38.5[a]	51.6[b]	7.82[a]	0.32	
Palm kernel oil	15.8	0.77[b]	2.96[b]	24.1[b]	13.0	40.9[c]	48.1[a]	8.83[a]	0.32	
Palm kernel/fish oil	14.9	0.68[b]	2.78[b]	24.0[ab]	12.9	40.5[c]	47.8[a]	8.73[a]	0.34	Hallenstvedt et al. (2010)
Control	NR	0.07	1.41	25.2[a]	12.6[a]	40.0[a]	48.4[a]	10.3[a]	0.26	
White grease	NR	0.07	1.39	24.1[b]	11.5[b]	37.6[b]	49.8[b]	11.2[b]	0.30	
High oil corn	NR	0.08	1.43	24.0[b]	10.6[c]	36.8[b]	47.7[a]	14.3[c]	0.39	
High oleic corn	NR	0.08	1.49	24.6[ab]	10.9[bc]	37.7[b]	51.6[c]	9.4[d]	0.25	Rentfrow et al. (2003)

* Marbling score; NR = not reported; HL = stated to be higher or lower; Within an experiment, means with different superscripts (a, b, c, d) differ ($P < 0.05$)

© Woodhead Publishing Limited, 2011

C16:0 and C16:1 and soyabean oil low in SFA. The proportion of C12:0, C14:0 and total SFA was highest for the palm kernel oil treatment while PUFA was highest for the soyabean oil treatment.

The inclusion of linseed, characterised by high PUFA rich in the omega-3 linolenic acid, increased the PUFA fraction (Guillevic *et al.*, 2009) and in particular the omega-3 fatty acids (data not shown). Fish oil, characterised by long carbon chain omega-3 fatty acids, has also been examined in pig rations. This had no effect on the major fat classes (Leskanich *et al.*, 1997; Hallenstvedt *et al.*, 2010) but did enrich muscle lipids in omega-3 fatty acids. In general the nutritional strategies reviewed suggest relatively small effects on the total SFA proportion or the proportions of C14:0 and C16:0 of pig muscle when ration lipid concentration is similar.

Chicken
Selected studies are summarised in Table 12.8. The mean SFA proportion of chicken intramuscular lipid is broadly similar to that outlined in Table 12.1, while the MUFA and PUFA proportions tend to be lower and higher, respectively. Crespo and Esteve-García (2002) offered broiler chickens a basal diet supplemented with olive oil, sunflower oil or linseed oil at 10% inclusion for 20 days before slaughter. The olive oil supplementation resulted in the highest proportion of MUFA, with sunflower oil and linseed oil supplementation resulting in the highest proportion of PUFA, and all plant oils decreased SFA. Within the PUFA sources sunflower oil resulted in the highest proportion of omega-6 PUFA and linseed the highest proportion of omega-3 PUFA. The site of deposition of C18:0 within the broilers differed with dietary fat source. Diets rich in C18:1 tended to deposit C18:0 in carcass fat other than abdominal, breast or thigh, while the diets rich in PUFA favoured deposition of C18:0 into the abdominal, breast and thigh fat. The decrease in SFA due to inclusion of linseed was also seen in the studies of Lopez-Ferrer *et al.* (2001a) and Azcona *et al.* (2008). Azcona *et al.* (2008) used flaxseed (linseed) and chia, a novel source of the omega-3 linolenic acid, and measured the fatty acid composition of white and dark meat. This study is interesting in that the reduction in SFA content was greatest with the chia seed diet, 9.1 and 12.8% compared with the control diet for the dark and white meats, respectively. The greater decrease in SFA for the white meat indicates a decreased conversion efficiency for the dark meat, compared with the white. The authors suggest that the difference may be related to variability in lipid manipulation between tissues. The concentration of SFA in bird tissues is related to its content in the ration, its oxidation rate, and its synthesis in the liver. Inhibition of fatty acid synthesis in the liver is greater during the digestion of unsaturated fats than of saturated fats. Thus, the greater reduction in SFA found with the chia seed diets compared with flaxseed could partially be attributed to different degrees of lipogenesis reduction brought about by lower PUFA absorption from flaxseed compared with chia seed (Azcona *et al.*, 2008).

In general, the effect of supplementation of chicken rations with lipid sources seems to be greater for the MUFA and PUFA fractions than for SFA. Recent studies on manipulating the fatty acid composition of poultry meat have focused on increasing the concentration of long-chain omega-3 PUFA. The most direct

© Woodhead Publishing Limited, 2011

Table 12.8 Influence of lipid sources on the fatty acid composition of chicken muscle

Source	Fat%	Fatty acid (g/100 g total fatty acids)							PUFA:SFA	Reference
		C14:0	C16:0	C18:0	C20:0	SFA	MUFA	PUFA		
Basal	11.1	0.77[b]	24.3[a]	6.5[ab]	0.12[b]	31.8[a]	45.4[c]	22.8[c]	0.72	Crespo and Esteve-Garcia (2002)
Tallow	13.2	2.01[a]	22.6[a]	7.6[a]	0.13[b]	32.7[a]	49.6[b]	17.8[d]	0.54	
Olive oil	12.7	0.44[c]	18.2[b]	5.1[bc]	0.14[b]	24.0[b]	57.5[a]	18.5[d]	0.77	
Sunflower oil	12.9	0.44[c]	13.6[c]	4.6[c]	0.03[c]	18.8[c]	28.8[d]	52.5[a]	2.79	
Linseed oil	12.5	0.39[c]	11.9[c]	3.7[c]	0.26[a]	19.8[bc]	29.9[d]	50.3[b]	2.54	
Tallow	NR	0.77	33.8[a]	8.5[a]	0.04[b]	43.8[a]	41.3[a]	14.9[c]	0.34	Lopez-Ferrer et al. (2001a)
2% linseed oil	NR	0.70	31.5[b]	9.0[a]	0.00[c]	41.7[b]	32.4[b]	25.4[b]	0.62	
6% linseed oil	NR	0.69	29.6[c]	6.4[b]	0.10[a]	37.5[c]	30.2[c]	32.1[a]	0.86	
Tallow	NR	0.77[c]	33.8[a]	8.54	0.04	43.8[a]	41.3[a]	14.9[c]	0.34	Lopez-Ferrer et al. (2001b)
2% fish oil	NR	1.26[b]	31.1[b]	9.42	0.02	43.6[a]	38.7[b]	17.5[b]	0.40	
4% fish oil	NR	1.47[a]	29.0[c]	8.54	0.05	39.8[b]	37.6[b]	22.2[a]	0.56	
Control	4.02[a]	0.45	15.48[a]	7.12[ab]	NR	23.05[a]	38.50[b]	35.18[b]	1.53[b]	Azcona et al. (2008, dark meat)
Flaxseed	2.34[b]	0.45	13.77[b]	7.76[a]	NR	21.98[ab]	36.46[bc]	37.08[b]	1.69[bc]	
Rapeseed	2.60[b]	0.45	14.68[ab]	6.69[b]	NR	21.82[ab]	43.71[a]	30.03[c]	1.37[a]	
Chia seed	2.51[b]	0.39	13.88[b]	6.69[b]	NR	20.96[b]	34.37[cd]	42.10[a]	2.01[d]	
Chia meal	3.04[ab]	0.45	14.53[ab]	7.22[ab]	NR	22.20[ab]	33.01[d]	40.14[a]	1.81[cd]	
Control	0.99	0.47[ab]	18.18[a]	7.28[ab]	NR	25.92[a]	36.58[b]	30.26[c]	1.17[a]	Azcona et al. (2008, white meat)
Flaxseed	0.94	0.42[b]	16.34[bc]	7.60[a]	NR	24.37[ab]	34.72[b]	33.80[b]	1.39[b]	
Rapeseed	1.03	0.51[a]	16.62[b]	6.80[ab]	NR	23.93[b]	44.09[a]	26.30[d]	1.10[c]	
Chia seed	1.24	0.43[b]	15.42[c]	6.76[b]	NR	22.60[b]	33.78[b]	38.16[a]	1.69[c]	
Chia meal	1.46	0.45[ab]	16.08[bc]	6.53[b]	NR	23.06[b]	33.95[b]	37.78[a]	1.63[a]	

NR = not reported; Within an experiment, means with different superscripts (a, b, c, d) differ ($P < 0.05$)

© Woodhead Publishing Limited, 2011

strategy is to supplement with fish oil (see review by Rymer and Givens, 2005). This strategy had a modest effect on SFA in the study of Lopez-Ferrer *et al.* (2001b).

12.4   Dietary effects on the fat content and fatty acid composition of milk

12.4.1   Influence of non-dietary factors

Genotype can influence the fatty acid composition of milk, for example milk from Jersey cows contains more fat than milk from Holstein cows and 'the proportion of C6:0 to C14:0 of total fatty acids has, irrespective of diet, been reported to be lower in milk from Holstein than Jersey cows' (Givens and Shingfield, 2006). Genetic selection for increased milk fat content also results in altered milk fatty acid composition, causing an increase in the proportion of short-chain fatty acids and a concomitant reduction in the amount of long-chain fatty acids.

Stage of lactation can also influence the fatty acid composition of milk. Irrespective of diet, the proportion of C4:0 to C12:0 is lower, and that of C18:0 and *cis*-9 C18:1 are higher in milk produced from cows in early lactation (< 30 days in milk) compared with mid (120 days) or late (210 days) lactation (Auldist *et al.*, 1998). The changes in milk fatty acid composition associated with advances in the stage of lactation appear to reflect the contribution of long-chain fatty acids mobilised from adipose tissue during the negative energy balance that occurs at peak lactation. Even though the stage of lactation, as related to the mobilisation of body fat stores, is an important determinant of milk fatty acid composition, these effects are relatively short-term and are mainly complete within the first four to six weeks of lactation.

12.4.2   Saturated fatty acids in milk

Milk fat content can be altered through nutrition (e.g. by total energy consumption). In countries where the pricing scheme for milk includes a premium for high fat content, nutritional strategies to decrease milk fat content and associated SFA content are not attractive to producers. In the United States in particular, the need to continue to increase milk yield without a decrease in fat content led to considerable research into the basis of milk fat depression. It became clear that there is a relationship between the effect of diet on milk fat content and on the fatty acid composition of milk fat. Milk fat depression appears to occur in at least two dietary situations: with rations that contain high levels of fermentable carbohydrate and low levels of fibre; and with rations that contain high concentrations of unsaturated oils. The extent of milk fat depression with such diets is modified by many factors, including associative dietary effects, feed management practices and animal physiological state (Harvatine *et al.*, 2009). Yields of fatty acids of all chain lengths are decreased during milk fat depression. However, *de novo* synthesised fatty acids are decreased to a greater extent and this

© Woodhead Publishing Limited, 2011

results in a shift in milk fatty acid profile such that the proportion of short- and medium-chain SFA are decreased and longer-chain and unsaturated fatty acids increased. It is not always clear therefore to what extent differences in milk fat content *per se* influence apparent effects of the type of ration on milk fatty acid composition, analogous to the issue of intramuscular fatness in meat animals!

The strategies examined to manipulate the fatty acid composition of bovine milk are, as might be expected, similar to those used to manipulate the fatty acid composition of beef and lamb. The earlier studies focused on increasing the PUFA proportion of milk fat while more recent studies have focused on increasing the omega-3 PUFA proportion. Progress on enhancing the fatty acid composition of cow's and goat's milk to provide foods more consistent with recommendations for improving health were recently reviewed (Givens and Shingfield, 2006; Chilliard *et al.*, 2006; Chilliard *et al.*, 2007). In this chapter only bovine milk fatty acid composition is considered and the studies chosen for illustrative purposes include some of those reviewed by Givens and Shingfield (2006) together with studies reported since that review was prepared.

Pasture or forage
As with beef production, grazed pasture is frequently a cheap ingredient in the diet of dairy cows. Because of a year-round demand for dairy products, milk production in most European Union countries is dependent also on the production of high-quality conserved forages. The influence of dietary forage on the fatty acid composition of milk has been reviewed (e.g. Dewhurst *et al.*, 2006; Lourenco *et al.*, 2008) and some examples are given in Table 12.9. There was no consistent effect of red or white clover silages on milk SFA (but clover silages increased PUFA at the expense of MUFA (Dewhurst *et al.*, 2003)). When compared with fresh pasture, offering cows a maize silage-based ration increased the proportion of C16:0 and total SFA (Kelly *et al.*, 1998). However, when compared to conserved grass, maize silage increased SFA ≤ C14:0 and decreased C16:0 without an effect on total SFA (Kliem *et al.*, 2008). These two studies illustrate the impact of the basal diet when comparing studies. Similarly, the method of grass conservation did not affect the SFA in milk of cows subsequently fed the conserved materials (Shingfield *et al.*, 2005).

From a statistical analysis of available data, Lourenco *et al.* (2008) concluded that milk from cows grazing botanically diverse pasture had lower short-chain (≤ C14:0) SFA, from which a decrease in total SFA can be calculated (Table 12.9). In general, where it is possible to adequately compare treatments, grazed herbage leads to a decrease in SFA in milk, the nature of the conserved forage has little effect and overall effects of forage *per se* on milk SFA are quite small.

Supplementation with unprotected lipids
The similar array of lipid sources used for beef, pigmeat and poultry meat production have also been examined in the context of milk production (Table 12.10). Responses to oil supplementation in dairy cow rations are also influenced by the proportion of concentrate in the ration and by duration of feeding

© Woodhead Publishing Limited, 2011

Table 12.9 Influence of forage on the fatty acid composition of bovine milk

Basal forage	Fatty acid (g/100 g total fatty acids)												Reference
	C4:0	C6:0	C8:0	C10:0	C12:0	C14:0	C16:0	C18:0	SFA	MUFA	PUFA	PUFA:SFA	
Fresh pasture	NR	1.8[a]	0.9[a]	1.7[a]	1.7[a]	6.7[a]	24.2[a]	13.2[a]	50.9	37.2	4.3	0.08	Kelly et al. (1998)
Maize and legume silages	NR	2.1[b]	1.2[b]	2.3[b]	2.6[b]	9.4[b]	30.7[b]	15.0[b]	64.1	28.6	3.3	0.05	
Perennial ryegrass silage	4.9	2.7	1.4	3.0	3.5	11.7	32.5	11.0	73.6	24.4	1.8	0.02	Dewhurst et al. (2003)
Red clover silage	5.8	3.0	1.4	2.8	3.3	11.3	30.6	11.6	72.9	23.5	3.3	0.05	
White clover silage	5.2	3.0	1.6	3.5	4.2	12.7	32.9	9.7	75.8	21.3	2.9	0.04	
Grass hay	2.5	2.2	1.5	3.4	4.0	13.3	34.5	9.2	74.3	22.8	2.9	0.04	Shingfield et al. (2005)
Grass silage untreated	2.9	2.2	1.5	3.3	3.8	12.9	34.7	9.8	74.5	22.6	2.6	0.03	
Grass silage + inoculant	2.9	2.3	1.5	3.4	3.9	13.1	33.8	10.0	74.3	22.7	2.6	0.04	
Grass silage + formic acid	2.6	2.2	1.5	3.4	4.0	13.2	34.2	10.0	74.6	22.4	2.5	0.03	
Grass silage	2.7	2.0	1.2	2.7	3.0	11.4	35.3	8.1	69.4	21.5	3.3	0.05	Kliem et al. (2008)
Maize silage – 1	2.7	2.1	1.3	3.0	3.4	12.0	35.2	7.9	70.9	20.3	3.3	0.05	
Maize silage – 2	2.6	2.2	1.3	3.2	3.6	11.9	33.5	7.9	70.4	20.7	3.5	0.05	
Maize silage – 3	2.7	2.3[L]	1.5[L]	3.6[L]	4.1[L]	12.3[L]	32.9[L]	7.8	70.3	20.4[L]	3.7	0.05	
Control pasture	3.8	2.3[a]	1.3[a]	2.8	3.4	10.3	26.8	9.2	59.9	21.6	2.7	0.05	Lourenco et al. (2008)
Botanically diverse pasture	3.9	2.0[b]	1.0[b]	2.7	2.7	9.0	26.0	9.0	55.5	23.8	3.7	0.07	

NR = not reported; L = linear effect of treatment; Within an experiment, means with different superscripts (a, b) differ (P < 0.05)

© Woodhead Publishing Limited, 2011

Table 12.10 Influence of lipid sources on the fatty acid composition of bovine milk: oils and oilseeds

Source	Fatty acid (g/100 g fatty acids)											PUFA:SFA	Reference
	C4:0	C6:0	C8:0	C10:0	C12:0	C14:0	C16:0	C18:0	SFA	MUFA	PUFA		
Control	3.3	2.3ab	1.3ab	2.7b	2.9b	10.0b	34.5a	9.8b	69.6a	22.7b	3.1	0.05	Givens et al. (2009)
Rapeseed oil	2.7	1.8c	0.9c	1.9c	2.2c	8.7c	19.8c	14.6a	55.6c	29.2a	4.4	0.08	
Whole rapeseeds	3.3	2.5c	1.5a	3.3a	3.6a	11.7a	31.1b	10.8b	71.7a	21.4b	3.1	0.04	
Milled rapeseeds	3.1	2.2b	1.2b	2.4b	2.6bc	9.6b	21.6c	15.5a	61.5b	27.7a	3.7	0.06	
Control	3.1a	2.2a	1.4a	3.4a	4.2a	12.6a	29.1a	8.3c	69.0a	26.1d	4.4c	0.06	Chilliard et al. (2009)
Crude linseed	3.1a	2.1a	1.2b	2.7b	3.2b	10.8b	25.0b	13.7a	66.3b	29.9c	3.5d	0.05	
Extruded linseed	2.8a	1.6b	0.9c	1.9c	2.4b	8.8b	19.6b	11.7ab	53.7c	38.6b	6.9b	0.13	
Linseed oil	2.1b	1.1c	0.5d	1.1d	1.5c	5.9d	15.9d	11.3b	42.4d	48.5a	8.5b	0.20	
Control	1.8	1.0	0.6	1.8b	2.7c	9.9b	40.2b	12.3c	73.6c	24.2	3.0a	0.04	Offer et al. (1999)
Linseed oil	1.8	1.0	0.6	1.5b	2.1a	8.8a	34.0a	15.6a	67.2a	29.9	2.8a	0.04	
Tuna orbital oil	1.8	1.0	0.6	1.7b	2.5bc	9.9b	39.5b	10.5b	69.7b	27.2	2.9a	0.04	
Fish oil	1.8	0.9	0.6	1.6a	2.4b	10.3b	39.6b	6.7b	66.1a	29.9	3.9b	0.06	
Control	4.6a	2.2a	1.1	2.2	2.4a	10.2a	24.7a	19.5a	71.0	26.0	2.5a	0.04	Shingfield et al. (2003)
Herring and mackerel oil	2.4b	1.7b	1.1	2.8	3.4b	13.3b	33.3b	4.4b	67.5	23.3	8.0b	0.12	
Control	4.1a	2.4a	1.2a	2.5a	2.9a	11.6a	30.6a	9.8a	66.9a	26.2	2.8	0.04	Bell et al. (2006)
Sunflower oil	2.8b	1.4b	0.6b	1.3b	1.5b	8.1b	18.7b	11.4a	47.0b	40.2	7.9	0.17	
Control	3.1	2.2	1.4	3.6a	4.5a	12.0a	31.1a	5.4c	67.7a	17.1a	4.0a	0.06	Collomb et al. (2004)
Ground rapeseed	3.1	2.3	1.4	3.3ab	3.8b	11.3ab	24.5bc	9.1ab	62.7b	23.7b	4.2ab	0.07	
Ground sunflower	3.0	2.2	1.4	3.1b	3.6b	10.9b	25.1b	8.8ab	62.0b	23.8b	5.1b	0.08	
Ground linseed	3.1	2.3	1.5	3.5ab	4.0ab	11.5ab	26.2b	8.7ab	64.9b	20.5c	4.6b	0.07	
Control	NR	NR	2.1	4.7a	4.8a	15.1a	34.9a	13.2c	72.1a	24.2c	3.8c	0.05	Bu et al. (2007)
Soyabean oil	NR	NR	1.7	3.8b	3.7a	12.6b	30.2b	14.8bc	66.5b	27.5b	6.2a	0.09	
Flaxseed oil	NR	NR	2.0	4.0b	3.8b	12.8b	27.2b	17.4a	63.6b	31.4a	5.1b	0.08	
Soya/Flax oil	NR	NR	1.8	3.8b	3.7b	12.2b	29.9b	16.0ab	66.3b	28.7ab	5.2b	0.08	
Control	5.1	2.5a	1.5a	3.2a	4.1a	11.7	36.0	6.8a	73.1a	22.4a	1.9a	0.03	Boeckaert et al. (2008)
Microalgae	3.6	1.4b	0.9b	2.0b	2.6b	11.3	34.0	1.2b	61.1b	29.0b	4.0b	0.07	

NR = not reported; Within an experiment, means with different superscripts (a, b, c, d) differ ($P < 0.05$)

© Woodhead Publishing Limited, 2011

(Dewhurst *et al.*, 2006). In general, supplements of plant oils or oilseeds rich in unsaturated C18 fatty acids reduce the proportion of short- and medium-chain fatty acids (C6:0–C16:0) and increase the proportion of C18:0. The result of these changes is a general decrease in SFA proportion in milk. These changes are thought to occur due to long-chain fatty acids (C16 and above) inhibiting *de novo* fatty acid synthesis in the mammary gland and because lipids increase the amount of circulating long-chain fatty acids available for incorporation into milk fat. In contrast, Odongo *et al.* (2007) included C14:0 in dairy cow rations and observed a marked increase in the C14:0 proportion of milk, a particularly undesirable result from a human health perspective, but a decrease in C16:0 and C18:0 and no effect on total SFA.

Because of ruminal biohydrogenation of dietary unsaturated fatty acids, C18:0 is the predominant long-chain fatty acid available for incorporation into milk fat. However, C18:1 secretion in milk exceeds mammary C18:0 uptake due to the activity of stearoyl CoA (*Δ*-9) desaturase activity in mammary secretory cells. The *Δ*-9 desaturase transforms proportionately 40% of C18:0 taken up by the mammary gland. It is therefore possible to exploit the endogenous conversion in the mammary gland to enhance milk fat C18:1 by supplementing diets with lipids rich in C18:0, but this strategy does not alter the C18:1:C18:0 ratio in milk fat (Givens and Shingfield, 2006). In a recent meta-analysis conducted on a database of 145 plant oil/oilseed supplementation experiments, Glasser *et al.* (2008) statistically confirmed the above observations, i.e. 'lipid supplementation induces a general increase in C18 percentage at the expense of the short- and medium-chain (fatty acids)'. Oils tended to decrease C6 to C16 SFA more than seeds while there was a greater increase in C18:0 due to consumption of C18:2 (non linseed) than C18:3 (linseed) rich oils. They further concluded that the effects on short-chain SFA were relatively small when compared with the fatty acid composition of milk from unsupplemented cows and with the effects on C18:0. Givens and Shingfield (2006), however, suggested that the decrease in milk production associated with feeding high levels of oilseeds would not be acceptable to producers unless a considerable premium was paid for milk of altered fatty acid composition.

The general trend for the effects of fish oil (or marine algae) supplementation was for a decrease in C18:0 proportion and total SFA (Table 12.10). Shingfield *et al.* (2003) observed an undesirable increase in C16:0 which was not evident in the study of Offer *et al.* (1999). The lack of consistency in the effect of fish oil supplementation on the proportion of C16:0 of milk lipids was previously highlighted by Kitessa *et al.* (2004).

Supplementation with protected lipids
The protection technologies used to prevent or decrease ruminal biohydrogenation of dietary lipids were described earlier. Examples of some of these approaches used in dairy cow ration formulation are given in Table 12.11. The effectiveness of the protection strategies varies and is frequently not reported. Moreover, the non-protected lipid source is rarely included in the control treatment, which makes assessment of the degree of protection impossible.

© Woodhead Publishing Limited, 2011

Table 12.11 Influence of lipid sources on the fatty acid composition of bovine milk: protected lipids

Source	Fatty acid (g/100 g fatty acids)												Reference
	C4:0	C6:0	C8:0	C10:0	C12:0	C14:0	C16:0	C18:0	SFA	MUFA	PUFA	PUFA:SFA	
Control	3.5	2.3[a]	1.5[a]	3.2[a]	3.5[a]	10.0[a]	25.9[a]	9.9[b]	59.8	20.6	2.0	0.03	
Ca–salts of rapeseed oil	3.0	1.5[b]	0.8[b]	1.6[b]	2.0[b]	7.6[b]	16.4[b]	12.9[a]	45.7	34.9	2.1	0.05	
Ca–salts of soyabean oil	3.4	1.6[b]	0.9[b]	1.6[b]	1.8[b]	6.9[b]	16.4[b]	13.3[a]	45.9	33.6	2.3	0.05	
Ca–salts of linseed oil	3.4	1.9[b]	1.0[b]	2.0[b]	2.1[b]	7.4[b]	16.2[b]	13.2[a]	47.1	30.0	2.7	0.06	Chouinard et al. (2001)
Control	5.1	3.7	1.8[a]	5.3[a]	4.7[a]	14.0[a]	32.1[a]	7.9[a]	74.6	21.5	4.0	0.05	
Rapeseed oil	5.5	3.1	1.3[b]	3.4[b]	3.0[b]	11.3[b]	21.4[b]	11.9[b]	60.9	34.5	4.6	0.08	
Amide of rapeseed oil[1]	5.4	3.3	1.4[b]	3.4[b]	2.9[b]	10.7[b]	21.4[b]	13.0[c]	62.4	33.5	4.3	0.06	Loor et al. (2002)
Control	3.5	2.2[a]	1.3[a]	2.9	3.2	10.5[a]	28.4[a]	12.2[a]	65.7[a]	28.7	4.0[a]	0.06	
Xylose-treated algae	3.5	2.0[b]	1.2[ab]	2.6	3.1	12.2[b]	31.0[b]	5.0[b]	61.6[b]	30.0	6.5[b]	0.11	
Marine algae	3.6	2.0[b]	1.1[b]	2.5	3.0	11.8[b]	33.0[c]	4.3[b]	62.7[b]	29.0	6.5[b]	0.10	Franklin et al. (1999)
Control	3.1	2.4	1.9	3.4	4.3[a]	11.8[a]	26.7[a]	7.1[a]	60.7	28.3	3.8	0.06	
Protected canola[2]	3.2	2.4	1.9	3.2	3.6[b]	9.5[b]	19.9[b]	9.2[b]	52.9	32.5	7.5	0.14	Ashes et al. (1992)
Control	4.2	2.4	1.3	2.4[a]	2.9[a]	9.8[a]	29.9[a]	9.9[a]	62.8	24.5	2.9	0.05	
Gel[4] (2010)	4.2	2.3	1.2	2.1[b]	2.4[b]	8.1[b]	24.8[b]	12.4[b]	57.5	26.5	7.6	0.13	Van Vuuren et al.
Control	NR	NR	1.2	2.2	2.2	9.2	31.6[a]	13.5[a]	59.9	26.4	6.0	0.10	
Protected HIDHA fish oil[3]	NR	NR	1.2	2.8	2.8	8.8	23.1[b]	3.6[b]	42.3	30.2	16.7	0.39	
Protected Max–EPA fish oil[3]	NR	NR	1.1	2.3	2.4	8.9	23.6[b]	2.8[b]	41.1	21.2	14.7	0.36	Gulati et al. (2003)
Control	NR	NR	1.4[a]	2.3[a]	2.4[a]	9.0	25.6[a]	14.7[a]	56.8[a]	29.9	3.7	0.07	
Protected tuna oil[3]	NR	NR	1.7[b]	2.8[b]	2.9[b]	8.8	23.0[b]	11.4[b]	52.0[b]	27.3	9.8	0.19	Kitessa et al. (2004)

[1] Prepared by reacting rapeseed oil with ethanolamine.
[2] Prepared by mixing full fat rapeseeds and using formaldehyde as a tanning reagent.
[3] Prepared by mixing with soyabean and fish oil and using formaldehyde as a tanning agent
[4] Whey protein soyabean oil emulsion
NR – not reported; Within an experiment, means with different superscripts (a, b, c) differ (P < 0.05)

© Woodhead Publishing Limited, 2011

Supplements of C18:1 protected as calcium salts (Chouinard *et al.*, 2001), formaldehyde treated whole seeds (Ashes *et al.*, 1992) or acyl amides (Loor *et al.*, 2002) increased milk fat C18:1 content (Table 12.11) with substantial decreases in SFA in milk fat. The pattern was as seen with unprotected plant oils, i.e. a decrease in SFA ≤C16:0 with an increase in C18:0. There were relatively few studies using protected plant lipids in the database compiled by Glasser *et al.* (2008) and a secure conclusion could not be reached on their effects on milk fatty acid composition. With regard to protected fish oil supplementation, there was a decrease in C16:0 and C18:0 leading to a substantial decrease in total SFA (Gulati *et al.*, 2003; Kitessa *et al.*, 2004). Protected fish oil did not have the negative effect on feed consumption observed for unprotected fish oil or plant oils and so may be a more acceptable tool to decrease SFA in milk lipids.

12.5   Influence of 'additives' on saturated fatty acids in meat and milk

While changes in the macro components of the diet of cattle, pigs and poultry can change the SFA concentration of meat and milk as reviewed in sections 12.3.2 and 12.4.2, there is some evidence that micronutrient inclusion can also have an effect. This is illustrated in Table 12.12. Most high-producing animals receive a supplement of minerals and vitamins to balance those supplied by the dietary ingredients. Engle *et al.* (2000) reported that consumption of copper by beef cattle in excess of that required for normal function decreased SFA in muscle. This response seems to be variable (Engle and Spears, 2004) and does not seem to have been reported by other groups. Siebert *et al.* (2006) reported that an increase in vitamin A consumption decreased intramuscular fat concentration but increased the SFA concentration in bovine adipose tissue. However, since forages generally contain more *β*-carotene (vitamin A precursor) than other feedstuffs, this observation is only relevant to production systems that either use feedstuffs with naturally low *β*-carotene/vitamin A concentrations or have available such feeds to substitute for forage. In this regard, Arnett *et al.* (2009) confirmed the observation of Siebert *et al.* (2006) that supplementing a low vitamin A ration with vitamin A decreased intramuscular fat concentration. However, no effect on beef muscle SFA proportion was detected.

Rumen fermentation modifiers, in particular ionophores, have been used for many years to improve productivity of growing and lactating cattle. The inclusion of monensin, the most studied ionophore, decreased SFA proportion in bovine milk (da Silva *et al.*, 2007), beef muscle (Marmer *et al.*, 1985) and lamb muscle (Gilka *et al.*, 1989), an effect not seen with non-ionophore antibiotics (Aldai *et al.*, 2008). More recently, *β*-adrenergic agonists have been developed which repartition absorbed dietary nutrients away from adipose and towards muscle tissue accretion. While there is a paucity of information on their effects on muscle fatty acid composition, there is some evidence that one *β*-agonist (approved for use outside the EU) decreases the SFA concentration in pig muscle when fed in

© Woodhead Publishing Limited, 2011

Table 12.12 Influence of selected micronutrients on the fatty acid composition of meat and milk

Species	Comparison	Fatty acid (g/100 g fatty acids)							SFA	MUFA	PUFA	PUFA:SFA	Reference
		C6:0	C8:0	C10:0	C12:0	C14:0	C16:0	C18:0					
Cows	Control	0.4	0.5	1.6	2.1	8.9	24.6[a]	18.8	58.2[a]	33.2	3.9	0.07[a]	de Silva et al. (2007)
	Monensin	0.4	0.4	1.4	1.9	8.3	23.3[b]	16.8	53.9[b]	35.2	4.2	0.08[b]	
Lamb[1]	Control	–	–	0.14[a]	0.18	3.9[a]	26.5	31.0	64.2	35.8	3.2	0.05	Gilka et al. (1989)
	Monensin	–	–	0.12[ab]	0.16	3.4[ab]	28.0	31.4	65.9	34.2	3.0	0.05	
	Lasalocid	–	–	0.15[a]	0.17	3.3[b]	29.3	30.4	65.9	34.1	3.4	0.05	
Beef[2]	Control	–	–	–	–	3.6	26.3[a]	10.0	43.4[a]	54.4[a]	1.8[a]	0.04	Siebert et al. (2006)
	Vitamin A	–	–	–	–	3.7	27.1[b]	10.4	47.0[b]	51.6[b]	1.5[b]	0.03	
Beef[1]	Control	–	–	–	–	3.4	27.7	13.6	52.2[a]	45.3	2.4[a]	0.05	Engle et al. (2000)
	Copper	–	–	–	–	3.9	27.0	11.3	49.6[b]	47.1	3.4[b]	0.07	
Pigmeat[1]	Control	–	–	–	0.04	0.83[a]	27.4[a]	11.6[a]	42.0[a]	44.5[a]	13.6	0.32	Cordero et al. (2010)
	CLA	–	–	–	0.06	1.28[b]	33.9[b]	14.7[b]	51.1[b]	35.9[b]	12.4	0.24	
Poultry[1]	Control	–	–	–	–	0.3[a]	19.5[a]	8.9[a]	29.0[a]	29.3[a]	41.1[a]	1.42	Szymczyk et al. (2001)
	CLA	–	–	–	–	0.6[b]	24.6[b]	13.7[b]	39.2[b]	23.4[b]	36.7[b]	0.94	
Beef[2]	Control	–	–	–	–	2.8[a]	25.7[a]	13.9	42.2[a]	49.8[a]	2.6[a]	0.06	Recalculated from Gillis et al. (2004)
	Protected CLA	–	–	–	–	3.5[b]	27.0[b]	14.5	44.9[b]	47.0[b]	2.9[b]	0.06	

[1] Muscle;
[2] Adipose tissue
Within an experiment, means with different superscripts (a, b) differ (P < 0.05)

© Woodhead Publishing Limited, 2011

combination with a source of PUFA (but not when fed with tallow) (Apple *et al.*, 2007). In contrast, in steers fed an unnamed β-agonist there was a shift towards SFA in muscle (Webb and Casey, 1995). Because of the prohibition on the use of growth-promoting antibiotics in food animal production in the EU, identification of alternatives is an area of active investigation, e.g. the EU 6th Framework funded project REPLACE. The focus of this project is on the discovery of plant compounds that may enhance livestock productivity including fatty acid composition of meat and milk. In this regard, Vasta *et al.* (2009) reported that dietary inclusion of quebracho powder (a source of tannins) decreased the proportion of SFA and MUFA in lamb muscle while increasing the proportion of PUFA. In contrast, Benchaar and Chouinard (2009) observed no effect of quebracho on bovine milk fatty acids but the level of dietary inclusion was one-tenth of that used by Vasta *et al.* (2009), so further study is required. Benchaar and Chouinard (2009) did observe a general decrease in the concentration of SFA in milk (albeit not statistically significant) when saponins were included in the ration of dairy cows.

While they are not components of the ration *per se*, anabolic steroids are used widely (outside the EU) in beef production. There is evidence that steroid implantation increases the percentage of SFA while decreasing the MUFA proportion of muscle fatty acids (Duckett *et al.*, 1999; Webb and Casey, 1995).

Conjugated linoleic acid (CLA) refers to a mixture of positional and geometric isomers of linoleic acid (C18:2 n-6). The *cis* 9, *trans* 11 form is believed to be the most common natural form of CLA with biological activity, but biological activity has been proposed for other isomers, especially the *trans* 10, *cis* 12 isomer. Conjugated linoleic acid has been shown to be an anticarcinogen, and to have antiatherogenic, immunomodulating, growth promoting, lean body mass enhancing and antidiabetic properties (Moloney, 2006). It is found in highest concentrations in fat from ruminant animals, where it is produced in the rumen as the first intermediate in the biohydrogenation of dietary linoleic acid. In the second step of the pathway, the conjugated diene is hydrogenated to *trans* 11 octadecenoic acid (trans-vaccenic acid) which is now thought to be a substrate for tissue synthesis of CLA via Δ-9 desaturase activity. Because of the potential health benefits arising from CLA consumption, there is considerable research effort directed to increasing the CLA content of ruminant-derived food. Since little CLA is synthesised in monogastric animals, inclusion of synthetic CLA in pig and poultry rations has been examined. Similarly, in dietary situations where the concentration of CLA in beef is likely to be low, supplementation with CLA could also be considered. Since CLA is hydrogenated in the rumen as described above, it must be protected to be effective. Because of the cost involved there are very few studies examining this approach in beef cattle. A consistent finding in the literature is that dietary inclusion of CLA, while increasing the concentration of CLA in tissue, leads to an increase in SFA concentration (examples are given in Table 12.12).

The *trans* 10, *cis* 12 isomer of CLA appears to be a potent inhibitor of milk fat synthesis (Bauman and Griinari, 2003). The feeding of commercially synthesised

© Woodhead Publishing Limited, 2011

lipid supplements high in *trans*-10, *cis*-12 CLA concentration may be a strategy to manipulate milk fat synthesis in the dairy cow (De Veth *et al.* 2005). When such products are fed, a decrease in milk fat concentration occurs which is accompanied by a general decrease in the proportion of short-chain SFA ($\leq$ C16:0) with an increase in C18:0. From de Veth *et al.* (2005), 59% and 52% SFA can be calculated for milk from control cows and cows supplemented with rumen-protected CLA, respectively. From the discussion in section 12.1 these responses could be considered positive from a human health perspective. In general the effects of dietary micronutrients in meat and milk SFA concentrations are small. Nevertheless, they are likely to be additive and so if incorporated into a meat or milk production system would enhance the healthiness of foods derived therefrom.

12.6   Future trends

The so-called 'lipid hypothesis' has guided medical advice for many years. This hypothesis is being increasingly criticised, particularly as ongoing research on lipid metabolism in humans and its relationship to health and disease yields data inconsistent with this hypothesis. Moreover, the hypothesis that a low-fat, high-carbohydrate diet is best for preventing the onset of cardiovascular disease and obesity is also being increasingly questioned (e.g. German and Dillard, 2004). Nevertheless, in many countries, reducing population SFA intake remains a public health priority. This will continue to put pressure on the agri-food industry to decrease the SFA concentration in animal-derived foods. Knowledge of the health risks to humans of consumption of the individual SFA found in meat and milk is incomplete and merits further investigation. This may allow 'rebranding' of animal-derived food products on the basis of the concentrations of SFA that are proven risks to human health, together with those other fatty acids such as MUFA and PUFA that are considered beneficial. The recent analysis of the human health impact of the high-MUFA milk produced by the inclusion of rapeseed in the diet of dairy cows merits highlighting in this regard. Givens (2008) demonstrated in a modelling exercise that replacement of milk containing 70% SFA and 20% MUFA with milk containing 55% SFA and 32% MUFA (and using the EU SFA consumption data from Hulshof *et al.*, 1999) would reduce the risk of coronary heart disease across the EU by an average of 2 to 4%, depending on the model used and the number of deaths from coronary heart disease, by 10 507 annually. Further analyses of this type, using modified meat products in addition to the modified milk, should be undertaken. The dietary modifications reviewed in this chapter did not consider in detail the *trans* fatty acid concentrations in meat and milk. Since *trans* fatty acids remain an issue of concern to the food industry and medical authorities the consequences of dietary modifications on this category of fatty acids in ruminant meat and milk need to be continually monitored.

As outlined earlier, much of the effort to date has focused on increasing the concentrations in milk and meat of MUFA and PUFA rather than decreasing SFA

© Woodhead Publishing Limited, 2011

per se, with varying degrees of success depending on the species examined. There are differing views as to the most appropriate strategies to pursue, i.e. enrichment with MUFA, with specific PUFA such as the omega-3 class or with CLA. Moreover, species would seem to differ in their suitability for different targets. Thus decreasing SFA seems a logical target for milk, while increasing the omega-3 proportion of muscle lipids would seem the most appropriate for poultry, since poultry meat is high in PUFA. Increasing MUFA would seem to be an achievable target for beef. Indeed it has been suggested that this is a more appropriate strategy than seeking to increase omega-3 PUFA. The discovery of CLA, together with the finding that ruminant fat is its primary natural source, is a positive advance for ruminant-derived food products. Increasing the concentration of CLA in meat and milk is a research target which may result in future meat and milk being considered a functional food, i.e. a food that has health benefits beyond basic nutrition. The view of Chilliard *et al.* (2006) in the conclusion to their article, that 'The aim of future research is to better understand the effects of using grass-based diets, new combinations of feedstuffs and nutrients in concentrates, and oilseed technology and processing, in order to increase more selectively fatty acids of interest to human nutrition, without increasing less desired fatty acids and without decreasing the sensory quality of dairy (and meat) products', is still very relevant.

Recent advances in molecular biology are likely to facilitate the selection of animals with a particular fatty acid genotype. For example, Zhang *et al.* (2008) reported the existence of single nucleotide polymorphisms in the bovine fatty acid synthase gene that are associated with beef fatty acid composition. The g.17924GG genotype had lower C14:0, C16:0 and total SFA and higher C18:1 and total MUFA than did other genotypes detected, raising the possibility of selecting for 'healthier' fatty acid composition. Similarly, Mele (2009) has discussed the possibilities for selection of dairy cows on the basis of a particular milk fatty acid composition. Such developments raise the possibility of a nutrigenomic approach to meat and milk production, i.e. a particular fatty acid genotype is chosen and then dietary strategies are designed to optimise expression of the genotype. However, exploitation of emerging nutritional and genomic information requires economic incentives. At present there are few, if any, fresh meat or milk products that are marketed on the basis of their fatty acid composition. This needs to happen soon to ensure momentum in this field is not lost. Moreover, a role for national governments could be envisaged on the basis that paying to maintain and enhance the health of the population is likely to be a more cost-effective strategy than paying to treat and care for the ill.

12.7   Sources of further information and advice

British Nutrition Foundation (1999) Meat in the Diet. Briefing paper. The British Nutrition Foundation, London, 24 p.
Gurr M I (1999) Lipids in Nutrition and Heath: A Reappraisal. Bridgwater, The Oily Press.
Taubes G (2007) Good calories, bad calories: challenging the conventional wisdom on diet, weight control and disease, New York, Alfred A Knopf.

© Woodhead Publishing Limited, 2011

McCance and Widdowson's The Composition of Foods (and supplements). The Royal Society of Chemistry and Ministry of Agriculture, Fisheries and Food.

Websites
British Nutrition Foundation: http://www.nutrition.org.uk
Conjugated linoleic acid references: http://fri.wisc.edu/cla.php
Healthfinder – Gateway to reliable Consumer Health Information: http://www.healthfinder.gov
Lipgene – Diet, genomics, and the metabolic syndrome: an integrated nutrition, agro-food, social and economic analysis: http://www.ucd.ie/lipgene
ProSafeBeef – Advancing beef safety and quality through research and innovation: http://www.prosafebeef.eu
U.S. Department of Agriculture, Nutrient data laboratory USDA. Nutrient database for standard reference: http://www.nal.usda.gov/fnic/foodcomp

12.8   References

Ahroni Y, Orlov A, Brosh A, Grant R and Kanner J (2005), Effects of soyabean oil supplementation of high forage fattening diet on fatty acid profiles in lipid depots of fattening bull calves, and their levels of blood vitamin E, *Anim Feed Sci Technol*, 119, 191–202.

Aldai N, Dugan MER, Kramer JKG, Mir PS and McAllister T (2008), Nonionophore antibiotics do not affect the *trans*-18:1 and conjugated linoleic acid composition in beef adipose tissue, *J Anim Sci*, 86, 3522–32.

Andrae JG, Duckett SK, Hunt CW, Pritchard GT and Owens FN (2001), Effects of feeding high-oil corn to beef steers on carcass characteristics and meat quality. *J Anim Sci*, 79, 582–8.

Apple JK, Maxwell CV, Galloway DL, Hutchison S and Hamilton CR (2009), Interactive effects of dietary fat source and slaughter weight in growing finishing swine: 1. Growth performance and longissimus muscle fatty acid composition, *J Anim Sci*, 87, 1407–22.

Apple JK, Maxwell CV, Sawyer JT, Kutz BR, Rakes LK, Davis ME, Johnson ZB, Carr SN and Armstrong TA (2007), Interactive effect of ractopamine and dietary fat source on quality characteristics of fresh pork bellies, *J Anim Sci*, 85, 2682–90.

Arnett AM, Dikeman ME, Daniel MJ, Olson KC, Jaeger J and Perrett J (2009), Effects of vitamin A supplementation and weaning age on serum and liver retinol concentrations, carcass traits, and lipid composition in market beef cattle, *Meat Sci*, 81, 596–606.

Ashes JR, St Vincent Welch P, Gulati SK, Scott TW and Brown GH (1992), Manipulation of the fatty acid composition of milk by feeding protected canola seed, *J Dairy Sci*, 75, 1090–6.

Ashes JR, Thompson RM, Gulati SK, Brown GH, Scott TW, Rich AC and Rich JC (1993), A comparison of fatty acid profiles and carcass characteristics of feedlot steers fed canola seed and sunflower seed meal supplements protected from metabolism in the rumen, *Aust J Agric Res*, 44, 1103–12.

Auldist MJ, Walsh BJ and Thomson NA (1998), Seasonal and lactational influences on bovine milk composition in New Zealand, *J Dairy Res*, 65, 401–11.

Azcona JO, Schang MJ, Garcia PT, Gallinger C, Ayerza Jr R and Coates W (2008), Omega-3 enriched broiler meat: the influence of dietary alpha linolenic omega-3 fatty acid sources on growth, performance and meat fatty acid composition, *Can J Anim. Sci*, 88, 257–69.

Bauman DE and Griinari JM (2003), Nutritional regulation of milk fat synthesis, *Ann Rev Nutr*, 23, 203–27.

© Woodhead Publishing Limited, 2011

Bell JA, Griinari JM and Kennelly JJ (2006), Effect of safflower oil, flaxseed oil, monensin and vitamin E on concentration of conjugated linoleic acid in bovine milk fat, *J Dairy Sci*, 89, 733–48.

Benchaar C and Chouinard PY (2009), Assessment of the potential of cinnamaldehyde, condensed tannins and saponins to modify milk fatty acid composition of dairy cows, *J Dairy Sci*, 92, 3392–6.

Boeckaert C, Vlaeminck B, Dijkstra J, Issa-Zcaharia A, Van Nespen T, Van Straalen W and Fievez V (2008), Effect of dietary starch or micro algae supplementation on rumen fermentation and milk fatty acid composition of dairy cows, *J Dairy Sci*, 91, 4714–27.

Bonanome A and Grundy SM (1988), Effect of dietary stearic acid on plasma cholesterol and lipoprotein levels, *New Eng J of Med* 318, 1244–128.

Bu DP, Wang JQ, Dhiman TR and Liu SJ (2007), Effectiveness of oils rich in linoleic and linolenic acids to enhance conjugated linoleic acid in milk from dairy cows, *J Dairy Sci*, 90, 998–1007.

Chilliard Y, Glasser F, Ferlay A, Bernard L, Rouel J and Doreau M (2007), Diet, rumen biohydrogenation and nutritional quality of cow and goat milk fat, *Eur J Lipid Sci Technol*, 109, 828–55.

Chilliard Y, Martin C, Rouel J and Doreau M (2009), Milk fatty acids in dairy cows fed whole crude linseed, extruded linseed, or linseed oil, and their relationship with methane output, *J Dairy Sci*, 92, 5199–211.

Chilliard Y, Rouel J, Ferlay A, Bernard L, Gaborit P, Raynal-Ljutovac K, Lauret A and Leroux C (2006), Optimising goat's milk and cheese fatty acid composition, in Williams C and Buttriss J (eds), *Improving the fat content of feeds*, Cambridge, Woodhead, pp. 281–312.

Chouinard PY, Corneau L, Butler WR, Chilliard Y, Drackley JK and Bauman DE (2001), Effect of dietary lipid source on conjugated linoleic acid concentrations in milk fat, *J Dairy Sci*, 84, 680–90.

Collomb M, Sollberger H, Bütikofer U, Sieber R, Stoll W and Schaeren W (2004), Impact of a basal diet of hay and fodder beet supplemented with rapeseed, linseed and sunflowerseed on the fatty acid composition of milk fat, *Int Dairy J*, 14, 549–59.

Cordero G, Isabel B, Menoyo D, Daza A, Morales J, Pineiro C and Lopez-Bote CJ (2010), Dietary CLA alters intramuscular fat and fatty acid composition of pig skeletal muscle and subcutaneous adipose tissue, *Meat Sci*, 85, 235–9.

Crespo N and Esteve-García E (2002), Nutrient and fatty acid deposition in broilers fed different dietary fatty acid profiles, *Poul Sci*, 81, 1533–42.

Da Silva DC, Santos GT, Branco AF, Damasceno JC, Kazama R, Matsushita M, Horst JA, Dos Santos WBR and Petit HV (2007), Production performance and milk composition of dairy cows fed whole or ground flaxseed with or without monensin, *J Dairy Sci*, 90, 2928–36.

Daley CA, Abbott A, Doyle PS, Nader GA and Larson S (2010), A review of fatty acid profiles and antioxidant content in grass-fed and grain-fed beef, *Nutr J*, 9, 10–12.

De Smet S, Raes K and Demeyer D (2004), Meat fatty acid composition as affected by genetics: a review, *Anim Res*, 53, 81–98.

De Veth MJ, Gulati SK, Luchini ND and Bauman DE (2005), Comparison of calcium salts and formaldehyde-protected conjugated linoleic acid in inducing milk fat depression, *J Dairy Sci*, 88, 1685–93.

Delgado CL (2005), Rising demand for meat and milk in developing countries: implications for grasslands-based livestock production. in McGilloway D, *Grassland: a global resource*, Wageningen, Wageningen Academic Publishers, 29–39.

Dewhurst RJ, Fisher WJ, Tweed JKS and Wilkins RJ (2003), Comparison of grass and legume silages for milk production 1. Production responses with different levels of concentrate, *J Dairy Sci*, 86, 2598–611.

Dewhurst RJ, Shingfield KJ, Lee MRF and Scollan ND (2006), Increasing the concentrations of beneficial polyunsaturated fatty acids in milk produced by dairy cows in high-forage systems, *Anim Feed Sci Technol*, 131, 168–206.

© Woodhead Publishing Limited, 2011

Duckett SK, Wagner DG, Owens FN, Dolezal MG and Gill OR (1999), Effect of anabolic implants on beef intramuscular lipid content, *J Anim Sci*, 77, 1100–4.

Engle TE and Spears JW (2004), Effect of finishing system (feedlot or pasture), high-oil maize, and copper on conjugated linoleic acid and other fatty acids in muscle of finishing steers, *Anim Sci*, 78, 201–69.

Engle TE, Spears JW, Armstrong TA, Wright CL and Odle J (2000), Effects of copper source and concentration on carcass characteristics and lipid and cholesterol metabolism in growing and finishing steers, *J Anim Sci*, 78, 1053–9.

Franklin ST, Martin KR, Baer RJ, Shingoethe DJ and Hippen AR (1999), Dietary marine algae (*schizochytrium sp*) increases concentrations of conjugated linoleic acid, docosahexaenoic and transvaccenic acids in milk of dairy cows, *J Nut*, 129, 2048–52.

French P, Stanton C, Lawless F, O'Riordan EG, Monahan FJ, Caffrey PJ and Moloney AP (2000), Fatty acid composition, including conjugated linoleic acid, of intramuscular fat from steers offered grazed grass, grass silage or concentrate-based diets, *J Anim Sci* 78, 2849–55.

German JB and Dillard CJ (2004), Saturated fats: what dietary intake, *Am J Clin Nutr*, 80, 550–9.

Gilbert CD, Lunt DK, Miller RK and Smith SB (2003), Carcass, sensory, and adipose tissue traits of Brangus steers fed casein-formaldehyde-protected starch and/or canola lipid, *J Anim Sc*, 81, 2457–68.

Gilka J, Jelinek P, Jankova B, Knesel P, Krejci, Masek J and Docekalova H (1989), Amino acid composition of meat, fatty acid composition of fat and content of some chemical elements in the tissues of male lambs fed monensin or lasalocid, *Meat Sci*, 25, 273–80.

Gillis MH, Duckett SK and Sackmann JR (2004), Effects of supplemental rumen-protected conjugated linoleic acid or corn oil on fatty acid composition of adipose tissues in beef cattle, *J Anim Sci*, 82, 1419–27.

Givens DI (2008), Impact on CVD risk of modifying milk fat to decrease intake of SFA and increase intake of *cis*-MUFA, *Proc Nutr Soc*, 67, 419–27.

Givens DI and Shingfield KJ (2006), Optimising dairy milk fatty acid composition, in Williams C and Buttriss J, *Improving the fat content of feeds*, Cambridge, Woodhead 252–80.

Givens DI, Kliem KE, Humphries DJ, Shingfield KJ and Morgan R (2009), Effect of replacing calcium salts of palm oil distillate with rapeseed oil, milled or whole rapeseeds on milk fatty-acid composition in cows fed maize silage-based diets, *Animal*, 3, 1067–74.

Glasser F, Ferlay A and Chilliard Y (2008), Oilseed lipid supplements and fatty acid composition of cow milk. A meta-analysis. *J Dairy Sci*, 91, 4687–703.

Guillevic M, Kouba M and Mourot J (2009), Effect of a linseed diet on lipid composition, lipid peroxidation and consumer evaluation of French fresh and cooked pork meats, *Meat Sci*, 81, 612–18.

Gulati DK, McGrath S, Wynn PC and Scott TW (2003), Preliminary results on the relative incorporation of docosahexaenoic and eicosapentaenoic acids into cows milk from two types of rumen protected fish oil, *Int Dairy J*, 13, 339–43.

Hallenstvedt E, Kjos NP, Rehnberg AC, Overland M and Thomassen M (2010), Fish oil in feeds for entire male and female pigs. Changes in muscle fatty acid composition and stability of sensory quality, *Meat Sci*, 85, 182–90.

Harvatine KJ, Boisclair YR and Bauman DE (2009), Recent advances in the regulation of milk fat synthesis, *Animal*, 3, 40–54.

Henderson L, Gregory J and Irving K (2003), The national diet and nutrition survey: Adults aged 19–64 years, London, HMSO.

Hulshof FAM, van Erp-Baart MA, Anttolainen M, Becker W, Church SM, Couet C, Hermann-Kunz E, Kesteloot H, Leth T, Martins I, Moreiras O, Moschandreas J, Pizzoferrato L, Rimstud AH, Thorgeirsdottir H, van Amelsvoort JMM, Aro A, Kafatos AG, Lanzmann-Peithory D and Van Poppel G. (1999), Intake of fatty acids in Western

© Woodhead Publishing Limited, 2011

Europe with emphasis on trans fatty acids: The TRANSFAIR study, *Eur J Clin Nutr*, 53, 143–57.

Hutchison S, Kegley EB, Apple JK, Wistuba TJ, Dikeman ME and Rule DC (2006), Effects of adding poultry fat in the finishing diet of steers on performance, carcass characteristics, sensory traits, and fatty acid profiles, *J Anim Sci*, 84, 2426–35.

Jakobsen MU, Overvad K, Dyerberg J and Heitman BL (2008), Intake of ruminant *trans* fatty acids and the risk of coronary heart disease, *Int. J. Epidemiol*, 37, 173–82.

Jordan E, Lovett DK, Monahan FJ, Callan J, Flynn B and O'Mara F (2006), Effect of refined coconut oil or copra meal on methane output and on intake and performance of beef heifers, *J Anim Sci*, 84, 162–70.

Joyce T, Wallace AJ, McCarthy SN and Gibney MJ (2008), Intakes of total fat, saturated, monounsaturated and polyunsaturated fatty acids in Irish children, teenagers and adults, *Pub. Health Nutr*, 12, 156–65.

Kelly ML, Kolver ES, Bauman DE, Amburgh Van ME and Muller LD (1998), Effect of intake of pasture on concentrations of conjugated linoleic acid in milk of lactating cows, *J Dairy Sci*, 81, 1630–6.

Kitessa SM, Gulati SK, Simos GC, Ashes JR, Scott TW, Fleck E and Wynn PC (2004), Supplementation of grazing cows with rumen-protected tuna oil enriches milk fat n-3 fatty acids without affecting milk production or sensory characteristics, *Brit J Nutr*, 91, 271–7.

Kliem KE, Morgan R, Humphries DJ, Shingfield KJ and Givens DI (2008), Effect of replacing grass silage with maize silage in the diet on bovine milk fatty acid composition, *Animal*, 2, 1850–8.

Lawrie RA (2006), Chemical and biochemical constitution of muscle, in Lawrie RA and Ledward DA, *Lawrie's meat science*, Cambridge, Woodhead, 75–127.

Leheska JM, Thompson LD, Howe JC, Hentges E, Boyce J, Brooks JC, Shriver B, Hoover L and Miller MK (2008), Effects of conventional and grass-feeding systems on the nutrient composition of beef, *J Anim Sci*, 86, 3575–85.

Leskanich CO, Matthews KR, Warkup CC, Noble RC and Hazzeldine M (1997), The effect of dietary oil containing (n-3) fatty acids on the fatty acid, physicochemical, and organoleptic characteristics of pig meat and fat, *J Anim Sci*, 75, 673–83.

Loor JJ, Herbein JH and Jenkins TC (2002), Nutrient digestion, biohydrogenation and fatty acid profiles in blood plasma and milk fat from lactating Holstein cows fed canola oil or canolamide, *Anim Feed Sci Technol*, 97, 65–82.

Lopez-Ferrer S, Baucells MD, Barroeta AC, Galobart J and Grashorn MA (2001a), n-3 enrichment of chicken meat. 2. Use of precursors of long-chain polyunsaturated fatty acids: linseed oil, *Poul Sci*, 80, 753–61.

Lopez-Ferrer S, Baucells MD, Barroeta AC and Grashorn MA (2001b), n-3 enrichment of chicken meat. 1. Use of very long-chain fatty acids in chicken diets and their influence on meat quality: fish oil, *Poul Sci*, 80, 741–52.

Lourenco M, Van Ranst G, Vlaeminck B, De Smet S and Fievez V (2008), Influence of different dietary forages on the fatty acid composition of rumen digesta as well as ruminant meat and milk, *Anim Feed Sci Technol*, 145, 418–37.

MAFF (Ministry of Agriculture, Fisheries and Food) (1998), Food Fatty Acids Supplement to McCance and Widdowson's The Composition of Foods. London, MAFF.

Marmer WN, Maxwell RJ and Wagner DG (1985), Effects of dietary monensin on bovine fatty acid profiles, *J Agric Food Chem*, 33, 67–70.

Mele M (2009), Designing milk fat to improve healthfulness and functional properties of dairy products: from feeding strategies to a genetic approach, *Ital J Anim Sci*, 8 (Suppl. 2), 365–73.

Miller MF, Shackelford SD, Hayden KD and Reagan JO (1990), Determination of the alteration in fatty acid profiles, sensory characteristics and carcass traits of swine fed elevated levels of monounsaturated fats in the diet, *J Anim. Sci*, 68, 1624–31.

© Woodhead Publishing Limited, 2011

Moloney AP (1998), Growth and carcass composition in sheep offered isoenergetic rations which resulted in different concentrations of ruminal metabolites, *Live Prod Sci*, 56, 157–64.

Moloney AP (2002), Growth and carcass composition in sheep offered low or high metabolisable protein supplemented with sodium propionate, *Proc Agric Res Forum*, 20–1.

Moloney AP (2006), Reducing fats in raw meat, in Williams C and Buttriss J (eds) *Improving the fat content of feeds*, Cambridge, Woodhead, pp. 313–35.

Moloney AP, Keane MG, Dunne PG, Mooney MT and Troy DJ (2008), Effect of concentrate feeding pattern in a grass silage/concentrate beef finishing system on performance, selected carcass and meat quality characteristics, *Meat Sci*, 79, 355–64.

Moreno T, Keane MG, Noci F and Moloney AP (2008), Fatty acid composition of muscle from Holstein-Friesian steers of New Zealand and European/American descent and from Belgian Blue x Holstein-Friesian steers, slaughtered at two weights, *Meat Sci*, 80, 157–69.

Noci F, French P, Monahan FJ and Moloney AP (2005a), The fatty acid composition of muscle fat and subcutaneous adipose tissue of pasture-fed beef heifers: Influence of duration of grazing, *J Anim Sci*, 83, 1167–78.

Noci F, O'Kiely P, Monahan FJ, Stanton C and Moloney AP (2005b), Conjugated linoleic acid concentration in *M. Longissimus dorsi* from heifers offered sunflower oil-based concentrates and conserved forages, *Meat Sci*, 69, 509–18.

Noci F, Monahan FJ, Scollan ND and Moloney AP (2007), The fatty acid composition of muscle and adipose tissue of steers offered unwilted or wilted grass silage supplemented with sunflower oil and fishoil, *Brit J Nutr*, 97, 502–13.

Odongo NE, Or-Rashid MM, Kebreab E, France J and McBride BW (2007), Effect of supplementing myristic acid in dairy cow rations on ruminal methanogenesis and fatty acid profile in milk, *J Dairy Sci*, 90, 1851–8.

Offer NW, Marsden M, Dixon J, Speake BK and Thacker FE (1999), Effect of dietary fat supplements on levels of n-3 polyunsaturated fatty acids, trans acids and conjugated linoleic acid in bovine milk, *Anim Sci*, 69, 613–25.

Owens FN, Gill DR, Secrist DS and Coleman SW (1995), Review of some aspects of growth and development of feedlot cattle, *J Anim Sci*, 73, 3152–72.

Rentfrow G, Sauber TE, Allee GL and Berg EP (2003), The influence of diets containing either conventional corn, conventional corn with choice white grease, high oil corn, or high oil high oleic corn on belly/bacon quality, *Meat Sci*, 64, 459–66.

Richardson RI, Hallett KG, Robinson AM, Nute GR, Enser M and Wood JD (2004), Effect of free and ruminally-protected fish oils on fatty acid composition, sensory and oxidative characteristics of beef loin muscle, in *Proceedings of the 50th international conference on meat science and technology*, Helsinki, Finland, 2.43.

Rymer C and Givens DI (2005), n-3 Fatty acid enrichment of edible tissue of poultry: a review, *Lipids*, 40, 121–30.

Scollan ND, Choi NJ, Kurt E, Fisher AV, Enser M and Wood JD (2001), Manipulating the fatty acid composition of muscle and adipose tissue in beef cattle, *Brit J Nutr* 85, 115–24.

Scollan ND, Enser M, Gulati S, Richardson RI and Wood JD (2003), Effect of including a ruminally protected lipid supplement in the diet on the fatty acid composition of beef muscle in Charolais steers, *Brit J Nutr* 90, 709–16.

Scollan N, Hocquette JF, Nuernberg K, Dannenberger D, Richardson I, Moloney A (2006a), Innovations in beef production systems that enhance the nutritional and health value of beef lipids and their relationship with meat quality, *Meat Sci*, 74, 17–33.

Scollan ND, Costa P, Hallett KG, Nute GR, Wood JD and Richardson RI (2006b), The fatty acid composition of muscle fat and relationships to meat quality in Charolais steers: influence of level of red clover in the diet, *Proc Brit Soc Anim Sci*, 23.

Shingfield KJ, Ahvenjärvi S, Toivonen V, Ärölä A, Nurmela KVV, Huhtanen P and Griinari JM (2003), Effect of fish oil on biohydrogenation of fatty acids and milk fatty acid content in cows, *Anim Sci*, 77, 165–79.

© Woodhead Publishing Limited, 2011

Shingfield KJ, Reynolds CK, Lupoli B, Toivonen V, Yurawecz MP, Delmonte P, Griinari JM, Grandison AS and Beever DE (2005), Effect of forage type and proportion of concentrate in the diet on milk fatty acid composition in cows fed sunflower oil and fish oil, *Anim Sci*, 80, 225–38.

Shingfield KJ, Salo-Vaananen P, Pahkala E, Toivonen V, Jaakola S, Piironen V and Huhtanen P (2005), Effect of forage conservation method, concentrate level and propylene glycol on the fatty acid composition and vitamin content of cows' milk, *J Dairy Res*, 72, 349–61.

Siebert BD, Kruk ZA, Davis J, Pitchford WS, Harper GS and Bottema CDK (2006), Effect of low vitamin A status on fat deposition and fatty acid desaturation in beef cattle, *Lipids*, 41, 365–70.

Sinclair LA (2007), Nutritional manipulation of the fatty acid composition of sheep meat. a review, *J Agric Sci*, 145, 419–34.

Steen RVJ and Robson A (1995), Effects of forage to concentrate ratio in the diet and protein intake on the performance and carcass composition of beef heifers. *J Agric Sci*, 125, 125–35.

Steen RWJ, Lavery NP, Kilpatrick DJ and Porter MG (2003), Effects of pasture and high-concentrate diets on the performance of beef cattle, carcass composition at equal growth rates, and the fatty acid composition of beef, *N Z J Agric Res*, 46, 69–81.

Steijns JM (2008), Dairy products and health: Focus on their constituents or on the matrix? *Int Dairy J*, 18, 425–35.

Stender S, Astrup A and Dyerberg J (2008), Ruminant and industrially produced *trans* fatty acids: health aspects, *Food and Nutr Res*, doi: 10.3402/fnrv52i0.1651.

Szymczyk B, Pisulewski PM, Szczurek W and Hanczakowski P (2001), Effects of conjugated linoleic acid on growth performance, feed conversion efficiency, and subsequent quality in broiler chickens, *Brit J Nutr*, 85, 465–73.

Teye GA, Sheard PR, Whittington FM, Nute GR, Stewart A and Wood JD (2006), Influence of dietary oils and protein level on pork quality. 1. Effects on muscle fatty acid composition, carcass, meat and eating quality, *Meat Sci*, 73, 157–65.

Van Vuuren AM, Van Wikselaar PG, Van Riel JW, Klop A and Bastiaans JAHP (2010), Persistency of the effect of long-term administration of a whey protein gel composite of soybean and linseed oils on performance and milk fatty acid composition of dairy cows, *Livest Sci*, 129, 213–22.

Vasta V, Mele M, Serra A, Scerra M, Luciano G, Lanza M and Priolo A (2009), Metabolic fate of fatty acids involved in ruminal biohydrogenation in sheep fed concentrate or herbage with or without tannins, *J Anim Sci*, 87, 2674–84.

Webb EC and Casey NH (1995), Fatty acids in carcass fat of steers treated with a β-adrenergic agonist individually or in combination with trenbolone acetate + oestradiol-17β, *Meat Sci*, 41, 69–76.

WHO (2003), Diet, nutrition and the prevention of chronic diseases. *Report of a joint WHO/FAO expert consultation.* WHO technical report series 916, Geneva, World Health Organization.

Wood JD, Enser M, Fisher AV, Nute GR, Sheard PR, Richardson RI, Hughes SI and Whittington FM (2008), Fat deposition, fatty acid composition and meat quality: a review, *Meat Sci*, 78, 343–58.

Woods VB and Fearon AM (2009), Dietary sources of unsaturated fatty acids for animals and their transfer into meat, milk and eggs: a review, *Livest Sci*, 126, 1–20.

Zhang S, Knight TJ, Reecy JM and Beitz DC (2008), DNA polymorphisms in bovine fatty acid synthase are associated with beef fatty acid composition, *Anim Gen*, 39, 62–70.

© Woodhead Publishing Limited, 2011

13

Reducing saturated fat in savoury snacks and fried foods

A. M. Kita, Wrocław University of Environmental and Life Sciences, Poland

Abstract: This chapter discusses different parameters influencing the quality of fried foods – especially savoury snacks. The chapter first reviews different types of frying oils and quality attributes of fried snacks: fat uptake, texture, acrylamide content and storage stability. The chapter then discusses changes in frying technologies – vacuum and microwave frying – and changes in the savoury snacks market.

Key words: frying oil, snacks, fat uptake, texture, acrylamide, vacuum frying, microwave frying.

13.1 Introduction

Manufactured from a wide spectrum of raw materials with the aid of different methods, savoury snacks comprise a large variety of products with specific sensory properties. Even though they differ noticeably in shape, colour and flavour, savoury snacks have one feature in common – the crispy and delicate texture. A major group of savoury snacks includes fried products, specifically potato crisps, and different kinds of snacks. Potato crisps are thin potato slices subjected to frying in fat or oil until the moisture content falls below two per cent. Fried snacks are obtained from ready-made, half-finished products, referred to as pellets, which require further frying. The pellets are obtained from a variety of components where starch-based substrates dominate. In the course of the frying process the pellets expand, and thus impart the specific crispy texture to the snacks (Lusas and Rooney, 2002).

In spite of being the least explored sensory property, the specific crispy texture ranks as the most significant indicator of the snack's quality. Another quality indicator of equal significance is fat content. Fat is not only a vehicle for the flavour and aroma of the finished product; it also makes a contribution to its

© Woodhead Publishing Limited, 2011

texture and significantly increases the calorific value of the snack. This is why the modification of the products by reducing their fat content has taken on a sense of importance, particularly in developed countries, where obesity is a widespread phenomenon and snacks have become a regular supplement to the daily diet. In addition, equal significance has to be attached to the quality of the fat used for frying, which is vitally important when assessing the nutritional value of the snacks, since they are generally consumed by children and young people.

13.2   Frying oils

For frying, use is made of a variety of vegetable and animal oils and fats. However, taking into account the specific character of deep frying, refined vegetable oils of fluid consistency are the preferred option. The majority of refined oils are practically devoid of a specific flavour and aroma, but cottonseed and peanut oils impart a characteristic nutty aroma to the fried products. The type of oil chosen depends largely on commercial availability and local preferences. The use of cottonseed and peanut oils as frying media has gained great popularity in the USA, while in Europe preference is given to sunflower and rapeseed oils. Owing to the high content of unsaturated fatty acids, the majority of vegetable oils are prone to undergo thermo-oxidation. This holds true primarily for oils rich in polyunsaturated fatty acids, which undergo thermo-oxidative changes at a remarkably faster rate than do oils with a high content of monounsaturated acids. The rate observed in linolenic acid oxidation, for example, is around 40 times that of the oxidation of oleic acid (Drozdowski, 2007). That is the reason why in many countries limits have been imposed on the linolenic acid content of frying oils (below 2%) (Brinkmann, 2000).

In order to minimize or remove the polyunsaturated acids that are present in the frying medium, use is made of the hydrogenation process. However, an inherent disadvantage to this process is the formation of geometrical *trans* isomers of fatty acids, despite the desired saturation of some part of the double bonds. The presence of *trans* isomers is also undesirable for nutritional reasons. That is why the past few years have witnessed attempts to reduce the use of hydrogenated fats, and some countries have introduced regulations on the content of *trans* isomers in edible fats, which should not exceed two per cent. The abandonment of the hydrogenation process in the production of frying fats triggers the necessity of replacing the oils being used with others. In recent years, palm oil and its fractions (specifically palm olein) have become alternatives to hydrogenated fats in the European countries (Matthäus, 2007). With an approximately 50% content of saturated fatty acids (which is considered high for vegetable fats), palm oil is a stable frying medium. Owing to the competitive price and the fact of being readily available (its production is continuing to rise), palm oil has found wide acceptance, particularly in the manufacture of snacks. However, since the composition of the fatty acids that are present in palm oil is not very promising in nutritional terms, increasing attention is currently being given to a new generation of oils obtained

© Woodhead Publishing Limited, 2011

Table 13.1   Fatty acid composition (%) of traditional and new-generation frying oils

	Palm olein	Hydrogenated rapeseed oil	High-oleic, low-linolenic rapeseed oil	High-oleic soybean oil	High-oleic sunflower oil
C16:0	39.1	5.1	6.5	7.3	7.0
C18:0	4.1	4.0	2.0	3.4	3.8
C18:1	42.4	59.3	73.2	85.1	76.4
C18:2	10.1	2.9	15.2	1.3	9.2
C18:3	0.2	0.3	2.4	2.0	0.1
Trans fatty acids	0.1	15.9	0.2	0.1	0.2

from genetically modified plants. In these oils the proportion of polyunsaturated acids has been reduced in favour of the monounsaturated (oleic) acid, with the intention to maintain a low content of saturated acids. Those modifications have produced new soybean, sunflower and rapeseed oils (Rossell, 2003; Normand *et al.*, 2006; Gerde *et al.*, 2007; Warner and Fehr, 2008), which, in the main, meet the requirements defined for a perfect frying oil (Table 13.1). Thus, a perfect frying oil should contain the lowest possible quantity of saturated acids, more than 75% of oleic acid, less than 10% of linoleic acid and less than 1% of linolenic acid; *trans* isomers should be absent.

With such a composition of fatty acids, as well as with their specific physicochemical properties, the modified oils display the thermo-oxidative stability desired and do not raise objections to their nutritional value. Further support for their stability comes from the addition of various antioxidants (Che Man and Tan, 1999; Houhoula *et al.*, 2003; Jaswir *et al.*, 2000; Kochhar, 2000; Lalas and Dourtoglu, 2003; Satyanarayana *et al.*, 2000; Warner and Gehring, 2009). A case in point is the *Good fry oil* obtained from sunflower oil (rich in oleic acid) and additives of rice oil and oat oil. On the one hand, the antioxidants that are present in rice and oat oils efficiently stabilize the new oil obtained via the above procedure, but on the other hand the procedure itself accounts for a considerable rise in the price of that oil. This is why, besides pure oils of a high oleic acid content, a variety of oil blends are in use as frying media. The use of such oils, often defined as 'healthy', has become increasingly common in the manufacture of fried savoury snacks and is beginning to penetrate some of the fast-food restaurant chains.

13.3   Effects of frying oils and frying parameters on the quality of fried foods

13.3.1   Fat uptake

The quantity of the fat absorbed in the course of frying is one of the major factors affecting the quality and calorific value of the finished products. Snacks constitute

© Woodhead Publishing Limited, 2011

a specific group of products characterized by a high fat content, which is not only an important contributor to their unique sensory properties, but also a key factor in the improvement of their storage stability.

The process of fat uptake is described taking into account two different mechanisms: (1) as continuous fat absorption due to partial mass exchange between the frying medium and the evaporating water; and (2) as a fat absorption process that occurs upon termination of frying (Saguy and Dana, 2003). According to the first mechanism, moisture loss induces changes in the cell structure of the material being fried, contributing to the formation of a matrix of small channels, which become occupied by the frying medium immediately after water vaporization. Most of the fat is taken up within the initial 20 seconds of frying (Moreira *et al.*, 1997). According to the second mechanism, the phenomenon of fat absorption occurs during cooling of the fried product after the frying process has been terminated. In the course of frying, a portion of the water which is present in the product evaporates and simultaneously induces some pressure. After that, the water is removed to the outside through a system of capillaries and channels in the cell structure. The oil that is present on the surface of the product being fried, or that partly penetrates this system, is expelled continually by the water vapour being formed in the course of frying. The process continues as long as water vapour is being produced and removed. While the product is being cooled, the internal subatmospheric pressure reduces as a result of condensation, thus producing the so-called 'vacuum effect', which enables the fat to penetrate into the product (the penetration depth being limited to approximately 1 mm) (Saguy and Dana, 2003).

The quantity of fat taken up in the course of frying depends on various factors regarding both the raw materials and the processing technologies applied. Those pertaining to the raw materials include the effect of the potato variety and chemical parameters, as well as the influence of the frying medium quality. Investigations into the effect of the chemical composition of the potato on the fat taken up by the crisps have revealed that the higher the dry mass content of the tuber, the lower the fat content of the crisps produced. As far as snacks are concerned, fat uptake in the course of frying largely depends on the composition of the blend from which the pellets have been prepared. The quantity of the fat absorbed is also strongly influenced by the shape and size of the pieces being fried. Analysis of the contribution of slice thickness to the extent of fat uptake has demonstrated that an increase in the thickness of potato slices is paralleled by a decrease in the quantity of the fat absorbed by the fried potato crisps (Mellema, 2003).

Analysis of pertinent data reported in the literature makes it clear that the extent of fat uptake also depends on the kind of frying medium used, and that the finished products may differ in the quantity of fat absorbed. In their experimental study on the contribution of the frying process and frying media (refined soybean and peanut oils; hydrogenated fat) to the quality of potato crisps, Rani and Chauhan (1995) observed that the highest uptake of the frying medium occurred when the crisps were fried in hydrogenated fat. Annapure and co-workers (1998), who related the fat content in fried snacks to the type of vegetable oils used for the

© Woodhead Publishing Limited, 2011

purpose of their study, have found that snacks fried in refined peanut oil were characterized by a higher fat content compared with hydrogenated oil.

The extent of fat uptake varies with each change in the properties of the frying medium. It has been reported that the lower the quality of the frying fat (which manifests in the high content of degradation products), the higher is the quantity of the fat taken up by the finished product (Dobarganes *et al.*, 2000; Kita, 2006). In the tests performed with refined rapeseed oil and hydrogenated fat as frying media such a relation held true only for the chips that were fried in modified fats. Chips fried in rapeseed oil were found to absorb the same quantity of fat regardless of the extent of frying medium degradation (Kita *et al.*, 2005). A similar relation was observed by Moreira and co-workers (1997) during deep frying of tortilla chips in fresh and degraded soybean oil. Although the chips fried in fresh oil took up larger quantities of the frying medium in the course of cooling, the oil content of the finished products was substantially the same.

Technological parameters, and the course of the frying process in particular, are also among the major contributing factors to the quality of the finished products. Fat uptake can be limited by the application of such treatment procedures as blanching and pre-drying, or by depositing edible coatings onto the surface before the product is fried, in order to reduce the quantity of the fat absorbed during frying (Debnath *et al.*, 2003; Mellema, 2003). It is essential to note that the larger the surface, or the higher the ratio of one load input to the volume of the frying oil, the higher is the fat content of the finished product. The data on the contribution of frying temperature to the extent of fat uptake by the product are inconsistent. Some investigators have demonstrated that when the frying temperature increases, so does the quantity of the fat absorbed by the product being fried (Krokida *et al.*, 2000). Others have observed a reverse relation – products fried at elevated temperature contained less fat (Pinthus *et al.*, 1995). Gamble *et al.* (1987), for example, claim that they failed to detect any relationship between frying temperature (over the range of 150 to 180°C) and the fat content of the finished product.

13.3.2   Texture

Of the sensory properties inherent in snacks, their specific crispy texture is considered the most important. The texture of the snack develops in the course of frying and is influenced by many different factors. So far, particular consideration has been given to the problem of how the chemical composition of the raw material impacts on the texture of the finished product (Kita, 2002b).

Apart from being affected by the parameters of the raw material used, the texture of the finished product is influenced by the parameters of the technological process. The texture of potato crisps produced from thin slices is more delicate and not as hard as that of crisps obtained from thick slices (Kita, 2002a). The extent of fat uptake during frying is another major factor affecting the texture of the finished product. Potato crisps of a high fat content (exceeding 40%) were found to display an oily texture, which was lacking in crispiness. Those of an

© Woodhead Publishing Limited, 2011

insufficiently high fat content were characterized by excessive hardness. In the case of both crisps and snacks an aspect of importance is the continuation of the frying process until the product has achieved the moisture content desired. If the moisture content is excessively high, the finished product fails to be either crispy or delicate. Low moisture content (as well as an appropriate texture) has a key role in the suitability of the finished products for storage.

Storage stability tests have revealed that with increase in moisture content the texture of the products being stored deteriorates. During storage, both crisps and snacks take up water, lose their specific crispiness and become harsh. The tests have also demonstrated that the rate at which those undesirable changes occur depends on the following factors: initial moisture content, type of ingredients (spices), type of wrapper, storage conditions and duration of storage (Kita, 2002a).

13.3.3 Acrylamide content

In the past few years it has been observed that the frying of carbohydrate-containing products is concomitant with the formation of acrylamide (AA), an undesired chemical compound, and that high acrylamide concentrations are detected in savoury snacks. Acrylamide has been synthesized on an industrial scale for many years, and its applications are manifold. It is used, *inter alia*, for the synthesis of polyacrylamide (a popular polymer made use of, for example, in the treatment of potable water), in wrapper manufacture, or in the textile industry (Friedman, 2003; Claeys *et al.*, 2005). Since acrylamide is classified as a chemical compound of potential carcinogenicity to humans (group 2A), limits have been imposed on its concentration primarily in potable water (0.5 µg AA/kg), as well as in products wrapped in plastics (10 µg AA/kg). The findings reported by some Swedish researchers in 2002 make it clear that acrylamide is detected in a variety of products at concentrations frequently exceeding the permissible values. Particularly large quantities of acrylamide were found to occur in products obtained from potatoes, i.e. chips (170 to 3700 µg/kg) and crisps (200 to 12 000 µg/kg) (Friedman, 2003). Since the origins of this carcinogenic compound are still far from being convincingly defined, a number of hypotheses have been put forward to elucidate the mechanism of acrylamide formation in food in the course of thermal processing, such as baking, frying or roasting. According to some researchers, the most probable mechanism underlying the formation of acrylamide entails the Maillard browning reactions (browning discoloration on the surface of potato products) (Zyzak *et al.*, 2003). Thus, acrylamide emerges in the course of the reaction of amino acids (asparagine) with a reactive carbonyl (glucose, fructose), through several stages including forming a Schiff base. Other investigators have increased the number of the reagents participating in the formation of acrylamide by the inclusion of acroleine, which forms either as a result of fat conversion or via degradation of amino acids and proteins (Gertz and Klostermann, 2002). Acroleine oxidizes to acrylic acid, which reacts with ammonia nitrogen and may account for the formation of acrylamide. Another mechanism reported in the literature suggests that acrylamide is the direct product

© Woodhead Publishing Limited, 2011

of the reactions of other nitrogen-containing compounds (e.g. alanins), with the exclusion of acroleine (Becalski *et al.*, 2003).

Researches into the mechanisms governing acrylamide formation in different food products were paralleled by investigations whose objective was to develop methods aimed at inhibiting (or blocking) the synthesis of acrylamide or for minimizing the quantity of the acrylamide formed. Among the methods that limit the formation of acrylamide in food products, two major groups can be distinguished. One of these includes methods where the content of acrylamide precursors is reduced in the raw material; the other group comprises methods that enable the synthesis of acrylamide to be inhibited or blocked by changing the technological parameters. As for the first group, focus is placed on the choice of appropriate potato varieties, which in the case of the products of interest should be characterized by a low content of reducing sugars. Such selection is made by the manufacturers of crisps and chips, who have established permissible values for the level of reducing sugars in the potato tuber, taking into account the coloration of the finished product. They have also determined the conditions (with emphasis on temperature) for the storage of the potatoes to be used for frying, in order to prevent the reducing sugars from accumulating in the tubers. It is, however, desirable that the raw material should contain a certain quantity of sugars because of their positive contribution not only to the coloration, but also to the specific flavour of the finished products. An efficient method has been patented, where use is made of asparaginase to remove another acrylamide precursor from the raw material being processed, i.e. asparagines (Elder *et al.*, 2004). Asparaginase has the ability to convert asparagine into asparaginic acid, which does not participate in the synthesis of acrylamide. Nevertheless, a large-scale application of this method has not been carried out because the costs involved are high (Friedman and Levin, 2008).

Although the potato varieties used as raw materials for crisps and chips are similar in the content of reducing sugars, it has been found that the finished products often differ in the content of acrylamide. This finding suggests that the course of the technological process also makes a significant contribution to the synthesis of this compound. The use of the popular blanching procedure fails to significantly reduce acrylamide content despite a partial extraction of the precursors (reducing sugars and asparagine). Jung and co-workers have observed (2003) that blanching or soaking in organic acid solutions (e.g. citric acid) is an effective operation, which inhibits the reaction of acrylamide formation owing to the decreased pH. Positive effects were also achieved when other amino acids than asparagine had been added into the reaction system. It is essential to note, however, that the key factors in acrylamide synthesis are the parameters and the course of the thermal process during which the reaction of acrylamide formation sets in. A decrease in frying temperature is one of the simplest methods for reducing the quantity of acrylamide in the finished products. Since acrylamide is synthesized at the final stage of frying, it is essential to determine the shortest possible, albeit sufficient, duration for the frying process (Gökmen and Palazoğlu, 2008). In their search for efficient methods of reducing the acrylamide content in

© Woodhead Publishing Limited, 2011

chips, Grob and co-workers (2003) have demonstrated that even the slightest extension of the frying time may greatly increase the amount of acrylamide in the finished product. Another decisive factor is the proportion of the one load input into the fryer to the volume of the frying oil used. In that particular case the 10% principle (frying oil volume/one load input volume of 10:1) was found to be the most efficient. The type of frying medium chosen may also influence the rate of acrylamide formation. Gertz and Klostermann (2002), who compared the quantities of acrylamide in chips fried in a variety of fats, revealed that the acrylamide content of the products fried in palm oil was higher compared to the other oils tested. Mestdagh et al. (2007) detected no relation between the type of frying oil used and the quantity of acrylamide produced. Some researchers reported that the amounts of acrylamide formed might depend on the extent of oil degradation (Zamora and Hidalgo, 2008); others found that acrylamide formation was favourably influenced by the products of fat oxidation (Capuano et al., 2010). Thus, when the product is fried in an oil with an increased capacity for oxidation (an increased degree of unsaturation), the quantity of the acrylamide synthesized may rise with the progress of the oxidation process. Another factor favouring the formation of acrylamide was found to be the addition of anti-foaming substances. Although the literature contains references to the effect of antioxidant addition on the synthesis of acrylamide, the results obtained are not consistent. Vattem and Shetty reported that the formation of acrylamide in fried potato slices increased when they were previously treated with phenolic antioxidants. However, other investigators claimed that antioxidant compounds could be effective tools to inhibit acrylamide production (Zhang et al., 2007; Napolitano et al., 2008).

13.3.4 Quality of frying oil and its effect on storage stability of fried products

Analysis of the fat breakdown products being formed in the course of frying has substantiated the occurrence of more than 400 chemical compounds. Among them more than 200 have been classified as volatile substances. Taking into account the category of some of these substances and potential health implications, many countries (mostly European) have established standards defining the permissible values for their concentrations in frying oil. In most instances they specify them as free fatty acids expressed as acid number (max. 2% or 2.5%), polar compounds (max. 25% or 27%), triacylglycerol polymers and dimers (max. 10%, Belgium and the Czech Republic; max. 16%, the Netherlands), and for the smoke point of the frying oil (not lower than 170 or 180°C) (Erickson, 2007).

Use is also made of other research methods for determining the frying quality of the fat. After analysing the changes observed in palm olein quality during industrial-scale manufacture of potato crisps, the methods that are in use have been ordered in the following way: variations in tocopherol content > dielectric constant > free fatty acid content > variations in tetrahydroquinone (TBHQ) > anisidine number > induction period determined by Rancimat. The first three methods are well correlated with the content of polar compounds; the determination of polar compounds was recommended as a method for the monitoring of oil properties in the course of frying. Since the frying process is dominated by oxidation and polymerization reactions, another parameter, the OSET index (100/ content of polymerized triacylglycerols), has been proposed as a thermal stability measure for frying fats, particularly when their properties are 'improved' by the addition of antioxidants (Kochhar and Gertz, 2004).

Fat conversion commences in the course of the frying process and continues in the fat portion of the finished products throughout their storage. This is of great significance to snack products, as they are made available to the consumer after varying periods of storage.

The changes observed in the fat taken up by the fried snack products, commonly defined as rancidity, are primarily due to hydrolysis and oxidation. Hydrolytic changes generally occur at a constant rate throughout storage. Changes induced by oxidation follow a different pattern. The rate of oxidative changes depends both on the kind of frying medium used (specifically on the degree of unsaturation) and on the storage conditions (*inter alia* on the exposure to light). When exposed to light during storage, the fat absorbed by the products oxidizes both under the influence of singlet oxygen and as a result of auto-oxidation. Since singlet oxygen reacts 1500 times as fast as does triplet oxygen, oxidation occurs at a noticeably faster rate in products exposed to light (Nawar, 1996). Although at the initial stage of storage the quantity of oxidation products may be small, their increment over the following weeks may be a logarithmic one.

The products of fat conversion during storage exert a direct effect on the sensory properties of the finished products. The flavour and aroma of rancid fat is attributable, in the majority of instances, to the presence of low-molecular-weight volatile substances, i.e. aldehydes, ketones and free fatty acids. Even very small amounts of low-molecular-weight free fatty acids suffice to make the rancidity of the fat perceivable. Rancid fat undergoes discoloration influenced by the changes in natural colourants and by the formation of new colourants (Petukhov *et al.*, 1999; Pangloli *et al.*, 2002).

13.4   Innovating technologies in frying and their impact on the quality of fried foods

The observation that the parameters of the frying process and the quality of the frying oil are the principal contributors to the properties of the finished product has triggered continuing efforts to modify the course of the frying process. When use is made of conventional submersion fryers in continuous processes, the products are placed on a special belt and then conveyed to the fryer, which has been filled with oil heated up to the required temperature. After that the products move through subsequent sections of the fryer – all submersed in the frying oil of a temperature chosen accordingly. The duration of the frying process, which depends on the size of the pieces and the type of product being fried, varies from several seconds (e.g. for snacks obtained from pellets) to more than ten minutes

© Woodhead Publishing Limited, 2011

(e.g. for chicken nuggets). Fryers of that type (particularly those of a large volume), where considerable amounts of oil are heated, have the disadvantage of being heavy in energy demand. They were also found to accelerate the process of oil degradation as a result of thermo-oxidative changes. Another troublesome drawback is the continuous filtration of large oil quantities.

A practical alternative appears to be the use of HeatWave® fryers (an invention of the company Heat and Control), where the product being fried circulates on a perforated metal belt to get in contact (several times or more) with curtains of hot oil. Oil curtains provide heat transfer more efficiently than does submersion. Oil passes over the product and through the conveyor, thus providing a fast removal of the fines from the fryer. The flowing oil and the wiping action of the conveyor belt remove the fines from the full width of the pan, while the total volume of the system oil circulates through the continuous filter within a few seconds. The time of contact between the product being fried and the frying medium, which has been reduced to the permissible minimum, enables an efficient heat transfer and mass exchange, yielding products with the quality attributes desired. The HeatWave technique is an ideal option for frying a variety of foods. As for portioned frozen food (especially when breaded), the use of the HeatWave fryer imparts an evenly fried surface to the finished products. Furthermore, owing to the direct removal of the fines, it is possible to minimize the accelerated degradation of the frying oil. The application of HeatWave fryers can also be a viable option for obtaining snacks by expansion from pellets, as this requires that the time of contact with the frying medium should be very short. The considerable reduction in the volume of the oil being used for frying offers the following benefits: a shorter time of oil exchange in the fryer, lower operating costs, and finished products of a fresh aroma and an ideal texture.

13.4.1 Vacuum frying

Vacuum frying is a comparatively new innovative technology for the manufacture of a new generation of snacks – frequently referred to as 'healthy' products. Vacuum-fried products are characterized by a lower fat content and a higher nutritional value, since fewer changes occur in the bioactive components of the raw material and in the frying oil. The raw materials used in this technology include a wide variety of fruits (e.g. mango, cassava, pineapple or apple) and vegetables (e.g. blue potato, green beans, carrots, broccoli or cauliflower), all rich in nutrients. Vacuum-fried products do not show such undesired properties as excessive browning or shrinkage. In the course of vacuum frying, the food is heated at reduced pressure (< 60 Torr ~8 kPa), which causes the boiling points to decrease both for the frying oil and for the water contained in the products being fried.

The benefits from vacuum frying are manifold. Compared to traditional frying, the process involves a lower temperature, its duration is shorter, and the finished product has the properties desired. The absence of air during frying is an inhibiting factor in the oxidation reactions (especially in the oxidation of fats) and at the same time has a protective effect against the degradation of the frying medium.

© Woodhead Publishing Limited, 2011

Seemingly, the absence of air is also a significant contributory factor in the inhibition of the enzymatic browning observed in the finished product. In sum, the inhibition of Maillard's browning reaction, as well as the decreased temperature of frying, may have significantly contributed to the colour of the finished products, which is lighter and more natural than the colour of the products obtained in a traditional fryer (Garayo and Moreira 2002; Mariscal and Bouchon, 2008).

Reduced fat content is a major quality attribute for vacuum-fried products. Garayo and Moreira (2002) have reported that vacuum frying permits the fat content of potato crisps to be reduced by 30%. Similar relations have been established by Yamsaengsung and Rungsee (2003) for potato crisps and guava slices processed by conventional and vacuum frying. The results reported by Da Silva and Moreira (2008) have revealed a reduced fat content only in vacuum-fried sweet potatoes (by 24%) and green beans (by 16%). For blue potatoes and mangoes the reverse was true: traditionally fried samples had a lower fat content than did the vacuum-fried ones. Also Troncoso et al. (2009) have observed that oil uptake by potato crisps was higher when they were vacuum-fried.

Fat uptake during vacuum-frying was found to depend not only on the process conditions applied but also on pressurization – the second stage of the vacuum-frying process. Although the course of the first stage in vacuum frying and that in conventional frying at atmospheric pressure are similar, heat transfer and mass exchange during vacuum frying proceed at a faster rate. This is what accounts for the key role of the pressurization stage, which commences when the product being fried has already left the frying medium. Pore pressure rises quickly, causing the oil adhering to the crisp surface to penetrate into the food (thus generating the 'sponge effect'), until the value of pore pressure and that of atmospheric pressure become equal. On analysing the distribution of fat in vacuum-fried potato crisps, Moreira et al. (2009) observed that immediately upon the termination of the frying procedure only 14% of the oil was retained in the inner part of the product while approximately 86% was found on its surface. Such a distribution of the frying fat suggests the application of a de-oiling process, which enables a comparatively easy removal of surface oil by centrifugation. De-oiling guarantees a 50% reduction in fat content on average, without detrimentally affecting the other quality attributes of the finished products, specifically their brittleness and fragility. Vacuum frying units are equipped with centrifuges designed for de-oiling the product after the termination of the frying process. The centrifuges are placed in a special vacuum dome, which is attached to the vacuum fryer.

There is a close relationship between the process of fat uptake and the texture characteristics of the finished product. Troncoso et al. (2009) have observed that vacuum-fried crisps display a more delicate texture and reduced hardness. Vacuum frying induces a greater collapse in the structural tissues of the product, which accounts for more shrinkage and a potential increase in porosity, strongly affecting the textural parameters of foods. Vacuum frying could enhance the puffing effect and thus improve the texture quality of the fried products. Vacuum frying was also found to positively influence the coloration of the finished products; they are in many instances lighter and capable of retaining their original colours as opposed

© Woodhead Publishing Limited, 2011

to the products obtained by traditional frying. This is attributable, on the one hand, to the limited Maillard's browning reactions as a result of the drop in temperature, and, on the other hand, to the noticeably poorer pigment degradation.

Some interesting observations emerged from the research reported by Da Silva and Moreira (2008), who compared the chemical compositions of several fruit and vegetable snacks fried under conventional and vacuum conditions. Their experimental study produced the following results: after vacuum frying, anthocyanin content was 60% higher in blue potato crisps; total carotenoid content was higher by 18% in green beans, by 19% in mango crisps, and by 51% in sweet potato crisps. The literature also contains references which demonstrate that vacuum frying yields finished products of a reduced acrylamide content. Granda, Moreira and Tichy (2004) have found that acrylamide concentration in vacuum-fried potato crisps was 97% lower than in traditionally fried crisps.

13.4.2   Microwave frying

Another alternative to the traditional process is microwave frying. Microwaves have the capacity for interacting directly with the polar water molecules in the food to generate heat throughout the volume of the food. In this way, heating time is reduced, and thicker food pieces are heated uniformly by microwaves (Venkatesh and Raghavan, 2004). Microwave frying has two energy sources, which not only heat the foods but also enable their simultaneous cooking: the interior of the foods is cooked by microwaves and the surface of the foods by hot oil. The product achieves the desired golden coloration and crispiness of the crusts. Microwaves significantly shorten the duration of the frying process, reduce lipid oxidation and minimize oil content (Chen *et al.*, 2009). They also improve the uniformity of the product, yielding unique microstructures and properties (Clark *et al.*, 2000). The research reported by Oztop *et al.* (2007) has substantiated the beneficial effect of microwave frying on the properties of potato slices. Again, the use of microwaves shortened frying time and reduced the fat content of the finished product. In contrast to traditional frying, no changes were observed in the colour or hardness of the fried products. Because of the significantly shortened frying time, the microwave process is recommended when large food pieces are to be fried (e.g. chicken or fish nuggets). Microwave frying guarantees that the finished product will retain the moisture content desired, and that the formation of the specific crispy texture on the external surface of the food will not be inhibited. In some studies it has been shown that microwave frying could also decrease acrylamide content in coatings of chicken portions (Barutcu *et al.*, 2009).

13.5   Changes in savoury snacks

Even though they top the lists of unhealthy food in many countries, snack products still enjoy widespread popularity. Nowadays many attempts are being made to

© Woodhead Publishing Limited, 2011

help the snacks establish a good reputation, e.g. by a careful choice of the raw material and technological improvements to the process, or by the introduction of new wrappers. There is growing interest in crisps obtained from jacket potatoes, where peel fragments are still present after frying. To produce such crisps, use is frequently made of thick potato slices, which are fried by submersion. Advertised by Kettle Chips (an American commercial enterprise) as handmade, they have become popular in the United States, and their equivalents are also manufactured in Europe. An important asset in the production of those crisps is the careful selection of the potato varieties that are to be used as raw material; they all are grown using organic or ecological farming techniques. The increase in the thickness of the potato slices reduces the fat content and slightly hardens the texture of the finished product as compared to the crisps obtained with traditional methods. It is worthy of mention that the 'slightly harder' texture has been promoted to the rank of a specific quality attribute for those crisps. Emphasis is also being placed on some positive aspects regarding the manufacture of this group of snack products: the use of high-oleic oils (predominantly sunflower oil) as frying fats; the flavouring method, where much consideration is focused on reducing the salt content of the finished products; and the use of parchment paper as a wrapper, which is to show close associations with nature and be indicative of a very low extent of processing.

Owing to the introduction of vacuum fryers, which have notably changed the technology of frying, the manufacture of potato crisps with a reduced fat content (by 50% on average) is increasing. There is also a trend to extend the range of the raw materials for the production of healthier snacks. As a result, carrot, celery or red-beet crisps have become available on the market in addition to potato crisps. A novelty on the European market is the supply of crisps with a purple coloration obtained from coloured potatoes. In other parts of the world a variety of fruits is used for the production of fried snacks, e.g. plantain, cassava or banana. A major asset of the new group of savoury snacks is the use of frying oils, specifically those characterized by a high oleic acid content. Traditional blends of flavours are replaced with new ones, where spicy flavours often dominate (American market). The European market gives preference to exotic flavours, which the consumers tend to associate with the meals they enjoyed while on holidays.

Changes also occur in the group of snacks obtained by extrusion. The past few years have witnessed a 'return to nature' – not only in the raw materials used but also in the look of the finished products. That is why snacks enriched with biologically active components (which largely add to their nutritional value) have gained in popularity. In recent years, wholegrain extruded snacks have appeared on the market. They need further frying, since the extrusion process involves low-pressure extruders, thus yielding a product whose moisture content varies between 15% and 18%. In the course of frying, the water content falls below 2%. Such snacks are characterized by a low fat content and retain their unrivalled sensory properties. For their manufacture, use is also made of high-oleic oils as frying media.

© Woodhead Publishing Limited, 2011

13.6   Future trends

In terms of health, interest in salty snack products that are organic or all-natural, low-calorie, low-fat, low-carbohydrate, low-sodium or offer some health-promoting benefit will remain high among consumers (Table 13.2). Although consumers are interested in healthier snack products, they are not willing to sacrifice flavour. Intense and full-flavour snacks will remain an important trend in the salty snack market.

Table 13.2   New product introductions (savoury snacks) in France, Germany, Italy, Netherlands, Spain and UK, with selected claims, as a % of total new product introductions

	2005	2006	2007	2008	2009	Total sample
No additives/preservatives	8	13	16	32	27	20
Low/no/reduced fat	18	21	17	19	14	18
Low/no/reduced sodium	3	3	3	1	2	2

Source: Data obtained on request from Mintel GNPD, May 2010

13.7   Sources of further information and advice

Organizations
American Oil Chemists' Society (AOCS): http://www.aocs.org
European Federation for the Science and Technology of Lipids (Euro Fed Lipid):
    http://www.eurofedlipid.org
European Snacks Association (ESA): http://www.esa.org.uk
Mintel GNPD: http://www.mintel.com
Snack Food Association (SFA): http://www.sfa.org

Trade shows
SNACKEX Europe and SNACKEX Asia: http://www.snackex.com
SNAXPOL: http://www.snaxpo.com

13.8   References

Annapure U S, Singhal R S and Kulkarni P R (1998), 'Studies on deep-fat fried snacks from some cereals and legumes', *J Sci Food Agric*, 76, 377–82.
Barutcu I, Sahin S and Summu G (2009), 'Acrylamide formation in different batter formulations during microwave frying', *LWT*, 42, 17–22.
Becalski A, Lau BP-Y, Lewis D and Seaman S W (2003), 'Acrylamide in food: occurrence, sources, and modeling' *J Agric Food Chem*, 51, 802–8.
Brinkmann B (2000), 'Quality criteria of industrial frying oils and fats', *Eur J Lipid Sci Technol*, 102, 539–41.
Capuano E, Oliviero T, Açar Ö Ç, Gökmen V, Fogliano V (2010), 'Lipid oxidation promotes acrylamide formation in fat-rich model systems', *Food Res Int*, doi:10.1016/j.foodres.2010.01.013.

© Woodhead Publishing Limited, 2011

Che Man Y B and Tan C P (1999), 'Effects of natural and synthetic antioxidants on changes in refined, bleached, and deodorized palm olein during deep-fat frying of potato chips', *J Am Oil Chem Soc*, 76, 331–9.

Chen S-D, Chen H-H, Chao Y-C and Lin R-S (2009), 'Effect of batter formula on qualities of deep-fat and microwave fried fish nuggets', *J Food Eng*, 95, 359–64.

Chung J, Lee Y and Choe E (2006), 'Effects of sesame oil addition to soybean oil during frying on the lipid oxidative stability and antioxidants contents of the fried products during storage in the dark', *J Food Sci*, 71(3), C222–6.

Claeys W L, Vleeschouwer K, Hendrickx E (2005), 'Quantification the formation of cancinogens during food processing: acrylamide', *Trends Food Sci Technol*, 16, 181–93.

Clark D E, Folz D C and West J K (2000), 'Processing materials with microwave energy', *Materials Sci Eng*, 287, 153–8.

Da Silva P F and Moreira R G (2008), 'Vacuum frying of high-quality fruit and vegetable-based snacks', *LWT*, 41, 1758–67.

Debnath S, Bhat K K and Rastogi N K (2003), 'Effect of pre-drying on kinetics of moisture loss and oil uptake during deep fat frying of chickpea flour-based snack food', *LWT*, 36, 91–8.

Dobarganes C, Màrquez-Ruiz G and Velasco J (2000), 'Interaction between fat and food during the frying process', *Eur J Lipid Sci Technol*, 102, 521–8.

Drozdowski B (2007), 'Lipidy', in Sikorski Z.E. Chemia żywności, Warszawa, WNT, 125 (In Polish).

Elder V A, Fulcher J G and Leong H K-H (2004), 'Method for reducing acrylamide formation in thermally processed foods', Patent WO/2004/026042.

Erickson M D (2007), 'Deep frying: chemistry, nutrition and practical applications', Urbana, Illinois, AOCS Press, 373–86.

Friedman M (2003), 'Chemistry, biochemistry, and safety of acrylamide. A review', *J Agric Food Chem*, 51, 4504–26.

Friedman M and Levin C (2008) 'Review of methods for the reduction of dietary content and toxicity of acrylamide', *J Agric Food Chem*, 56, 6113–40.

Gamble M H, Rice P and Selman J D (1987), 'Relationship between oil uptake and moisture loss during frying of potato slices from c.v. Record U.K. tubers', *Int J Food Sci Technol*, 22, 233–41.

Garayo J and Moreira R (2002), 'Vacuum frying of potato chips', *J Food Eng*, 55, 181–91.

Gerde J, Hardy C, Fehr W and White P J (2007), 'Frying performance of no-trans, low-linolenic acid soybean oils', *J Am Oil Chem Soc*, 84, 557–63.

Gertz Ch and Klostermann S (2002), 'Analysis of acrylamide and mechanism of its formation in deep-fried products', *Eur J Lipid Sci Technol*, 104, 762–71.

Gökmen V and Palazoğlu T K (2008), 'Acrylamide formation in foods during thermal processing with a focus on frying', *Food Bioproc Technol*, 1, 35–42.

Granda C, Moreira R G and Tichy S E (2004), 'Reduction of arylamide formation in potato chips by low-temperature vacuum frying', *J Food Sci*, 69, 405–11.

Grob K, Biedermann M, Biedermann-Brem S, Noti A, Imhof D, Amrein T, Pfefferle A and Bazzocco D (2003), 'French fries with less than 100 μg/kg acrylamide. A collaboration between cooks and analysts', *Eur Food Res Technol*, 271 (3), 185–94.

Houhoula D P, Oreopoulou V and Tzia C (2003), 'Antioxidant efficiency of oregano during frying and storage of potato chips', *J Sci Food Agric*, 83, 1499–503.

Jaswir I, Che Man J B and Kitts D D (2000), 'Use of natural antioxidants in refined palm olein during repeated deep-fat frying', *Food Res Int*, 33, 501–8.

Jung M Y, Choi D S, Ju J W (2003), 'Novel technique for limitation of acrylamide formation in fried and baked corn chips and French fries', *J Food Sci*, 68, 1287–90.

Kita A (2002a), 'Factors affecting potato chips texture during storage', *Acta Agroph*, 7, 23–32.

Kita A (2002b), 'The influence of potato chemical composition on crisp texture', *Food Chem*, 76, 173–9.

© Woodhead Publishing Limited, 2011

Kita A, Lisińska G and Powolny M (2005), 'The influence of frying medium degradation on fat uptake and texture of French fries', *J Sc Food Agric*, 85, 1113–18.

Kita A (2006), 'The effect of some technological parameters on the quality of fried snack products', *Zesz Nauk AR Wroc, Rozprawy CCXL*, 537 (in Polish).

Kita A, Pęksa A, Zięba T and Figiel A (2002), 'The influence of pellets moisture and dietary fiber addition on some potato snacks properties', *Acta Agroph*, 7, 33–42.

Kochhar S P (2000), 'Stabilization of frying oils with natural antioxidative components', *Eur J Lipid Sci Technol*, 102, 552–9.

Kochhar S P and Gertz Ch (2004), 'New theoretical and practical aspects of the frying process', *Eur J Lipid Sci Technol*, 106, 722–7.

Krokida M K, Oreopoulou V and Maroulis Z B (2000), 'Water loss and oil uptake as a function of frying time', *J Food Eng*, 44, 39–46.

Lalas S and Dourtoglu V (2003), 'Use of rosemary extract in preventing oxidation during deep-fat frying of potato chips', *J Am Oil Chem Soc*, 80 (6), 579–83.

Lusas E W and Rooney L W (2002), 'Snack food processing', CRC Press Boca Raton, London, New York, Washington, DC, 1–629.

Mariscal M and Bouchon P (2008), 'Comparison between atmospheric and vacuum frying of apple slices', *Food Chem*, 107, 1561–9.

Mestdagh F, De Meulenaer B and Van Peteghem C (2007), 'Influence of oil degradation on amounts of acrylamide generated in a model system and in French fries', *Food Chem*, 100, 1153–9.

Matthäus B (2007), 'Use of palm oil for frying in comparison with other high-stability oils', *Eur J Lipid Sci Technol*, 109, 400–9.

Mellema M (2003), 'Mechanism and reduction of fat uptake in deep-fried foods', *Trends Food Sci Technol*, 14 (9), 364–73.

Moreira R G, Da Silva P J and Gomes C (2009), 'The effect of a de-oiling mechanism on the production of high quality vacuum fried potato chips', *J Food Eng* 92(3), 297–304

Moreira R G, Sun X and Chen Y (1997), 'Factors affecting oil uptake in tortilla chips in deep-fat frying', *J Food Eng* 31, 485–98.

Napolitano A, Morales F, Sacchi R and Fogliano V (2008), 'Relationship between virgin olive oil phenolic compounds and acrylamide formation in fried crisps', *J Agric Food Chem*, 56, 2034–40.

Nawar W W (1996), 'Lipids', in Fennema, O R (ed.) *Food chemistry*, New York, Basel, Hong Kong, Marcel Dekker Inc., p. 260.

Normand L, Eskin N A M and Przybylski R (2006), 'Comparison of the frying stability of regular and high-oleic acid sunflower oils', *J Am Oil Chem Soc*, 83, 331–4.

Oztop M H, Sahin S and Summu G (2007), 'Optimization of microwave frying of potato slices by using Taguchi technique', *J Food Eng*, 79, 83–91.

Pangloli P, Melton S L, Collins J L, Penfield M P and Saxton A M (2002), 'Flavor and storage stability of potato chips fried in cottonseed and sunflower oils and palm olein/sunflower oil blends', *J Food Sci*, 67(1), 97–103.

Petukhov I, Malcolmson L J, Przybylski R and Armstrong L (1999), 'Storage stability of potato chips fried in genetically modified canola oils', *J Am Oil Chem Soc*, 76(8), 889–96.

Pinthus E J, Weinberg P and Saguy I S (1995), 'Deep-fat fried potato product oil uptake as affected by crust physical properties', *J Food Sci*, 60 (4), 770–2.

Rani M and Chauhan G S (1995), 'Effect of intermittent frying and frying medium on the quality of potato chips' *Food Chem*, 54 (4), 365–8.

Rossell J B (2003), 'Developments in oils for commercial frying', *Lipid Technol*, 1, 5–8.

Saguy I S and Dana D (2003), 'Integrated approach to deep fat frying: engineering, nutrition, health and consumer aspects', *J Food Eng*, 56, 143–52.

Satyanarayana A, Giridhar N, Joshi G J and Rao D G (2000), 'Ascorbyl palmiate as an antioxidant for deep fat frying of potato chips in peanut oil', *J Food Lipids*, 7, 1–10.

Troncoso E and Pedreschi F (2009), 'Modeling water loss and oil uptake during vacuum frying of pre-treated potato slices', *LWT*, 42, 1164–73.

© Woodhead Publishing Limited, 2011

Vattem D A and Shetty K (2003), 'Acrylamide in food: a model for mechanism of formation and its reduction', *Inn Food Sci Emerg Technol*, 4, 331–8.

Venkatesh M S and Raghavan G S V (2004), 'An overview of microwave processing and dielectric properties of agri-food materials', *Biosystems Eng*, 88, 1–18.

Warner K and Fehr W (2008), 'Mid-oleic/ultra low linolenic acid soybean oil: a healthful new alternative to hydrogenated oil for frying', *J Am Oil Chem Soc*, 85, 945–51.

Warner K and Gehring M M (2009), 'High-temperature natural antioxidant improves soy oil for frying', *J Food Sci*, 74, C500–5.

Yamsaengsung R and Rungsee S (2003), 'Vacuum frying of fruits and vegetables', Manuscript 1-2003, Hat Yai, Songkhla.

Zamora R and Hidalgo F J (2008), 'Contribution of lipid oxidation products to acrylamide formation in model system', *J Agric Food Eng*, 56, 6075–80.

Zhang Y, Chen J, Zhang X, Wu X and Zhang Y (2007), 'Addition of antioxidant of bamboo leaves (AOB) effectively reduces acrylamide formation in potato crisps and French fries', *J Agric Food Chem*, 55, 523–8.

Zyzak D, Anders R, Stokanovic M, Tallmadge D, Ebehart B, Ewald D (2003), 'Acrylamide formation mechanism in heated foods', *J Agric Food Chem*, 51, 4782–7.

© Woodhead Publishing Limited, 2011

14

Saturated fat reduction in biscuits

G. Atkinson, AarhusKarlshamn UK Ltd, UK

Abstract: This chapter looks at the technology involved in the manufacture of biscuits and the role of saturated fats in the recipe and processing of various types of biscuits including short dough biscuits, semi-sweet biscuits, crackers and wafers. It then considers options for reducing the level of saturates and considers the impact that these changes may have on the quality of the biscuit and the processing. Techniques considered include simple fat reduction, replacement with fats having a lower saturates content, fat replacers and fat substitutes.

Key words: saturated fat reduction in biscuits, fat replacers, biscuit quality, biscuit processing, healthy biscuit.

14.1   Introduction

Fat – and especially saturated fat – has traditionally been one of the key ingredients in the formulation and development of any biscuit-type product. It provides key characteristics such as flavour, structure and shortness in the end product along with good handling and processing characteristics through the manufacturing operations. The challenge for product development professionals therefore is to maintain those key characteristics that consumers expect in the end product while reducing the levels of fat and calories in the biscuit in order to meet the target guideline reductions given by various governmental agencies and the World Health Organisation (for example see FSA, 2010). The challenge for process development and operational staff is to keep the manufacturing processes working efficiently with the new products, as these new recipes will potentially have very different handling characteristics to the traditional ones which have been in use for many years.

In this chapter we will examine the general trends in consumption and the levels of fats in biscuits; the types of fats, ingredients, techniques and processes used in the manufacture of various types of biscuit products; and the way in which

© Woodhead Publishing Limited, 2011

these can be manipulated to achieve the required reduction of saturated fats. We will then consider future trends which could further influence the development of biscuit products.

Consideration will also be given to the secondary systems in biscuits that contribute to the overall fat content. These include systems such as filling creams, coatings, barrier fats and oil sprays. Although these are relatively minor components they can have a significant impact on the saturated fat content of the products, especially as the level of fat in the base product decreases.

14.2   Types of fat used in biscuits

Although a small amount of animal fats and also butter was and indeed still is used in biscuit making, for many years, up until around 2004, biscuit dough fats were primarily based on hydrogenated vegetable fats, the base oils being typically palm or rapeseed oil in Europe, and the key factor for any change was price. Because the process of hydrogenation was so flexible the properties of the base oil could be modified to allow both sources to be used depending on which was the most cost effective at the time. After around 2004, when health concerns relating to high levels of *trans* fats in certain types of hydrogenated fats were becoming more prevalent (NDA, 2004), there was a very rapid move to the use of non-hydrogenated fats as dough fats, and because of the requirement for a certain percentage of solid, high-melting fat to provide functionality in the biscuit (as can be seen in Fig. 14.1) the fat of choice became palm oil, which is the only commercially available solid fat in the UK.

Moving to non-hydrogenated palm oil did indeed remove the *trans* fats from the biscuits but it also resulted in an increase in saturated fat levels to compensate

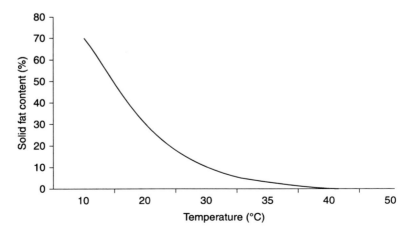

Fig. 14.1   Solid fat content profile of a typical dough fat.

© Woodhead Publishing Limited, 2011

Table 14.1   Saturated fat content as a percentage of total fat

	1998	2006
Cream cracker	40.8	51.2
Digestive	44.3	47.0

1998 data: McCance and Widdowson (based on composite data collected in 1992)
2006 data: Food Standards Agency processed foods database

Source: Talbot, 2008

for the loss of *trans* fats, which supplied some of the functionality in the fat as shown in Table 14.1. A hydrogenated dough fat may typically have had saturated fat levels of around 41–44% but a non-hydrogenated palm oil based dough fat would have saturated fat levels of around 49–50%.

Palm oil has dominated the biscuit industry in recent years as the fat of choice for use as a dough fat but this is now changing with the push to reduce saturates, and more specialist fats with more liquid oil and specialist palm fractions are being used. The technical requirement for these fats still remains and these will be discussed in more detail later in this chapter.

14.3   The technology of biscuits

In this section we are going to consider various types of biscuits individually, firstly looking at the fat sources, content and types in typical recipes, and the influence and function of saturated fat in the product and production methods for what could be classed as 'standard' products. This will form the basis of discussions later in the chapter when we consider ways of reducing the levels of saturated fat and the influence this can have on the end product and production methods. The classifications used for the following sections are based on those described by Manley (2000, Chapter 20).

14.3.1   Crackers

The term 'crackers' could refer to many different types of biscuit but the most common are cream crackers, puff biscuits and savoury crackers such as 'Ritz' (United Biscuits) or 'TUC' (Jacob Fruitfield Food Group). The products are all laminated but differences are down to the way that the recipe is formulated and the dough is handled. Each type will be described in more detail below.

Cream crackers
These biscuits were first produced around 1885 by the Irish firm of Jacob's and have remained very popular as a snack cracker in the UK. They contain two primary

© Woodhead Publishing Limited, 2011

sources of fat. The first is in the base dough, which typically contains around 11% by weight of fat (approx. 16% on flour weight). The second is from the filling that is dusted onto the sheeted dough before it is laminated. This dust contains approx. 25% fat by weight (approx. 33% on flour weight) and the fat needs to have a relatively high melting point to give it the flaky, blistered appearance that is typical of cream crackers. The higher proportion of fat (approx. 85–90%) is formulated into the base dough and so the possibilities of reducing levels of saturates are in favour of doing so in the base dough. The baked final product will typically contain around 14% fat by weight, of which 6–7% is saturated fat.

Puff biscuits
These biscuits are again manufactured via a lamination process but differ from cream crackers in that they are not fermented and are much more akin to a standard puff pastry product in that a laminating fat or margarine is used to form the typical flaky, layered structure with slightly more lift than is seen with other types of laminated crackers. Again there are two key sources of fat in the product: the dough fat and the laminating fat. In this type of product the higher proportion of fat (approx. 80–85%) comes from the laminating fat, with a relatively small amount in the base dough. This means that the biggest potential gain in terms of saturates reduction will come from a change to the laminating fat. The structure of this fat is, however, most critical as the melting profile will determine the eating quality of the end product. Too high melting and the biscuit will taste 'waxy'; too low a melting point (too little saturated fat) and the structure of the biscuit will be affected adversely as the fat will not function effectively to give the lift required during baking. The final baked product will typically contain around 32% fat, of which 17–18% will be saturated fat.

Savoury crackers
In common with the previous two products in this section, savoury crackers are also laminated and can be either fermented like cream crackers or non-fermented like puff biscuits. What defines a biscuit as a savoury cracker is the addition of a flavouring ingredient, usually onto the surface of the cracker prior to baking. These are typically materials such as coarse salt or seeds such as sesame or poppy. These seeds themselves can contain relatively high levels of oil (45–50% by weight), but the oil is relatively low in saturates and so does not contribute to high levels of saturated fats.

Many of the formulation and processing characteristics described in earlier sections can also be applied to savoury crackers with recipes being many and varied, but the key difference as far as fat content in savoury crackers is concerned is the addition of an oil-spraying step after baking to seal the surface of the biscuit, improve the mouthfeel and improve the overall appearance of the cracker. Although the amount of oil which is incorporated in this step seems relatively small, traditionally the oil that is used is one which is very high in saturates such as coconut or palm kernel oil (approx. 92% and 82% saturated fats respectively). The reason for choosing these types of fats is the requirement for the oil to be

© Woodhead Publishing Limited, 2011

stable to oxidation and so not develop any rancidity or off-flavours during the life of the biscuit. This oil spray is particularly susceptible to oxidation due to the high surface area of the biscuit exposing it to high levels of air. Because of the high levels of saturates in these oils, they are solids at normal UK ambient temperatures and so must be melted and sprayed warm onto the biscuits. The act of melting and holding the oils above the melting point also increases the chance of oxidation; another reason for the use of high-stability saturated fats. These products will typically contain around 27% fat in the baked end product, of which up to around 22% can be saturated fat.

14.3.2   Hard sweet and semi-sweet biscuits

This is a broad category of biscuits incorporating some types which are seldom seen outside of the UK, such as Marie, Rich Tea and Morning Coffee, although similar recipes are used throughout Europe, but with different processing conditions leading to biscuits with different characteristics to those mentioned above.

In this type of product the fat is primarily from a single source, the dough fat, and is typically incorporated into the dough at levels of around 10% weight for weight (17% on flour weight). Because of the particular processing of the dough for this type of biscuit, where the mixing takes place at around 40°C, the composition of the fat is less important than in other types of biscuits and so allows some flexibility in the choice of fat to allow a reduction in the level of saturates. The end baked product will have levels of fat around 15–16%, of which saturates will be around 7–8%.

A special type of biscuit based on the above that incorporates currants as a filling between two sheets of semi-sweet dough is known as a Garibaldi. The level of currants in the final baked biscuit are around 35–40% of the product by weight and hence, by the simple principle of dilution, the biscuits are lower in fat than their basic counterparts with levels of fat typically around 9%, of which saturates are around 4–5%.

14.3.3   Short dough biscuits

This group of biscuits are by far the most widespread commercially and are also the most varied in terms of recipe, encapsulating such products as digestives, shortbread, ginger nuts and shells for creamed biscuits such as custard creams or Bourbons.

The recipes can vary in fat content very significantly. High-fat products such as shortbread will typically contain 25–35% by weight of fat in the dough coming from a single source, the dough fat, which can be either vegetable fat/margarine or, more traditionally for this type of biscuit, butter. Lower fat products are typically those that are to be chocolate coated. These biscuits will have fat contents in the region of 15–20% by weight in the dough (20–27% on flour weight), of which 7–10% would typically be saturated fat. This fat will again come solely from the dough fat. Being lower in fat will help to prevent migration of fat between the coating and the biscuit causing discolouration or bloom on the product.

© Woodhead Publishing Limited, 2011

A special class of short dough biscuits is known as the deposited or soft dough type. The name describes them well as the doughs are very fat rich (up to 40% by weight of the dough) and very soft, allowing them to deposited more like a cake batter. Because these products are very fat rich and the process allows for very intricate shapes to be formed, they are often classed as luxury items and as such are also often made with butter, driving the saturates level higher than with vegetable fats, up to around the 22% mark. Typical examples of this type of product would be Viennese biscuits, which are also often chocolate coated and/or sandwiched.

14.3.4   Wafers

Wafer biscuits are a special case and differ from other biscuits discussed here in a number of ways. They are made from a batter (containing up to about 60% moisture) rather than the more usual dough and they are low in fat, containing only 1 or 2% of fat in the batter, equating to 2–3% of the baked wafer. Because it has very little functionality in the biscuit other than to help prevent it sticking during baking, it is entirely possible to use a liquid vegetable oil such as rapeseed or sunflower oil rather than a specially formulated dough fat. This means that the scope for saturates reduction in this type of product is negligible as the levels of saturates in liquid oils are the lowest for any fat product at around 8–10% by weight. Any significant amount of fat which is present in the end product on the shelf would come from either a filling or chocolate coating.

14.3.5   Sandwich/filled biscuits

This is another very popular type of biscuit, based around the short dough biscuit shell described in section 14.3.3. The fillings are usually described as creams but are often based on non-dairy vegetable fats in combination with sugars such as icing sugar and glucose. The type of fat used for this application needs to have properties that allow it to aerate during mixing and also to melt quickly when eaten so as not to feel 'waxy' in the mouth. These two properties require the fat to have what is called a steep melting curve, where the aeration requires a relatively firm fat at ambient temperatures to hold the air from the mixing but the 'non-waxy' mouthfeel requires the fat to soften and melt quickly at temperatures close to body heat (37°C). To achieve this, the fat is often a combination of fats, one of which is a lauric fat (coconut or palm kernel oil), which is naturally low melting. However, this type of fat is very high in saturates, meaning that these filling or cream fats, as they are often called, do tend to be high in saturated fats, typically around 85–90%.

14.3.6   Coated biscuits

Although there are many potential coatings for biscuits, the two most popular are fondant and chocolate, with chocolate products far outstripping the others, and so we will focus on this key area.

© Woodhead Publishing Limited, 2011

When a biscuit is chocolate coated then this will of course lead to an increase in fat content of the biscuit, with the chocolate coating typically comprising around 25–30% by weight of the biscuit. The chocolate itself will contain around 25–35% fat by weight, of which around 15–21% will be saturated fat, usually from a combination of cocoa butter, milk fat and vegetable fat. Commission Directive 2000/36/EC specifies minimum standards for the composition of chocolate in the European Union with a minimum total fat content of 25%, minimum cocoa butter content of 18%, and up to 5% vegetable fat is allowed to be added to chocolate in the European Union as outlined in Chapter 16. The relatively low level of vegetable fat in the chocolate gives only limited scope for saturates reduction and there is no change possible to the cocoa butter element of the chocolate. This makes any change to the overall saturates level of the chocolate coating almost insignificant.

14.4   Techniques for saturates reduction

A number of techniques are available to the developer to allow a reduction in the level of saturates in biscuit products. The general merits or demerits of each technique are discussed below.

14.4.1   Reduction in the total fat content

This is perhaps the simplest and preferred route for many formulators as it allows development using standard, well-known and understood ingredients with modification to an existing, established recipe. It also offers the potential for cost savings as fat can often be one of the most expensive ingredients in a biscuit recipe. It can be applied across all ranges of products and is applicable to all fats, including dairy fats such as butter and not just vegetable fats and margarines. It also offers the advantage of not only reducing the level of saturated fat but also the overall calorific value of the end product as fat will be the highest-calorie ingredient in the biscuit. This aligns well with the aims of the UK Food Standards Agency, who in their guidelines for baked goods (FSA, 2010) have asked for not only a reduction in the level of saturated fats but also an accompanying reduction in calories 'unless a technical case can be made that this is not achievable'.

Although this may seem to be the simplest route forward, in many cases it is the one with the most potential impact on the end product as a reduction in overall fat level often has to be accompanied by increased levels of water and/or sugar. This in itself has the potential to impact upon key parameters of product quality such as the eating quality, texture, flavour delivery and shelf-life. The impact of simple fat reduction in relation to each area of fat use in biscuits is outlined below.

Dough fat
The impact of any change to the dough fat is without doubt the most critical factor in any type of biscuit production because of the vital role that it plays in controlling the quality of the processing characteristics and final quality of the biscuit.

© Woodhead Publishing Limited, 2011

Since around 2004 the main fat that has been used as a dough fat in biscuits has been refined deodorised palm oil. The reason for this is that it can supply the level of high-melting-point fat required to provide the necessary structure in the biscuit without requiring the fat to be partially hydrogenated as had previously been the case. Around this time the relatively high level of trans-fatty acids (*trans* fats) in partially hydrogenated fats was being questioned because of their potentially detrimental health effects (BMJ, 2006). This change to non-hydrogenated palm oil has, however, resulted in a general increase in the level of saturated fats as hydrogenated variants typically had levels of saturates lower than the 49–50% found in palm oil.

The key role of the dough fat is to coat the gluten (wheat protein) in biscuit doughs (Lawson, 1981) and so prevent water being absorbed by the gluten during mixing. This is important because when the gluten is wetted it becomes elastic and extensible, and whereas this is vital in bread-type products, where this extensibility is necessary to get the lift required during proofing and baking, in biscuits it simply leads to a biscuit which is tough and chewy to eat. This can happen if the level of fat is reduced too far without making any other significant changes to the recipe as the fat simply becomes too widely dispersed in the dough and there is not enough present to coat all of the gluten.

Reduced-fat biscuits which have been on the market to date and used this simple reduction technique, such as McVitie's Light Digestives, typically have levels of fat which are 70–75% of the standard level of fat (source: tesco.com, May 2010). To compensate for this, levels of sugar are generally increased to bulk out the biscuit and maintain the texture. Although this technique results in a lower fat content and a corresponding reduction in the level of saturates, it does tend to have only a very small effect on the overall energy level of the biscuit because of the increased sugar level.

Apart from the general quality issues arising from a reduction in overall fat content in biscuit doughs, there is also an impact on the processing properties of the biscuit dough. As the fat content is reduced the dough becomes tougher, there is more of a tendency for the biscuit to shrink during baking and there would typically be less colour development during the baking process. To compensate for these factors it is necessary to make some significant changes to the product and process including increasing the water content of the dough, increasing the baking time and temperature and possibly using a release agent on the oven band to prevent the biscuit sticking. This makes this simple removal option less favourable than it may at first seem.

Although it is not commercially available at the moment, there is one technology under investigation which may prove useful in the future when using this strategy of fat reduction. This is a technique known as 'cryo-crystallisation', which was patented by the company BOC (British Oxygen Company), now part of the The Linde Group (BOC, 2010), and involves the rapid cooling of molten fat in a stream of liquid nitrogen. The molten fat is atomised to form small droplets and then this comes into contact with a stream of liquid nitrogen at −196°C, which instantly cools the fat droplets, forming a powder that can be collected for use in a variety of bakery applications. This is illustrated in Fig. 14.2.

© Woodhead Publishing Limited, 2011

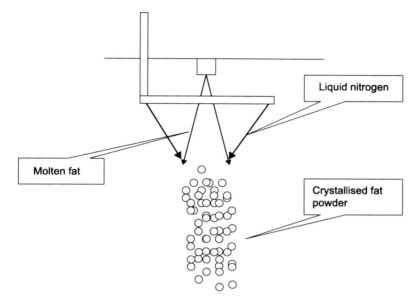

Molten fat

Liquid nitrogen

Crystallised fat powder

Fig. 14.2   Cryo-crystallisation.

The interest in this technique when compared to traditional methods of crystallising fats is that initial work done by AAK Bakery Services (Atkinson, 2010) indicates that a reduction of up to 20% in fat content may be possible. Although this work is still in its early stages and the reasons behind this improved functionality are not fully understood, the indications are that the rapid crystallisation gives rise to large number of very small fat crystals, which in turn increases the level of solid fat at a given temperature. As has been discussed previously, it is the solid (high melting) fat which provides much of the functionality in biscuit applications and the possibility of producing a fat with a higher level of solid fat with the same level of saturates is of significant interest to developers. One note of caution with this technology which needs to be considered is the potential expense, as the liquid nitrogen coolant is lost to waste in the process and this has the potential for adding significantly to the manufacturing costs, making it perhaps less favoured at this time than other potential options.

Laminating fat
Reduction in the amount of fat used in laminated biscuits such as cream crackers is somewhat limited as this can have a major change on the structure of the biscuit. Reducing the amount of laminating fat will result in a cracker which displays much less of the typical 'blistered' appearance seen on such products, as the fat will be absorbed more easily into the biscuit and not perform its function in trapping steam during the baking process and providing the lift which gives the structure. The proportion of fat used in laminating is typically only 10–15% of the

© Woodhead Publishing Limited, 2011

total fat content and so a reduction of 10% of the total laminating fat would only result in a change in saturates levels of around 0.5% in the total fat and less than 0.1% in the baked biscuit.

Coating fat
There are limits on the options with coatings for both technological and legislative reasons. Legislation is in place which dictates the minimum fat content of chocolate products and so to drop the fat content below this minimum level is not possible. Technically it is also difficult to reduce the fat content in a chocolate coating as the level of fat is a key factor in controlling the viscosity of the chocolate, as shown in Fig. 14.3.

The chocolate will need a low viscosity to allow it to effectively coat the product through a standard enrober. The fat content of chocolate will be typically around 30%, and reduction to less than 27% can significantly increase the viscosity, which will in turn lead to a poor coating on the biscuit as the chocolate will not flow over the surface. A more viscous coating will almost inevitably lead to a thicker coating, which will in turn increase the saturated fat content of the biscuit. Some work has been done on mechanical handling methods for higher viscosity chocolate coatings, which involve spraying the chocolate (Nestec, 2009) instead of the additional enrobing method. This indicates possible reductions of up to 40% in fat content, which would reduce the saturated fat levels from 18.5% to 11%, a significant reduction, and this is a technology that would be worth exploring further.

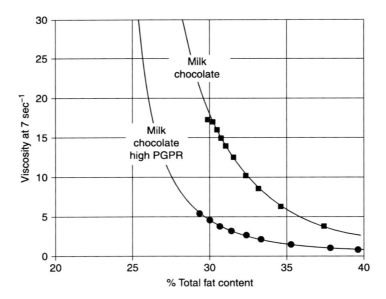

Fig. 14.3   Influence of fat content on the viscosity of chocolate PGPR = polyglycerol polyricinoleate. (Reproduced from Wells, 2009).

© Woodhead Publishing Limited, 2011

Spray oils

As with chocolate coatings, any reduction in the weight of oil and hence the saturated fat level applied to the surface of the biscuit lies primarily with the technology used to apply the oil. The requirement is for a very light film and this requires very fine droplets of oil. Traditionally a spinning disc applicator has been used for this and the speed of rotation of the discs needs to be high to give the best oil droplet. More recently, electrostatic or airless spray systems have been able to produce finer droplets, giving more effective coverage and so less oil requirement.

14.4.2   Use of fats with lower levels of saturates

This route is potentially the most productive for developers as it offers an opportunity to reduce the level of saturated fat without making any major changes to the recipe, as it is a simple substitution of one type of fat for another. This approach does, however, have its disadvantages, such as that it will not necessarily help with the calorific reduction requested by the UK Food Standards Agency and it has the potential to require major changes to the processing/manufacturing systems not only for the biscuit manufacture itself but also for the materials handling side. These changes may require potentially large investments in product development and modifications to processing equipment or to install bulk handling systems for new lower saturate fats. This could preclude a number of businesses from pursuing this route simply because they cannot afford the investment. This approach has been most publicly taken by United Biscuits, as since 2008 they have reduced the saturated fat levels in their McVitie's brand plain biscuits (Digestive, Rich Tea and HobNobs) in stages to a level of approximately 75% of the values from 2008 (UB, 2010) as can be seen in Table 14.2.

This reduction has not been without its cost. It has been reported that since the programme of work started in 2005 it has cost McVitie's approx six million pounds in ingredients and investments in the manufacturing facilities to deliver a high-quality product based on the new recipe (FDF, 2009).

As a general principle the reduction of saturate levels in a fat is brought about through an increase in the level of liquid oil in the product, as it is these liquid oils, such as rapeseed oil or sunflower oil, that have the lowest levels of saturated fats. This could be through the use of such a liquid oil by itself, although this presents

Table 14.2   Saturated fat content of McVitie's plain biscuits

	Total fat content (g per 100 g)	Saturated fat content (g per 100 g)		
		2008	2009	2010
McVitie's Digestives	21.3	10.1	4.8	2.0
McVitie's Rich Tea	15.5	7.3	3.5	1.5

© Woodhead Publishing Limited, 2011

significant technical challenges, as can be highlighted by the investment made by McVitie's. A more common and perhaps a more realistic approach for companies who cannot afford such an investment is through the use of so-called pumpable or fluid shortenings. These are manufactured through a simple blending process of the liquid oil with higher melting point/higher saturate fats or through a more complex process such as interesterification, where the liquid and solid fats are combined chemically to produce a new fat with properties different from the starting components. Products such as this are often supplied in what is known as a pre-crystallised state to provide product in the optimal format to supply maximum functionality and minimise the impact of saturate reduction. Here the higher melting component in the shortening has been rapidly crystallised, typically in a scraped-surface heat exchanger, and this forms a crystal matrix which can encapsulate the liquid oil component and bind it into the system, thus imparting the functionality of the higher saturates fat while offering a reduced saturates end product. When considering this route for reducing saturates there are a number of factors that need to be taken into consideration.

The first of these is the shelf-life of the end product. When replacing saturated fats with more liquid oils which contain more unsaturated fats there is an increased risk of oxidation of the fats and the development of rancidity in the biscuit during storage. For this reason the oil of preference when taking this approach is now high-oleic sunflower oil, as this has one of the lowest saturates levels of any oil (approx. 9%) but is also approximately two or three times more oxidatively stable than its closest counterpart, rapeseed oil with around 7% saturates. This increase in oxidative stability allows shelf-life to be maintained in the vast majority of cases.

The second factor is oil migration. As more liquid oil is incorporated into a recipe then there is more chance that oil will migrate from the biscuit into either the filling or particularly the coating, causing a softening of the filling or discolouration (fat bloom) on a chocolate coating. The mechanism for this is well understood (Ziegleder, 1997) and is exactly the same as is seen with bloom on chocolates with praline centres where the soft/liquid fat migrates into the chocolate, increasing the mobility of the triglycerides in the chocolate and allowing the fat crystals formed during the tempering of the chocolate to change into a different form which unfortunately often gives rise to fat bloom. This effect can also be exaggerated in biscuits where the thickness of the coating is reduced as another method of reducing the saturated fat content. Thicker chocolate coatings can absorb more liquid oil before the texture becomes unacceptable. Fortunately, several methods of preventing this phenomenon of oil migration are potentially available to the developer. One of these is to apply a layer of high-melting-point fat to the biscuit prior to applying the coating or filling to form a physical barrier to the migration. The fat is sprayed onto the biscuit surface when molten and must be completely set before the filling or coating is applied, otherwise the barrier will be compromised. The fat must be applied in a thin continuous coating to maximise the barrier properties and minimise the effects on mouthfeel and any increase in saturated fats. The design of such a fat is important

© Woodhead Publishing Limited, 2011

as it must be able to crystallise rapidly to allow good processing and ideally should be designed so that the triglycerides are similar to those in the coating, so that should any oil migration occur then the effect on the chocolate will be one of dilution rather than recrystallisation. Other materials such as shellac and a number of hydrocolloids have also been proposed (Duffy, 1993) as non-fatty barriers to perform a similar function in forming a physical barrier to the oil.

The third issue for consideration is the change that a more liquid fat will cause to the consistency of the biscuit dough and the effect that this will have on the handling and processing of the dough through the whole of the processing. This can start at the hoppers that hold the dough, where it may be necessary to reduce the weight of dough held in the hopper as pressure on the dough may physically squeeze liquid oil out. If the dough is too soft then pattern definition from a moulded soft-dough biscuit may be lost. During baking, biscuit spread may increase and colour may be affected, requiring changes to the baking profile in the oven to compensate. The type of release agent (if any) on the oven band may also need to be changed to compensate for the change in the dough to control the spread of the biscuit. These changes to the processing of the dough perhaps offer the biggest challenges for the smaller manufacturer who does not have the capital available to change their equipment or indeed the time to dedicate to such changes.

For laminated biscuits like cream crackers the potential to reduce the saturates in the lamination fat is limited as significant reductions in the saturated fats will result in a fat which is too soft and will be absorbed into the biscuit, becoming part of the base rather than trapping the steam during baking and giving the biscuit the flaky lamination that is expected. However, new, more technologically advanced fats from fractions of palm oil subjected to further processing techniques such as interesterification are being developed and it is hoped that these will allow more liquid oil inclusion by working as effective 'oil absorbers' and providing the reduction in saturates but maintaining functionality

From an economic perspective, when compared to the option of reducing the total fat content as described in section 14.4.1 this option is perhaps less preferable as these lower saturate products tend to be more expensive. This is because liquid oils, especially the more stable high-oleic sunflower oil, tend to be more expensive than their higher saturate counterparts like palm oil and they can also require more processing to get them to the appropriate quality.

14.4.3 Fat replacers
The term 'fat replacer' is a generic term which covers a very wide variety of materials such as starches, proteins, emulsifiers, hydrocolloids, fibres, etc. Over the years many claims have been made about the effectiveness of these types of systems, some more realistic than others, but it is fair to say that as technology has moved on then a number of these products are becoming much more viable as at least partial fat replacers in many products, including biscuits. Each of the types of fat replacer works in a different way and the key points for each of the major groups are highlighted below.

© Woodhead Publishing Limited, 2011

Starches

The technology allowing the use of starches to be used as fat replacers is not new. There have been significant developments in recent years which have made the use of these ingredients more practical. Back in the 1990s a class of products such as Paselli SA2 (Avebe) and N-Lite (National Starch) were introduced. These were based on low-DE (dextrose equivalent) maltodextrins and often required some pre-processing of the starch before use, e.g. dispersion in water and cooling to form a 'fat-like' paste which was then added to the dough mix. This obviously adds an additional processing step and complexity that is not desirable. Although these types of products were effective in some applications (Sudha *et al.*, 2007) there was a negative impact on biscuit qualities such as texture and dough consistency. As starch technology has progressed and more work has been done to understand the way that these materials affect the microstructure of the products, starches have been developed which much more closely mimic the properties of fat, such as thermoreversible gelling, i.e. liquefying on heating and solidifying on cooling to allow much more flexibility in the use of the materials. Examples of these new generations of products include the 'Etenia' range from Avebe, the 'N-Dulge' range from National Starch and the 'Delyte' range from Ulrick & Short. Some of the products are designed for manufacturers of ingredients such as margarines to allow them to reduce the fat content and this will then cascade into the biscuit manufacturers' recipes, whereas others are for direct addition into the biscuit dough or filling cream by the biscuit manufacturers themselves. Reductions in fat content of 25% or more are being claimed (Ulrick, 2008) and it is likely that this starch-based technology will become ever more important in driving down saturate levels in biscuits.

Emulsifiers

Although they have become less favoured in recent years as there has been a general move within the food industry to remove artificial additives from foods, emulsifiers have had a role to play in reduced-fat biscuits for many years, be it in reducing fat levels in the recipes for soft-dough biscuits or stabilising the filling creams. However, as the level of fat and particularly saturated fat is pushed lower and lower it is likely that their use will become increasingly important.

Emulsifiers contribute to reduced-fat biscuit recipes in a number of key areas including texture, volume and dough consistency, but behind all of these is the basic function of the emulsifiers to improve the distribution of fat in the biscuit dough. This effect is often known as 'fat sparing' as it involves a more even distribution of reduced levels of fat, allowing the fat to basically become more effective in its functionality of coating the gluten in biscuit dough, as has been described earlier in this chapter. The emulsifiers also have other functions, which will be touched upon later in this section, but fat sparing is the most important and is brought about through the inherent properties of emulsifiers to reduce surface tension and so allow the fat be to be broken up into smaller particles or droplets than would be possible without the emulsifiers being present. This allows smaller amounts of fat to more effectively coat the gluten in the flour as illustrated in Fig. 14.4.

© Woodhead Publishing Limited, 2011

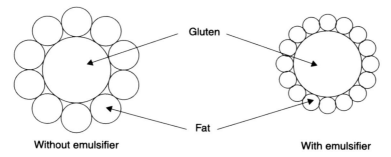

Fig. 14.4   Effect of emulsifier on fat coating of gluten.

Many different types of emulsifier are available to the formulator of biscuit products but the most important ones are lecithin (E322), diacetyl tartaric esters of mono and diglycerides, also known as DATEM (E472e), and sodium stearoyl lactylate, also known as SSL (E481). All of these contribute significantly to the fat-sparing effect described above but they also offer other functionality, each one different. Lecithins are perhaps most commonly used in wafer biscuits, which are low in fat anyway but the addition of lecithin also significantly improves the release of the wafers from the irons after baking. This effect can also be seen with other biscuit types but to a lesser degree. DATEM emulsifiers tend to soften the dough and improve its homogeneity, also leading to some low-level aeration of the dough during mixing, which can lead to improvements in the texture and volume of the biscuit; one of the problems associated with lowering the fat content. Typical addition levels are around 0.2 to 0.4% of the dough weight and can offer up to 20% fat reduction (Burt and Thacker, 1981). SSL works in a similar way to DATEM but has a different effect on the dough in that it tends to make the dough drier and more crumbly but still leading to an easy-to-mould, crisp and crunchy biscuit (Danisco, undated).

Hydrocolloids
This class of ingredient includes products such as guar gum, carrageenan, xanthan gum and carboxy methyl cellulose (CMC). There is less of a defined role for hydrocolloids in reduced-fat biscuits to date with less work seemingly being undertaken particularly in the biscuit doughs themselves, but the key properties imparted by all such ingredients are moisture retention and control over dough rheology. These functions can be important in reduced-fat biscuits because, as has been highlighted previously, reducing the fat content leads to a dough which is more difficult to process along with a harder biscuit after baking. Because these materials work within the water phase of the biscuit they can also help to control the crystallisation of the dissolved sugar during and after the baking process, preventing the formation of large agglomerates of sugar which can lead to biscuits being too hard.

Fibres
This category to some degree is similar to that of hydrocolloids in that the amount of work that has been done is much more limited than areas such as

© Woodhead Publishing Limited, 2011

emulsifiers and starches, although interest in dietary fibres as possible fat replacers has increased in recent years as more sophisticated products have been developed. Examples of these include 'Z Trim' (http://www.ztrim.com), 'Vitacel' (http://www.jrs.de), 'Oatrim' and 'Orafti' (http://www.orafti.com). Again, they all work to mimic the function of fat in areas such as lubricity in the mouth, binding water and building structure through the formation of a gel which is supposed to be 'fat-like'. Many of these fibres, such as 'Oatrim', also offer the advantage of additional dietary health claims where components such a β-glucan offer heart health benefits (FDA, 2003).

14.4.4   Fat substitutes

The logic behind fat substitutes is to take the basic structure of a fat or triglyceride and try to modify this to reduce the calorific impact of the molecule on body. This can be done in three ways.

Change the backbone of the fat

Fat is based on a backbone of glycerol, which has three possible linkages to a fatty acid. Increasing this number of linkages decreases the absorption of the fat into the body (Mattson and Volpenhein, 1972) and so 'Olestra' was developed by Proctor and Gamble with a backbone of sucrose giving eight linkages. This material was given initial US FDA approval in 1996, but even though it is still approved has fallen out of favour due to side effects relating to high consumption causing some gastrointestinal disease (CSPI, 2003). Olestra is banned in a number of countries, including the UK.

Change the fatty acids

In this option the backbone of the fat is kept as glycerol but the connected fatty acids are changed to move them away from the normal range of 12 to 18 carbon chain lengths that form the bulk of most fats. The fatty acids are substituted with a combination of long chain length (18–22 carbon chain), medium chain length (6–10 carbon chain) and short (2–4 carbon chain) saturated fats. This change to the fatty acids affects the way that the body metabolises these materials and this means that rather than supplying nine calories per gram like a standard fat they only supply five calories per gram. These types of products, known as 'Salatrim', were approved for use in the EU in 2003 (EC, 2003). Although the product does offer some calorific reduction and so would go some way to helping meet the FSA targets on calorific reduction it is much higher in saturated fats (>90% saturated fats) than a typical biscuit dough fat such as palm oil and so may not be considered to be of great interest to our challenge of reducing saturated fats in food. However, the saturated fatty acids present will be either very long chain, and so not metabolised fully, or short to medium chain and metabolised by a different route from the more common C12–C18 fatty acids. These metabolic differences could make the use of such fats interesting even though the absolute saturates level is high.

© Woodhead Publishing Limited, 2011

Reduce the number of fatty acids
This technique involves modifying the standard triglyceride backbone to cleave or remove one of the fatty acids, leaving what is known as a diacylglycerol or DAG-Oil. The advantage of these materials is that they are lower in calories than standard triglyceride fats (only two-thirds of the fatty acids) and the same applies to the saturated fat content. There is also evidence that this type of material is useful in controlling certain metabolic conditions relating to fat (Matsuo, 2001). This product was approved by the UK Novel Foods Committee in 2006 for a variety of uses including bakery products (EU, 2006) and commercialised by ADM (Archer Daniels Midland) under the brand name 'Enova', but never received mass acceptance in the market, although the technology is still interesting and may become more so as the quest for reduced saturates increases. DAG oils are considered in more detail in Chapter 8.

14.5   Future trends

Technology is progressing rapidly in relation to saturated fat reduction in biscuits and new techniques, materials and processing equipment are becoming available all of the time, many of which have been discussed in this chapter. The most likely scenario is that no single technology will provide an industry-wide answer to this issue but different solutions will be applicable to different products and, as is often found, a combination of technologies will provide the most effective results.

14.6   Sources of further information and advice

AAK Bakery Services: http://www.aak-uk.com
AAK 'Global' magazine 'Saturated fat reduction in food and confectionery', accessible online at http://www.aak.com/Global/Magazines/Global/Global_June_2010.pdf (accessed 9 December 2010).
Manley D (2000) *Technology of biscuits, crackers and cookies* (Third edition), Cambridge, Woodhead Publishing.
Talbot G (2009) *Science and technology of enrobed and filled chocolate, confectionery and bakery products*, Cambridge, Woodhead Publishing

14.7   References

Atkinson G (2010) 'Applications of cryo-crystallised fats in bakery products for saturates reduction', Internal report, AAK Bakery Services.
BMJ (2006) 'Trans fatty acids and coronary heart disease, *British Medical Journal*, 333 (7561): 214.
BOC (2010) Brooker BJ *et al.* 'Cryogenic crystallisation of fats', US patent 20100055278.
Burt DJ, Thacker D (1981) 'Use of emulsifiers in short dough biscuits', *FMBRA Bull*, 2: 55.
Commission Directive 2000/36/EC of the European Parliament and of the Council of 23 June 2000 relating to cocoa and chocolate products intended for human consumption, Official Journal L197 of 03/08/2001 (as amended).

© Woodhead Publishing Limited, 2011

CSPI (2003) 'Olestra linked to gastrointestinal disease', available at http://www.cspinet. org/new/200307151.html (accessed 13 June 2010).

Danisco (undated) 'New textures with emulsifiers in rotary moulded biscuits' Technical Memorandum TM 1038-2e.

Duffy BF (1993) 'Method of inhibiting fat and oil migration from an oily substrate of a food product into a coating layer of a food product', US patent 5202137.

EC (2003) '2003/867/EC: Commission Decision of 1 December 2003 authorising the placing on the market of salatrims as novel food ingredients under Regulation (EC) No 258/97 of the European Parliament and of the Council (notified under document number C(2003) 4408) Official Journal L 326, 13/12/2003 P. 0032-0034

EU (2006) '2006/720/EC: Commission Decision of 23 October 2006 authorising the placing on the market of diacylglycerol oil of plant origin as a novel food under Regulation (EC) No 258/97 of the European Parliament and of the Council (notified under document number C(2006) 4971)' OJ L 296, 26.10.2006, p. 10–12.

FDA (2003) 'Health Claims; Soluble dietary fiber from certain foods and coronary health disease' Federal Register 68 FR 44207 July 2008 accessible from http://frwebgate. access.gpo.gov/cgi-bin/getdoc.cgi?dbname=2002_register&docid=02-25067-filed.pdf (accessed 9 December 2010).

FDF (2009) United Biscuits (UB) – reformulation case studies. Available at http://www. fdf.org.uk/industry_casestudies/reformulation_ub.aspx (accessed 13 June 2010)

FSA (2010) 'Food Standards Agency voluntary recommendations on saturated fat reductions for biscuits, cakes, buns and chocolate confectionery added sugar reductions in soft drinks, and portion size availability, for chocolate confectionery and soft drinks'. UK Food Standards Agency March 2010 accessible from http://www.food.gov.uk/ multimedia/pdfs/satfatrecommendations (accessed 9 December 2010).

Lawson R, Miller AR, Thacker D (1981) 'Rotary moulded short dough biscuits: Part II. The effects of the level of ingredients on the properties of Lincoln Biscuits', *Flour Millers and Baking Research Association Report*, 93: 15–20.

Manley D (2000) *Technology of biscuits, crackers and cookies* (Third edition), Cambridge, Woodhead Publishing.

Matsuo N (2001) 'Diacylglycerol oil: an edible oil with less accumulation of body fat', *Lipid Technology*, 13, 129–33.

Mattson FH and Volpenhein RA (1972) 'Rate and extent of absorption of the fatty acids of fully esterified glycerol, erythritol and sucrose as measured in thoracic duct cannulated rats', *J. Nutr.* 102: 1177–80.

NDA (2004) 'Opinion of the Scientific Panel on Dietetic products, nutrition and allergies [NDA] related to the presence of trans fatty acids in foods and the effect on human health of the consumption of trans fatty acids' request number EFSA-Q-2003-022 adopted on 8 July 2004.

Nestec (2009) Leas A *et al.* 'Reduced fat chocolate coatings formed by spraying', US Patent CA2703269 (A1).

Sudha ML *et al.* (2007) 'Fat replacement in soft dough biscuits: its implications on dough rheology and biscuit quality', *Journal of Food Engineering*, 80(3), 922–30.

Talbot G (2008) 'Reduction of Saturated Fat in Bakery Products', Report to the UK Food Standards Agency, 3 December.

Ulrick (2008) 'Ulrick & Short adds to tapioca starch fat replacement range' available at http://www.foodnavigator.com/Financial-Industry/Ulrick-Short-adds-to-tapioca-starch-fat-replacement-range (accessed 13 June 2010).

Wells M (2009) 'Controlling the rheology of chocolate and fillings' in Talbot G (ed.) *Science and technology of enrobed and filled chocolate, confectionery and bakery products*, Cambridge, Woodhead Publishing, p. 267.

Ziegleder G (1997) 'Fat migration and bloom', *Manuf. Confect.* 77 (February) 43–4.

© Woodhead Publishing Limited, 2011

15

Saturated fat reduction in pastry

B. de Cindio and F. R. Lupi, University of Calabria, Italy

Abstract: Pastries are baked goods mainly produced to complement the flavor of the fillings and to provide them with a casing. The main kinds of pastry, short and puff, are produced with hard fats hydrogenated with catalytic processes in order to match the rheological properties of the dough. Unfortunately, these processes lead to the formation of *trans* fats dangerous for consumers' health. Therefore, the use of hydrogenated fats is nowadays reduced in favor of natural added fat sources. This chapter gives an overview of pastry characteristics, also looking at the new frontiers in healthy food production based on rheological modeling.

Key words: pastry, shortenings, margarines, structured emulsions, natural fats.

15.1 Introduction

15.1.1 General definitions

The name 'pastry' is used to define various kinds of baked goods obtained by mixing flour, water, fats (e.g. margarines, butter, shortening), baking powder and eggs. Different products can be produced by changing the processing conditions involving the mixing of dough with fats. The main properties of these pastry products are, for different reasons, due to the use of saturated fats, particularly during their preparation. A simple and direct saturated fat reduction, eventually up to their complete substitution, leads to poor-quality products (bad filling, low puffing, etc) that do not respond to consumer requirements and expectations. Limited knowledge of the link between structure, ingredients and process conditions has led to the production of pastry that is almost restricted to the use of saturated fat (where there is already a strong technological expertise). In the last few decades, the association of the presence of saturated fats with health problems has begun to push the market towards 'healthy' pastry. Consequently this has renewed the interest of technologists in developing new expertise in this area. It should be stated that this is a rather difficult skill, requiring a new view of the

© Woodhead Publishing Limited, 2011

whole production process, because of the central role played by the fat in the structure development of the pastry. To tackle this problem a deeper understanding of the mechanical/rheological properties of the main ingredients (flour and fat) is needed in order to realize a so-called rheological matching between them during all the process steps.

15.1.2   Pastry classification: mixing action

When classified on the basis of the mixing action, most bakery products can be categorized in two classes: extensible dough (bread or puff pastry) and flowable or friable mixtures, used in the preparation of batters. Compared to simple dough-based products, pastries, because of their high fat content, are characterized by a particular crumbly and aerated texture, which makes them flexible and flaky, but also strong enough to be resistant to fillings and to the weight of other ingredients.

Different kinds of pastries can be distinguished depending on their preparation procedure, ingredients and final use, such as:

- shortcrust pastry
- choux pastry
- puff pastry
- yeast-leavened product: Danish pastries
- pastry-based products
  ○ croissant, cornetto, pain au chocolat
  ○ filled pastries.

For these products, the process variation involves just a proper fat/dough matching procedure, the final sheeting/lamination process being the same in all cases.

Shortcrust pastries are mainly used as a bottom for pies, tarts or petit fours made with a certain amount of fat and water, according to the 'half-fat-to-flour' ratio. These kinds of pastries are prepared by mixing solid fat, flour and salt, and gradually adding water to obtain the consistency for rolling the dough into the desired shape.

In other types of pastry – puff pastry, Danish pastry, croissants or Italian 'cornetto' – the characteristic flaky texture is achieved by repeatedly folding and rolling out the dough together with a solid fat in a sheeting process. In particular, puff pastry consists of as many as 700 layers of paper-thin pastry separated by butter and air, giving a light, crisp, and rich system (Harte, 2003).

The leavening in laminated dough-like puff pastry is due to the vapor released by either butter or dough during the cooking step. In the case of Danish or croissant pastries, a small amount of yeast is added to the ingredients to aid the leavening. Therefore puff pastry, when produced without leavening agents, requires a higher percentage of butter and a more elaborate folding process in order to release a greater quantity of vapor.

All the pastries are commercialized in the form of laminated sheets, and sheeting is, in several cases (i.e. puff or Danish pastries), the main process step in which fat/dough rheological matching is achieved. In these cases the lamination process has to be carried out by taking into account some important aspects.

© Woodhead Publishing Limited, 2011

Table 15.1   Classification of pastries according to the fat/dough matching process and ingredients

Pastry	Process for fat/dough matching	Main ingredients
Yeast-leavened pastry (Danish)	Mixing* and sheeting/lamination	High-protein flour/pastry flour, butter/margarine/shortenings, yeast, milk solids, eggs (optional), salt
Puff pastry	Mixing* and sheeting/lamination	Fat (shortenings), high-protein flour, water, salt
Choux pastry	Mixing/extrusion	Fat, flour, water, eggs, salt
Shortcrust pastry	Mixing	Fat, flour, water and salt

* In the industrial process the mixing phase is different according to the method (French, English or Scottish)

The dough must have a well-developed gluten network, allowing the gas expansion to be supported and the subsequent structure collapse to be avoided, but in addition it must be capable of creating a soft and flaky product after cooking. Therefore the gluten network strength has to reach a good compromise between these two required characteristics. To accomplish this, the butter must be solid-like and have similar rheological characteristics with respect to the dough when laminating (Simovic *et al.*, 2009) (showing a greater elastic modulus with respect to the loss modulus in a frequency sweep test). It has to be able to be rolled out easily without breaking into pieces but firm enough not to squeeze out of the edges of the dough layers. The butter and dough should be approximately at the same temperature and the layers must remain distinct from each other, otherwise the end product will resemble a brioche more than a delicately layered and flaky laminated dough.

The pastry types defined above may then be classified from a process point of view, according to the method used to match the fatty phase with the dough, as shown in Table 15.1, which also lists the classical ingredients that are used.

15.1.3   Pastry ingredients: the role of fats

It should be noted that pastries use solid fats such as margarines, shortenings or butters as ingredients. These are water-in-oil (W/O) emulsions, structured in the oil phase to guarantee a rheological matching with the dough. Margarines used in pastry production derive their consistency from a fat crystal network of fully saturated triglycerides (TAGs) (Cavillot *et al.*, 2009). TAGs allow a better molecular interaction and packing to give a more ordered structure. Traditionally, saturated TAGs can be obtained by hydrogenation, which also produces *trans* fatty acids (TFAs). TFAs in particular are responsible for an increased risk of coronary heart disease. Because of this, there is a growing amount of research, mainly focused on the development and design of new pastries produced with a

© Woodhead Publishing Limited, 2011

low saturated fat content, and, most of all, without TFA (Simovic *et al.*, 2009). To achieve this, it appears that a deeper rheological study is necessary because of the role played by fat in structure development during processing.

15.2   The dough/fat matching process in pastry

15.2.1   Mixing as the dough/fat matching process: shortcrust pastry

Shortcrust pastry is a rich dough containing a large amount of fat, water, flour and, when necessary, eggs and sugar. This pastry is mainly used for biscuits, tarts, pies and the bottom and sides of fruit pies, flans and cheesecakes, and it can be considered the simplest and most common pastry. As already mentioned, its production process includes mixing of the fat and flour, adding water, and rolling out the paste.

In both sweetcrust (sweetened) and shortcrust pastry, fat and flour have to be blended thoroughly before liquid is added, ensuring an adequate coating of flour granules with fat in order to reduce the likelihood of a gluten network to be completely developed (this guarantees the expected final textural characteristics of the product). The energy required for the mixing phase has to be enough to achieve this. In fact, overworking the dough is considered hazardous because it elongates the gluten strands, creating a 'chewy' product, while low-energy mixing can make the system unstable. It is fairly easy to define saturated fats that respond to those technological requirements, because there is much experience in this area. Fat that does not cover the flour granules is present as lumps that may melt during cooking, creating voids that are responsible for the texture. Saturated fat reduction must be achieved in such a way as to maintain the same degree of deformation of the dough matrix in order to avoid gluten extension. This can be achieved by using structured fat emulsions instead of saturated fat showing approximately the same rheological behavior when subjected to a small-amplitude oscillatory test. The choice of this particular test is due to the fact that the pastry mixing phase is well defined by the material parameters determined under the rheological equilibrium conditions of the test (Baldino, 2007).

15.2.2   Mixing/extrusion as the dough/fat matching process: choux pastry

Choux pastry is a kind of pastry often filled with creams or prepared in decorative shapes for garnishing. Its main composition consists of 150–200 parts of eggs, 100 parts of flour, 100 parts of shortening (butter) and approximately 200 parts of water (Harte, 2003).

In the traditional preparation procedure, mixing is different from the other pastries: flour is quickly stirred into a mixture of the above-mentioned liquids, followed by seasoning and fat, and, finally, eggs. The fat must be completely dispersed in hot water in order to form an emulsion and heated to boiling, then the flour together with seasoning or sugar and other powders can be added. The mixture has to be stirred until a smooth and gelatinized paste is produced. After

© Woodhead Publishing Limited, 2011

the mixture has cooled, the eggs are beaten into the choux mix one or two at a time, mixing well after each addition. Finally, the soft paste can be extruded to obtain the final choux shape. To obtain a smooth consistency and maximum pastry volume, a small amount of chemical leavening can be added to the liquid phase. The paste is spooned or piped onto parchment-paper-lined pans and baked at 215–226°C until crisp.

Industrially, choux pastry can be prepared by a continuous extrusion process. The extruder is a screw system within a tube or barrel, which conveys the dough towards a die (Fig. 15.1 shows extruder-cooking equipment for cereal mixtures). In the confined space of the barrel, the dough is compressed and heated to high temperatures at high pressures before being extruded through the dies into the atmosphere. During extrusion cooking many transformations take place in the dough, mainly due to mixing, kneading, starch gelatinization, protein coagulation, formation of amylose-lipid complexes and development of non-enzymatic browning and homogenization: these transformations should be taken into account in order to accomplish a proper process for choux pastry production (Peressini *et al.*, 2002).

In this case rheological matching is achieved by characterizing the materials with small-amplitude oscillatory flow. However, because a shear flow is observed into the extruder, a flow curve is necessary to link ingredient changes to process parameters. Very often a temperature rheological matching is needed, and a so-called 'time cure test', an oscillatory test made at fixed frequencies of oscillation and cooling/heating rates, is helpful in defining temperature dependency in view of the melting and coagulation reactions occurring during the cooking step.

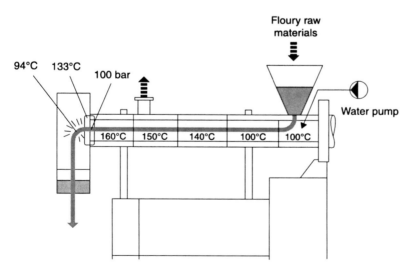

Fig. 15.1   Extruder-cooking equipment for cereal goods (from de Cindio *et al.*, 2002, with permission).

© Woodhead Publishing Limited, 2011

15.2.3 Lamination as the dough/fat matching process: puff pastry and Danish pastry

Puff pastry, also called *pâte feuilletée* or *pâte feuilletage*, is a dough which is spread with solid fats and repeatedly folded and rolled out. Thus it consists of alternating layers of dough (wheat flour and water) separated by alternating layers of a solid-like fat, margarine, designed to obtain the proper rheological matching. The matching between fat and dough can be achieved with different methods: the more common are French, Scottish and English.

The French method is the most popular but it is complicated and difficult to produce under high-speed commercial manufacturing processes. In this method, a portion of the fat is rubbed into the flour, and the remaining part is rolled within the dough. After the dough is completely mixed up to the proper fat amount, it is sheeted into a rectangle with a thinner external border and the remaining fat is rolled to the size of the dough. After the fat is placed on it, its thinner parts are folded over on the thicker dough and fat in the form of pockets and rolled according to the three-fold pastry preparation technique (Fig. 15.2). The subsequent folding and rolling steps allow the formation of links between the different layers of pastry, giving a closed and uniform aerated structure.

As far as the English method is concerned, the dough is sheeted into a rectangular shape and it is spread over two-thirds of the area with solid fats. The alternate dough/fat layers are then produced by the three-fold pastry preparation technique. In the Scottish method, which is widely used commercially, all the pastry fat is broken into lumps (5 cm) and mixed in the flour to lubricate the gluten. The remaining ingredients are then added to form a lumpy dough. The rolling procedure follows the three-fold pastry technique with the addition of one extra half-turn.

In the case of the Scottish method, careful timing is critical in the mixing phase: in fact, the overmixing of fat with the dough can lead to system instability preventing the 'puffing' process.

In Fig. 15.3 the distinction of alternate layers is clearly shown thanks to the microstructural image of a commercial puff pastry (Buitoni, Italy) performed by an NMR analysis on a Bruker Avance 300 (Bruker, Germany) wide-bore spectrometer equipped with a standard micro-imaging probe (Lupi, 2009).

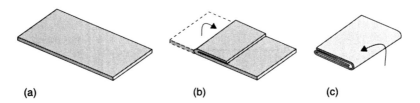

(a)   (b)   (c)

Fig. 15.2 Three-fold pastry production: (a) the dough is sheeted into a rectangle; (b) one end is folded two-thirds of the way down the rectangle; (c) the opposite end is folded to cover the first one.

© Woodhead Publishing Limited, 2011

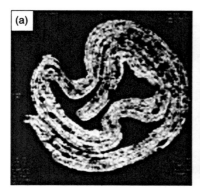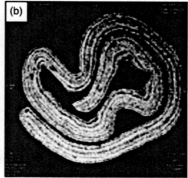

Fig. 15.3 NMR image analysis of a commercial puff pastry: (a) an MRI (magnetic resonance image) obtained with a GEFI experiment; (b) an MRI image 'weighed on T_2', obtained by MSME experiments on the puff pastry (from Lupi, 2009).

According to the impulse sequence used to observe the proton signal, the intensity of the pixel brightness of the image can be related to the water quantity of the material (gradient-echo fast imaging, GEFI tests) or alternatively to the transverse relaxation time T_2 (multi-slice-multi-echo, MSME tests). Figure 15.3(a) shows a magnetic resonance image (MRI) image of an axial section of puff pastry dough obtained with a GEFI experiment. The signal intensity is proportional, in this case, only to the proton density differences. As can be seen, the image shows the structure of the pastry, revealing the structural composition. Figure 15.3(b) shows an MRI image 'weighed on T_2', obtained by MSME experiments on puff pastry. In this case the stratification of the aqueous dough is more evident with respect to the fat phase.

Danish pastry is a rich pastry prepared with a lamination process and, as previously explained, including a fermented, sweetened dough. Therefore the puffing process is improved by the baking ingredients producing CO_2 as a leavening gas together with steam. Usually the dough is made with high-protein flour (11.5–12%), often combined with up to 30% pastry flour for easier lamination. The total amount of fat can range up to 50% of the dough.

Danish pastry preparation can be performed with two different methods: (a) conventional or short mixing time, and (b) the lamination or the long mixing time method, mostly used in the industrial sheeting processes. In the conventional three-fold method, all the ingredients are combined with the exception of the fat (Harte, 2003). A large portion of fat is distributed over two-thirds of the dough previously sheeted alone, and the rectangle is folded as shown in Fig. 15.2. In the four-fold or book-fold technique the fat is distributed over the centre of the dough and folded as shown in Fig. 15.4.

In commercial lamination, Danish pastry is produced by layering the shortening between two pieces of dough. This can be accomplished by extruding dough around the shortening, or high-speed pumping of the shortening between two continuous dough sheets.

© Woodhead Publishing Limited, 2011

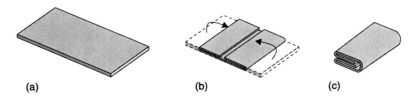

Fig. 15.4   Four-fold pastry production: (a) the dough is sheeted into a rectangle; (b) both ends of the dough are folded; (c) one folded end is turned to cover the opposite one.

As far as these pastries are concerned, the main process, from a rheological point of view, may be subdivided into two different steps: mixing/lamination and puffing. During the first step a squeezing flow predominates, while during puffing elongational flow must be considered. Saturated fats, as already observed, tend to have a more plastic behavior (elastic component predominates above fluid component), therefore lump formation is favored. On the contrary, fats with low saturated components, for instance olive oil, are usually more liquid and tend naturally to lubricate the layers. In this respect, at a first glance, the saturated fat reduction seems to be unacceptable because layers will each slip over the other and a poor texture will result. To avoid this, a structured fat emulsion can again be used to make a proposed reduced saturated fat system more 'consistent'. Oscillatory and shear flow rheological characterization is therefore a good start to match the dough and fat, but this is not enough because the puffing effect must be controlled too and needs a more difficult approach, as shown in the following section.

15.3   Process rheological modeling

15.3.1   Bubble expansion in a viscoelastic matter

As mentioned above, in some cases pastries are subjected to an expansion due either to the presence of a leavening agent or just to the water directly present in the dough and in fat (about 20% by weight). During mixing, a certain amount of air is entrapped inside the dough, forming small gas bubbles, the volumes of which increase as an effect of process temperature or gas development. Since the bubble-dough may be assumed to be a thermodynamically closed system, evaporated water remains entrapped as vapor inside the bubble, thus approaching an equilibrium state. Evaporating water availability is linked to the binding effect of the ingredients (de Cindio, 2004). The presence of leavening agents will supply the gas bubble by diffusion within the dough. The final gas bubble dimensional distribution is assumed to be mainly responsible for the texture of the goods. Fats may be considered as the ingredients of the dough that greatly influence either its capability to entrap gas or its expandability. In fact, they form a sort of membrane at the gas–dough interface avoiding gas loss, but, at the same time, they allow a greater or lesser volume increase according to their lubrication effect on the rheological properties. In this respect the use of different fats may alter significantly

© Woodhead Publishing Limited, 2011

the final texture. Thus any fat substitution must be very carefully considered. It has been found (Baltasavias *et al.*, 1997) that these doughs are not only fat-continuous but also bi-continuous systems. In fact, by reducing fat content or replacing solid fat with oil, it is possible to obtain a fat-dispersed system. The non-fat phase is mainly a solution of saturated saccharose connected to a particle of flour/starch that contributes to conferring a greater resistance at high deformation, while gluten is responsible for the strain-hardening behavior. From a mechanical point of view bubble volume increases following a bi-extensional flow. Thus the puffing effect may be depressed if the fat inserted into the pastry is not properly chosen in terms of its rheological properties when subjected to an elongational flow, because shear or oscillatory properties are not helpful in making a correct choice. To avoid a trial-and-error approach, which can be very expensive and often unsuccessful, an innovative technique based on rheological modeling and process simulation has been proposed (Baldino, 2007). The result is something that is capable of predicting the final distribution of voids when changing ingredient and/or recipe by knowing the main physical properties and particularly the rheological equation. Several publications are available in the open literature to handle this problem that can be set in a simple form only if the approximation to a single bubble expanding in a infinite medium is applied (Bird *et al.*, 1977), even if some attempt to treat the coalescence of bubbles has been reported (de Cindio *et al.*, 2003). Essentially the system is modeled as shown in Fig. 15.5. The radius R of the bubble is obtained by a classical mechanical approach assuming as reference the moving boundary of the bubble surface against an infinite mass of viscoelastic matter.

In this case, continuity equation under incompressibility hypothesis assumes the following form:

$$V(r,t) = \frac{R^2}{r^2}\dot{R} \qquad\qquad\qquad [15.1]$$

where $V(r,t)$ is the radial velocity at any point $r>R$. The velocity at the interface is the time derivative of R, indicated by $\dot{R}$.

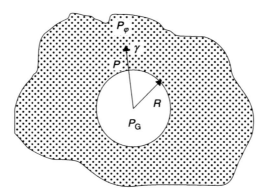

Fig. 15.5   Sketch of a gas bubble immersed in an infinite medium.

© Woodhead Publishing Limited, 2011

The force balance at the dough–gas interface, R, is given by:

$$P_G = \frac{2\gamma(T,x_i)}{R} + P_\infty - \int_R^\infty 3\frac{\tau_{rr}}{r}dr \qquad [15.2]$$

where γ is the interfacial tension and the rheological contribution (third term of the right side of Eq. 15.2) takes into account the bi-extensional deformation through a viscoelastic time dependent modulus G. By assuming current time t as reference and applying a superposition principle, Eq. 15.3 is obtained:

$$\int_R^\infty 3\frac{\tau_{rr}}{r}dr = \int_0^t G(s,T,x_i)\dot{R}(s)\cdot\frac{R^2(s)}{R^3(s)-R^3}\ln\frac{R(s)}{R}ds \qquad [15.3]$$

where s indicates the past time deviation from current time, T is the absolute temperature and x_i is the content of the i-component. As far as the time dependency is concerned, it is actually found that a weak gel, two-parameter constitutive equation (Gabriele *et al.*, 2001) seems to be a good representation for food systems

$$G(t) = S \cdot t^{-n} \qquad [15.4]$$

By substitution into Eq. 15.2 and 15.3 it is possible to follow the void fraction increase when time elapses in terms of internal pressure P_G, thus finding the final apparent volume by the ideal gas law. Therefore when substituting fats, or other ingredients, it is necessary to determinate the three material parameters γ, S and n by proper experimental techniques, and make a simulation at the process conditions.

A more complex model is needed when bubble coalescence occurs, but few results are available in this field (Baldino, 2007) and they do not seem to be relevant for short dough.

15.3.2   Lamination process modeling

The same rheological approach may be used for the lamination or sheeting step. In this case the material is subjected to a pre-eminent shear flow between two rollers (see Fig. 15.6).

The process is modeled by applying the lubrication theory, consisting of finding velocity and pressure profiles referred to a plane stationary rectangular flow. In such a way material trajectories are almost parallel and a local solution can be found easily as for a shear flow. The material is subjected to a drag flow according to the rotation velocity of the rollers, and the pressure firstly increases, reaching a maximum value approximately at the minimum gap, and subsequently decreases until it reaches the zero exit value. The material is accelerated along the x-axis and as a consequence is extended, i.e. laminated. The effectiveness of lamination is mainly governed by shear rheological properties, thus time-dependent properties are not evidenced or at least may be neglected due to the governing kinematics of deformation. If a power law is assumed to represent the rheological behavior

$$\tau = k \cdot \dot{\gamma}^n \qquad [15.5]$$

© Woodhead Publishing Limited, 2011

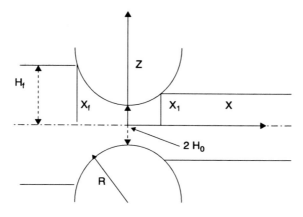

Fig. 15.6   Sketch of sheeting.

where k and n are respectively the consistency and the flow index, the value of the pressure at any position inside the two rollers is then found (Tanner, 2000)

$$P(x') = \left(\frac{2n+1}{n}\right)^n \cdot k \cdot \left(\frac{H_0}{U}\right)^{-n} \cdot \sqrt{\frac{2R}{H_0}} \int\limits_{-x'}^{x'_l} \frac{\left|x'^2_l - x'^2\right|^{n-1}\left(x'^2_l - x'^2\right)}{\left(1+x'^2\right)^{2n+1}} \, dx' \qquad [15.6]$$

where x', x'_f and x'_l are, respectively, x, x_f and x_l (see Fig. 15.6) adimensionalized with respect to $\sqrt{2RH_0}$ and U is the peripheral velocity of the rolls.

If the value of P is assumed to be zero at the exit, from the solution of Eq. 15.6 the value of x_l is found, and therefore, the value of the final thickness. Thus, if the ratio $H_f/H_0 > 10$ HOLDS, a more 'flowable' fat (i.e. less saturated) corresponds to lower values of n, ($n < 1$) and a thicker lamination is expected. However the use of Eq. 15.6 allows the result to be predicted when any change in the formulation is proposed. For instance, for any given n-value, when increasing k a proportional increase of the pressure exerted by the material to the rolls is evidenced. This implies that the laminate may swell to relax the normal stresses. Similarly, for any given k-value, the final laminate thickness changes with n owing to flow pattern drastic variations. Unfortunately, scarce literature data are available about this latter argument.

Therefore, according to this equation, proper fat characteristics should be achieved in order to obtain the rheological matching with dough, and consequently, the desired laminate thickness.

15.4   Margarine and shortenings for reducing saturated fats

The production of all pastries is achieved with shortenings or margarines as the fatty phase. Various approaches have been taken to reduce the calorie and the TFA content of the laminating materials. Carbohydrate-based fat replacers are

© Woodhead Publishing Limited, 2011

unsuitable because of their hydrophilic properties that prevent and avoid water vapor entrapping during baking (Lupi, 2009). Therefore it is necessary to use an oil-soluble, restructured lipid to form a water-insoluble barrier. For this reason, structuring W/O emulsions is a well-known technique for the production of shortenings for pastries. Margarines are W/O-structured emulsions with a dispersed phase ratio of less than 20_{wt}%. If the water phase amount is higher than this threshold limit, W/O emulsions, called 'spreads', which cannot be considered as margarines, can be commercialized as spreadable shortenings (Borwankar et al. 1992).

The taste of margarines and food spreads is due to water-soluble flavors, oil-soluble flavors and salt in the water phase (Blanco Muñoz, 2004). Their rheological characteristics are given by the high melting point of saturated fats in the oil phase. Crystals interact and form a three-dimensional network surrounding water droplets and stabilizing the biphasic system. Thus the high consistency of margarine is obtained with a certain amount of TAGs that allow a better molecular interaction and, as a consequence, a better packing, giving a more ordered structure. The traditional process employed to saturate the TAGs is generally hydrogenation, which also can produce trans isomers (TFAs). In general, fats containing a majority of SFA are solid at room temperature, and those containing mostly cis unsaturated fatty acids (oils) are usually liquid at room temperature (Ghotra et al., 2002).

Different data indicate that TFAs are not metabolically equivalent to the natural cis isomers and that they promote the development of arteriosclerosis and predispose to coronary heart disease and other health risks (Blanco Muñoz, 2004). The substitution of TFAs with different ingredients giving the same rheological characteristics but producing at the same time healthy foods is one of the most relevant problems for food designers (Norton et al., 2009).

Three different methods are currently employed in the food industry in order to obtain a hardening of the oil phase:

• partial hydrogenation of vegetable oils
• catalytic interesterification of vegetable oils and completely saturated fats
• addition of solid fats to the starting liquid oil.

Historically, the most common technique among those listed above has been the catalytic hydrogenation of the double bonds of unsaturated fatty acids chains. Industrial hydrogenation of vegetable oil (and, occasionally, fish oil) is a process involving three phases (gas–solid–liquid) carried out in a batch autoclave over a nickel-based catalyst as a slurry at 110–190°C, 30–70 psi H_2 pressure, with $0.01–0.15_{wt}$% Ni (Singh et al., 2009).

As already stated, this process can promote the development of TFAs. Their formation can be minimized by increasing pressure, decreasing temperature and increasing agitation to address mass transfer limitations. Precious metal catalysts are active at considerably lower temperatures and can thus produce less TFAs compared to conventional Ni catalysts, but they cannot completely avoid their formation. The order of catalytic activity of precious metal catalysts is Pd>Rh>Pt>Ru (Singh et al., 2009).

© Woodhead Publishing Limited, 2011

An alternative process that does not produce TFAs is catalytic interesterification between a fully hydrogenated fat and a natural *trans*-free vegetable oil (Criado *et al.* 2007; Hee Lee *et al.*, 2008). Interesterification is an exchange of fatty acids between the two TAG molecules participating in this reaction, thereby causing a rearrangement of the fatty acid residues in both of these molecules. This reaction can be intramolecular if the exchange of fatty acids happens between two chains in the same TAG molecule or intermolecular if two TAGs are involved. Therefore the SFA chains of a fully hydrogenated TAG source can replace the unsaturated chains of TAGs naturally present in a vegetable oil. These rearrangements are accompanied by a concomitant change in the properties of the original physical mixture. The final properties of the semi-solid fat product are strongly influenced by both the relative proportions of reactants in the original starting mixture and the type of catalyst used. Normally in this process, a chemical catalyst such as sodium metal or sodium alkoxide is used to promote acyl migration among glyceride molecules, but owing to its toxicity different enzymes have been used to promote the reaction. Macrae (1983) suggested using lipases to produce useful glyceride mixtures which cannot be obtained by conventional chemical interesterification processes. Kim *et al.* (2009) used the same enzyme, immobilized on silica granules in order to interesterify olive oil with palm stearin.

If the oil phase is continuous, the structure of the final biphasic system could be improved by adding fat crystals. In fact, one of the methods that could be applied to enhance their mechanical characteristics is the addition of hard fats in the liquid oil phase with a suitable emulsifier and stabilizing agent. Jahaniaval (2005) in his patent suggests a preparation of healthy margarine and butter substitutes based on liquid oils (at room temperature) like olive oil and phospholipids as stabilizers. The final consistency of the resulting margarine is increased by mixing at a high temperature the oil and added hard fat like cottonseed stearin, palm and canola stearins and intermediate melting point triglycerides such as interesterified fats, cocoa butter or cocoa butter substitutes and/or any fractionated fat with a melting point of 34–40°C. Skogerson *et al.* (2007) propose an interesting patent relating to a glyceride emulsifier with a high diglyceride content, which is especially useful in preparing puff pastry products. Mono- and diglycerides of fatty acids are very common emulsifiers widely employed in the food industry. They are produced by the reaction of glycerol with vegetable oils and fats, the compositions of which strictly depend on the characteristics of the starting fruit from which the oil is obtained (Clogston *et al.*, 2000). This emulsifier is lipophilic and its hydrophilic–lipophilic balance (HLB) value, about 3.7, should allow the formation of W/O emulsions (Constantinides and Yiv, 1994; Friberg, 1997).

Commercial mono- and diglycerides usually contain 40–60% monoglycerides, 38–45% diglycerides, 8–12% triglycerides and 1–7% free glycerol. In accordance with their patent, the authors suggest increasing the diglyceride portion preferably to about 75% (on a weight basis) by vacuum distillation, with the remaining monoglyceride portion being about 10% and the triglyceride portion of the order of 15%. Therefore, the resulting W/O emulsion recipe could be prepared by admixing, on a w/w basis, from about 10% to about 16% of the high-diglyceride

© Woodhead Publishing Limited, 2011

Table 15.2   Some brands of olive oil shortenings in various markets

Brand	Made in	Name	% olive oil
Biona	USA	Organic Olive Extra Spread	12.7
Migros	Switzerland	Margarine Sanissa Olive	15
Kaiku-Benecol	Spain	Margarina con Aceite de Oliva	15
Flora (Unilever)	Spain	Margarina Oliva	20
Bertolli	Italy	Spread Olive Oil	21

emulsifier, from about 55% to about 65% of vegetable oil, and from about 13% to about 25% of saturated fat.

The growing consumer demand for healthy foods is pushing research to substitute dangerous and unhealthy additives with better-known and natural ingredients. Olive oil and products based on it are recognized worldwide as healthy foods and promoted as part of the Mediterranean diet, which is currently viewed as making a favorable dietary contribution. Therefore, in this respect, olive oil can be recommended in the diet, and has a positive image in terms of consumer appeal.

Although the product 'margarine with olive oil' already exists, the maximum percentage of olive oil contained in these original recipes is 21 w/w%. In Table 15.2 some different brands of shortenings containing olive oil are listed; the total amount of olive oil is reported on a weight basis.

Recent literature focuses on the production of olive-oil-based shortenings as puff pastry roll-fat substitutes. In fact, following the suggestion of Jahaniaval (2005), different W/O emulsions were prepared by Lupi *et al.* (2010) by using cocoa butter as added hard fat and mono- and diglycerides of fatty acids as emulsifiers. The authors found that a fast cooling rate of the warm oil phase (mainly composed of olive oil and with a certain percentage of pure cocoa butter) followed by a subsequent emulsification with water produced emulsions having rheological properties very similar to those of commercial margarines (Lupi *et al.*, 2010).

15.5   Conclusions

The technological problems arising when saturated fats are reduced in pastry have been discussed, from which it is possible to conclude that it is better to avoid operating on a trial-and-error basis, because the solution may not even be possible to be reached, owing to the complex way in which different ingredients interact with one another. It has been recognized that a very important role is played by the change of rheological properties that are mainly responsible for the texture of the pastry. Thus, a proper rheological characterization is required to prepare the same food but with reduced saturated fats, ranging from shear to bi-elongational to oscillatory equilibrium tests depending on the particular application. If process

© Woodhead Publishing Limited, 2011

modeling is coupled with a rheological equation of state, a predictive model is obtained capable of simulating the transformations occurring into the product. It may be suggested that this innovative approach should be used to predict the texture of pastry goods when reducing saturated fats by matching material rheology.

15.6   Future trends

Pastry production is a typical food industry challenge. The growing demand from consumers for healthy foods is driving research to substitute dangerous and unhealthy additives with better-known and natural ingredients. The importance of designing healthy everyday foods without *trans*-fats can be clearly understood from looking at the recent literature. In the last International Symposium of Food Rheology and Structure (Zurich, 15–18 June 2009) a lot of interesting works were published in the proceedings; an example is the plenary lecture given by Ian T. Norton *et al.* (2009). Thus, the problem of substituting TFA in margarines or shortenings is a huge problem treated differently by research and discussed as a future challenge.

The study of emulsions prepared with a high oily phase concentration is, therefore, very relevant in order to produce new pastry products with improved characteristics. The basic knowledge about the structural properties of an emulsion is progressing, but the inherent complexity of such materials permanently raises a variety of fundamental questions at the frontier between physics, chemistry and biology. Two phenomena of potential relevance to the formulation of novel functional and structured emulsions for pastry products are *droplet attractive interactions* and the *formation of a polymer network* in the continuous phase. These topics should give interesting results allowing the production of *trans*-free and healthy structured emulsions.

Moreover, another interesting challenge should be the addition of natural, healthy ingredients for pastry production, like olive oil, as the main constituent of the continuous phase of margarines or shortenings. The oily phase should then be structured by the addition of natural hard fats and emulsifiers.

Recent development of rheological inspections of modified dough (produced with proper flour mixtures) and the gradual acquisition of knowledge about non-Newtonian fluid mechanics is improving the modeling of the sheeting process.

15.7   Sources of further information and advice

de Cindio B., Correra S. (1995). Mathematical modelling of leavened cereal goods. *Journal of Food Engineering*, **24**, 379–403.
de Cindio B., Gabriele D., Pollini C. M., Peressini D., Sensidoni A. (2002). Filled snack production by co-extrusion-cooking: 2. Effect of processing on cereal mixtures, *Journal of Food Engineering*, **54**, 2002, 63–73.

© Woodhead Publishing Limited, 2011

Sliwinski E. L., Kolsterb P., van Vliet T. (2004). On the relationship between large-deformation properties of wheat flour dough and baking quality, *Journal of Cereal Science*, **39**, 231–45.
Steffe J. F. (1996). *Rheological methods in food process engineering*, Freeman Press, Michigan.

15.8   Acknowledgments

Thanks are due for its support to the Food Science & Engineering Interdepartment Centre of the University of Calabria and to L.I.P.A.C., Calabrian Laboratory of Food Process Engineering (*Regione Calabria APQ-Ricerca Scientifica e Innovazione Tecnologica I atto integrativo, Azione 2 laboratori pubblici di ricerca mission oriented interfiliera*). The authors are also grateful to Dr Cesare Oliverio Rossi for assistance with the experimental work on NMR analysis.

15.9   References

Azadmard-Damirchi S. (2007). Olive Oil – Phytosterols, Tracing of Adulteration with Hazelnut Oil and Chemical Interesterification, Doctoral thesis, Swedish University of Agricultural Sciences, Uppsala, *Acta Universitatis Agriculturae Sueciae* **36**.
Baldino N. (2007). Rheological study of aerated systems. Doctoral thesis in 'Chemical Engineering and Materials', University of Calabria.
Baltasavias A., Jurgens A., van Vliet T. (1997). Rheological properties of short doughs at small deformation. *Journal of Cereal Sciences*, **29**, 33–42.
Bird R. B., Armstrong R. C., Hassanger H. (1977). *Dynamics of polymeric liquids*. Vol. 1. Wiley, New York.
Blanco Muñoz M. A. (2004). Olive oil in food spreads, *Grasas y Aceites* **55**, 92–4.
Borwankar R.P., Frye L. A., Blaurock A.E., Sasevich F.J. (1992). Rheological characterization of melting of margarines and tablespreads, *Journal of Food Engineering* **16**, 55–74.
Cavillot V., Pierart C., Kervyn De Meerendré M., Vincent M., Paquot M., Wouters J., Deroanne C., Danthine S. (2009). Physicochemical properties of European bakery margarines with and without trans fatty acids, *Journal of Food Lipids*, **16**, 273–86.
Clogston J., Rathman J., Tomasko D., Walker H., Caffrey M. (2000). Phase behaviour of a monoacylglycerol (Myverol 18–99K)/water system, *Chemistry and Physics of Lipids* **107**, 191–220.
Constantinides, P. P., Yiv S. H. (1994). Particle size determination of phase-inverted water-in-oil microemulsions under different dilution and storage conditions, *International Journal of Pharmaceutics* **115**, 225–34.
Criado M., Hernández-Martín E., López-Hernández A., Otero C. (2007). Enzymatic interesterification of extra virgin olive oil with a fully hydrogenated fat: characterization of the reaction and its products, *Journal of American Oil Chemists Society* **84**, 717–26.
de Cindio B. (2004), Coalescenza e collasso di bolle in fluidi semi-solidi, *Panta Rei* **0**, 14–18 (in Italian).
de Cindio B., Gabriele D., Pollini C. M., Peressini D., Sensidoni A. (2002). Filled snack production by co-extrusion-cooking: 2. Effect of processing on cereal mixtures, *Journal of Food Engineering* **54**, 2002, 63–73.
de Cindio B., Gabriele D., Migliori M., Celot F., Cicerelli L., Rolston R.M. (2003). Proceed. AERC1, Guimaraes (P), pp. 11 and 18.

Friberg S. E. (1997). 'Emulsion Stability', in S.E. Friberg, K. Larsson, *Food Emulsions*, 3rd ed., Marcel Dekker Inc, New York.

Gabriele D., de Cindio B., D'Antona P. (2001). A weak gel model for foods. *Rheol. Acta* **40**, 120–7.

Ghotra B. S., Dyal S. D., Narine S. S. (2002). Lipid shortenings: a review, *Food Research International* **35**, 1015–48.

Harte J. B. (2003). 'Pastry Products/Types and Production' in Caballero B., Trugo L., Finglas P., *Encyclopaedia Of Food Science And Nutrition*, Academic Press, Amsterdam, pp. 4407–12.

Hee Lee J., Akoh C. C., Himmelsbach D. S., Lee K-T. (2008). Preparation of interesterified plastic fats from fats and oils free of trans fatty acid, *Journal of Agricultural and Food Chemistry* **56**, 4039–46.

JahanJaval F. (2005). Process for preparing high liquid oil, no trans, very low saturates, regular margarine with phospholipids, patent US 2005/0233056 A1, international classification A23D007/00.

Kim I.-H., Lee S.-M., Lee B.-M., Park H.-K., Kim J.-Y., Kwon K.-I., Kim J.-W., Lee J.-S., Kim Y.-H. (2009). Interesterification of olive oil with a fully hydrogenated fat in a batch reactor using step changes in temperature, *Journal of Agriculture Food Chemistry* **56**, 5942–6.

Lupi F. R. (2009). Rheology of highly-concentrated-in-oil emulsions, Doctoral thesis in 'Environment, Health and Eco-sustainable process', Department of Engineering Modeling, University of Calabria.

Lupi F. R., Gabriele D., Migliori M., de Cindio B. (2010). Analisi reologica di emulsioni strutturate a base di olio d'oliva, XI Congress of the Italian society of rheology, Trieste (I), 23–26 May, Grassi M., Lapasin R. (eds), edi.europa Franco Raja, Peschiera Borromeo (MI), pp. 57–62 (in Italian).

Macrae A. R. (1983). Lipase-catalyzed interesterification of oils and fats, *Journal of the American Oil Chemists Society* **60**, 291–4.

Norton I. T., Spyropoulos F., Alex E., Heuer K., Le Reverend B. J. D., Cox P. W. (2009). Microstructure engineering of healthy everyday foods, Proceedings of the 5th International Symposium on Food Rheology and Structure, Zurich 15– 18 June, pp. 10–16.

Peressini D., Sensidoni A., Pollini C. M., Gabriele D., Migliori M., de Cindio B. (2002). Filled-snacks production by co-extrusion-cooking. Part 3. A rheological-based method to compare filler processing properties, *Journal of Food Engineering* **54**, 227–40.

Rodríguez-Abreu C., Lazzari M. (2008). Emulsions with structured continuous phases, *Current Opinion in Colloid & Interface Science* **13**, 198–205

Simovic D. S., Pajin B., Seres Z., Filipovic N. (2009). Effect of low-trans margarine on physicochemical and sensory properties of puff pastry, *International Journal of Food Science and Technology* **44**, 1235–44.

Singh D., Rezac M. E., Pfromm P. H. (2009). Partial hydrogenation of soybean oil with minimal trans fat production using a Pt-decorated polymeric membrane reactor, *Journal of American Oil Chemists Society* **86**, 93–101.

Skogerson L., Boutte T., Robertson J., Zhang F. (2007). Non-hydrogenated vegetable oil based margarine for puff pastry containing an elevated di-glyceride emulsifier, USPTO Patent Application 20070148313, Class: 426602000 (USPTO).

Tanner R. I. (2000). *Engineering Rheology*. 2nd Edition, Oxford University Press, New York.

© Woodhead Publishing Limited, 2011

16

Reducing saturated fat in chocolate, compound coatings and filled confectionery products

G. Talbot, The Fat Consultant, UK

Abstract: The types of fats used, particularly in chocolate and chocolate-like (compound) coatings, are high in saturated fat in order to achieve the hard structure at ambient temperatures that is necessary for the product to be properly produced and satisfactorily consumed. The limitations imposed on chocolate formulations by legislation restrict the reductions in saturates that could be achieved. There are potentially greater possibilities for saturates reduction in coatings outside the scope of chocolate legislation. The greatest scope for saturates reduction in confectionery is in the fillings. There the problems of increased oil migration become an issue. Ways of overcoming this while allowing a reduction in saturates are described.

Key words: chocolate, compound coatings, fillings, oil migration, saturates reduction, chain length effects.

16.1　Introduction

Chocolate and confectionery form one of the 'dilemma' sectors with regard to saturated fat reduction. On the one hand, they are seen as occasional indulgences and luxuries; on the other, we are encouraged to eat a couple of squares of dark chocolate a day because of the health benefits of the flavanols present in the cocoa. Coupled with that there is a school of thought (German and Dillard, 2004; Sanders and Berry, 2005) that some of the saturated fatty acids in cocoa butter may not be that injurious to health, particularly in terms of cardiovascular disease (CVD).

Before looking at what can be done to reduce saturated fats in chocolate and confectionery it is useful to consider exactly what materials we are considering and what the extent of the 'problem' is in terms of annual consumption. As far as this chapter is concerned the sector has been divided into three parts.

© Woodhead Publishing Limited, 2011

a) Chocolate. This is any material that conforms to the definition of chocolate within the legislation of the major consuming countries and, in that regard, I have chosen to consider EU chocolate legislation, US chocolate legislation and the guidelines for chocolate composition laid down by Codex Alimentarius. As far as the fats present in chocolate are concerned, these are limited to cocoa butter, (cow's) milk fat and some well-defined vegetable fats (in countries where these are permitted).
b) Compound coatings. These are coatings (or, indeed, tabletted bars) that look like chocolate but do not conform to the definition of chocolate as laid down in legislation. This is usually because of the types of fat used in the product. Compound coatings contain less cocoa butter than does chocolate and more non-cocoa vegetable fat.
c) Filled confectionery. These are composite products with at least two phases – a coating and a filling. The coating can be either chocolate or a compound. The filling can be almost anything that is (i) edible and (ii) suitable for coating in chocolate. Although the filling can be relatively free from fat, e.g. Turkish Delight, this chapter will focus on fat-rich and often fat-continuous fillings such as pralines and truffles.

CAOBISCO, the association of chocolate, biscuit and confectionery industries of the European Union, publishes annual consumption statistics (CAOBISCO, 2009). Consumption trends for chocolate confectionery from 2005 to 2007 for the major consuming countries are shown in Fig. 16.1. Although there has been a small increase in the European countries in 2007 compared with 2006, consumption levels are fairly static, indicating that this is a mature market. Within individual

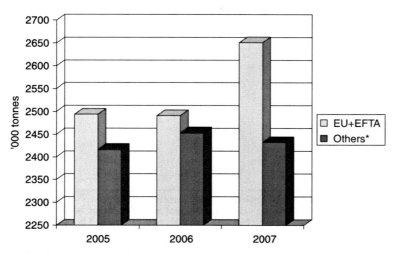

* USA, Brazil, Australia, Canada, Japan, China

Fig. 16.1 Chocolate confectionery consumption trends 2005–2007 (from CAOBISCO, 2009).

© Woodhead Publishing Limited, 2011

countries, however, there are considerable differences in per capita consumption of chocolate confectionery. In 2007, Ireland had the greatest per capita consumption at 11.85 kg/head, followed by Switzerland (10.82 kg/head) and the United Kingdom (10.10 kg/head) (CAOBISCO, 2009). Indeed the top ten chocolate confectionery consuming countries in the world in 2007 were all northern European countries. Following them were Australia (5.64 kg/head) and the USA (5.18 kg/head). China consumed only 0.12 kg/head in 2007 but, as in other markets, this is expected to grow significantly in the future.

There is clearly a temperature effect in chocolate consumption. Consumption levels are greater in those countries with a cooler ambient temperature profile. Consumption levels in warmer, Mediterranean European countries are significantly lower. Seligson *et al.* (1994) also found that, in the USA, chocolate was consumed by more people in the winter than at other times of the year. Both these geographical and seasonal trends are probably due to the fact that chocolate softens and eventually melts at higher ambient temperatures.

In the United Kingdom, DEFRA (Department of the Environment, Food and Rural Affairs) publishes annually a report, 'Family Food', which details expenditure on the full range of food groups. The figures for the household purchases of chocolate confectionery are detailed in Table 16.1. Although there are year-to-year variations, these figures are fairly constant at between 82 g/person/week and 90 g/person/week, apart from in 1996/97 when this rose to

Table 16.1   Household purchases of chocolate confectionery in the United Kingdom

Year	Grams per person per week		
	Chocolate confectionery	Solid chocolate	Chocolate coated bars/sweets
1994	83**	26	57
1996–97	97		
1999	89**	26	63
2000–01	112		
2001–02	85		
2002–03	83		
2003–04	86**	27	59
2004–05	90**	30	60
2005–06	82*		
2006	82*		
2007	88*		

* For these years, figures for total confectionery were quoted of 123 g/person/week, 123 g/person/week and 129 g/person/week respectively. These included amounts of mints, boiled sweets and other confectionery. In previous years these had been separately listed and ranged from 37–44 g/person/week with a mean of 40.75 g/person/week. To enable a comparison for chocolate confectionery composition to be made 41 g/person/week was subtracted from the figures quoted in DEFRA (2007)
** For these years chocolate confectionery was divided into solid chocolate and chocolate coated bars and sweets. To enable a comparison for chocolate confectionery to be made these two figures have been added together to give a total chocolate confectionery figure.

Source: DEFRA, 2002, 2003, 2005, 2007

© Woodhead Publishing Limited, 2011

97 g/person/week and in 2000/01 when it reached a peak of 112 g/person/week. Taking a typical level of about 90 g/person/week and scaling this up to a full year gives a total of 4.68 kg/person. This is less than half of that quoted for the UK by CAOBISCO (2009), suggesting that a major proportion of expenditure on chocolate confectionery in the UK is as a result of impulse buying.

How much of a problem, then, is chocolate confectionery in terms of both total fat and saturated consumption? We can gather together information from various (but a limited number of) sources to help answer this. Lambert (2008) gives figures to show that 3% of total calories and 3% of total fat in a UK adult's diet comes from chocolate. This contrasts with only 1% of calories and 1% of total fat from chocolate in a French adult's diet. The UK National Diet and Nutrition Survey (Henderson *et al.*, 2002) also showed that 3% of total fat in a UK adult's diet comes from chocolate confectionery but also that 5% of total saturated fat comes from chocolate confectionery. Chocolate confectionery results in 0.6% of daily energy from saturated fat. The DEFRA Family Food Report for 2007 (DEFRA, 2007) indicates that the percentage of total fat and saturated fat per person per day from household purchases of confectionery has risen to 4% and 6% respectively. As this figure also includes contributions from mints and boiled sweets that are low in fat, the actual contribution from chocolate confectionery could be higher than this. All of this shows that chocolate confectionery falls into a category of moderate concern in terms of saturated fatty acid consumption – one that is worth trying to make changes to. The rest of this chapter will look at the potential to make these changes within technical and legislative limitations.

16.2   Chocolate

Chocolate is a well-defined material in terms of its composition. The legislative constraints will be described in the next section but, suffice to say at this point, from a fat point of view it is made from cocoa butter, milk fat and, in countries that permit them, non-cocoa vegetable fats. All of these components contain significant levels of saturated fatty acids.

Cocoa butter is rich in palmitic, stearic and oleic acids, the ratios of which are dependent upon the geographical origin of the cocoa butter. Typical fatty acid compositions of different origin cocoa butters are shown in Table 16.2. Cocoa butters from Brazil tend to be lower in total saturates than do cocoa butters from West Africa or Malaysia – but that also makes them softer. While cocoa butters from West Africa and Malaysia are similar in terms of total saturates they differ in the ratio of stearic acid (C18:0) to palmitic acid (C16:0), this ratio being higher in Malaysian cocoa butters than in West African cocoa butters.

Milk fat is also rich in saturated fatty acids but, in this case, they cover a much wider range of fatty acid chain lengths and can also include some saturated branched chain acids. Shukla (1994) quotes levels of *unsaturated* fatty acids in milk fat from New Zealand cows that range from about 23% in the summer to about 25% in the winter. He also indicates that the stearic acid content of milk fat in the Northern

© Woodhead Publishing Limited, 2011

Table 16.2   Fatty acid composition of cocoa butter from different origins

Origin	C16:0	C18:0	C18:1	C18:2	C18:3	C20:0	C22:0	Total SAFA
Brazil	25.1	33.3	36.5	3.5	0.2	1.2	0.2	59.8
Ivory Coast	25.8	36.9	32.9	2.8	0.2	1.2	0.2	64.1
Malaysia	24.9	37.4	33.5	2.6	0.2	1.2	0.2	63.7

Source: Lipp and Anklam, 1998

Hemisphere is at its highest in the spring and summer and at its lowest in the winter. In the Southern Hemisphere (Australia and New Zealand) oleic acid reaches a peak during the winter months. Jensen *et al.* (1962) give total saturates in June milk fat of 62.0% and in December milk fat of 63.5%. Variations in cattle feed will also have an effect on the saturated fatty acid content. Since ways of reducing saturates in milk and milk fat are being considered in other chapters this will not be considered further here except to say that reducing the saturates in milk fat will also reduce its hardness and, consequently, the hardness of the chocolate.

Where vegetable fats other than cocoa butter are permitted (see section 16.2.1 for further information on this), they are sometimes restricted to a small number of plant sources. The EU, for example, has defined six vegetable oils that can be used in chocolate (European Union, 2000). Although not all countries that permit the use of vegetable fats in chocolate have this restriction, it is unusual to find fats other than the six permitted in the EU being used in this way. The six oils permitted by the EU are:

- Palm oil   *Elaeis guineensis* and *Elaeis olifera*
- Illipé   *Shorea stenoptera*
- Sal   *Shorea robusta*
- Shea   *Butyrospermum parkii*
- Kokum gurgi   *Garcinia indica*
- Mango kernel   *Mangifera indica.*

All of these oils contain significant levels of SOS (saturated-oleic-saturated) triglycerides with the saturated fatty acids being mainly palmitic and stearic acids (although moderate levels of arachidic acid – C20:0 – are found in sal fat). The main triglycerides found in cocoa butter are also of this type, cocoa butter being typically composed of 18–19% POP, 38–40% POSt and 26–30% StOSt[1] (Chaiseri and Dimick, 1989). Talbot (2006) quotes slightly different levels of 16% POP, 37% POSt and 26% StOSt but it needs to be remembered that there is a natural variability in the triglyceride composition of cocoa butter. These are compared with the triglyceride compositions of the basic vegetable oils used in chocolate in Table 16.3.

It is clear that some of these oils (palm oil, shea butter and mango kernel oil in particular) contain significantly lower levels of total SOS than those found in cocoa butter. The vegetable fats used in chocolate are also known as cocoa butter

---

[1] P = palmitic acid, St = stearic acid, O = oleic acid; POP denotes 1,3-dipalmitoyl – 2-oleoylglycerol, POSt denotes 1-palmitoyl-2-oleoyl-3-stearoylglycerol, StOSt denotes 1,3-distearoyl-2-oleoylglycerol.

© Woodhead Publishing Limited, 2011

Table 16.3   Triglyceride composition of basic vegetable oils permitted in EU chocolate

Triglyceride	Cocoa butter[a]	Palm oil[b]	Illipe butter[b]	Sal oil[c]	Shea butter[a]	Kokum gurgi[a]	Mango kernel oil[a]
POP	16	26	7	5	< 1	< 1	6
POSt	37	3	34	16	6	6	13
StOSt	26	< 1	45	36	30	72	18
Total SOS	79	29	86	67*	36	78	37

* includes 9% StOA and 1% AOA
[a] Talbot (2006); [b] Jurriens (1968); [c] Sridhar and Lakshminarayana (1991)
 P = palmitic acid; St = stearic acid; O = oleic acid; S = total saturated acids

equivalents (CBEs) and, as their name implies, they are equivalent to cocoa butter in both their physical characteristics and chemical composition. To bring the SOS content of oils such as palm, shea and mango kernel up to the level found in cocoa butter it is necessary to fractionate them. This means holding the oils themselves or in solution in an organic solvent such as acetone at a temperature at which they are partially crystalline. The crystals (or stearine fraction) are separated from the liquid (oleine fraction) by filtration. The stearine fraction is generally the fraction that is rich in SOS triglycerides. Palm oil, however, contains a significant proportion of very high-melting, almost fully saturated triglycerides. These do not contribute any functionality to CBEs (indeed they are detrimental in terms of rheological properties) and so these are also removed by fractionation, leaving a mid-fraction as the one to be used in CBEs.

The triglyceride compositions of the fractions generally used in CBEs are shown in comparison to that of cocoa butter in Table 16.4.

Although functionally it is the triglycerides in cocoa butter and CBEs that are of the greatest importance, nutritionally it is the balance of fatty acids that is of greatest importance. The fatty acid compositions of cocoa butter, the six basic vegetable oils and, where these differ, the fractions used in CBEs are shown in Table 16.5.

Table 16.4   Triglyceride compositions of vegetable fats and fractions used in EU chocolate

Triglyceride	Cocoa butter	Palm mid-fraction	Shea stearine	Illipe butter	Sal stearine	Kokum gurgi fat	Mango kernel stearine
POP	16	66	1	7	< 1	< 1	1
POSt	37	12	7	34	10	6	16
StOSt	26	3	74	45	60	72	59
Total SOS	79	81	82	86	81*	78	76

* includes 11% StOA
Source: Talbot, 2006

P = palmitic acid; St = stearic acid; O = oleic acid; S = total saturated acids

© Woodhead Publishing Limited, 2011

Table 16.5 Fatty acid composition of cocoa butter and vegetable oils and fractions permitted in EU chocolate

	Cocoa butter[a]	Palm oil[b]	Palm mid-fraction[c]	Shea oil[d]	Shea stearine[e]	Illipe butter[f]	Sal oil[g]	Sal stearine[c]	Kokum gurgi[f]	Mango kernel oil[h]	Mango kernel stearine
C14:0		1.1	0.8		0.3				1.0		0.2
C16:0	25.8	44.0	56.5	3.3	4.9	19.3	6.3	4.3	4.0	10.0	4.5
C18:0	36.9	4.5	4.1	44.3	57.3	43.5	44.6	48.4	53.0	40.0	58.8
C20:0	1.2	0.4	0.3	1.3	0.4	1.3	5.7	6.9		1.0	3.5
C22:0	0.2										
C18:1	32.9	39.2	34.4	45.6	32.2	35.3	41.6	38.5	40.0	44.0	32.1
C18:2	2.8	10.1	3.7	5.5	3.5	1.0	1.7	1.2	2.0	5.0	0.9
C18:3	0.2	0.4									
Total sats	64.1	50.0	61.7	48.9	62.9	64.1	56.6	59.6	58.0	51.0	67.0

[a] Ivory Coast cocoa butter (Lipp and Anklam, 1998)
[b] Tan and Oh (1981)
[c] Wong Soon (1991)
[d] Sawadogo and Bézard (1982)
[e] Vereecken et al. (2009)
[f] Bracco et al. (1970)
[g] Bhattacharyya and Bhattacharyya (1991)
[h] Sridhar and Lakshminarayana (1991)

© Woodhead Publishing Limited, 2011

It is clear from this that the levels of total saturates in cocoa butter and CBEs are very similar, and not only that, they are also similar to the level of total saturates found by Jensen *et al.* (1962) in milk fat. This means that there is no scope for reducing saturates in chocolate by changing the balance between the individual fat components. Any reduction that can be achieved must be made by modifying the components themselves. However, this must be done within the scope of national legislation.

16.2.1   Legislative constraints

Chocolate is subject to quite restrictive legislation. In the European Union it is defined by Directive 2000/36/EC (European Union, 2000). In the United States, it is covered by the Code of Federal Regulations (CFR). Title 21 of the CFR is concerned with Food and Drugs; Part 163 of this title defines the composition of cocoa and chocolate products. Outside of these two regions there are many individual national regulations. However, the Codex Alimentarius Commission of Codex was set up in the 1960s by the World Health Organisation and the UN Food and Agriculture Organisation to define world-wide standards for different foodstuffs. Standard STAN 87-1981, Rev. 1-2003 is the standard for cocoa and chocolate products.

These three standards differ in a number of ways, some of which will affect the ability of a chocolate manufacturer to reduce the level of saturates in chocolate while still staying within the definition of chocolate. The United States standard, for example, does not permit the use of vegetable fats other than cocoa butter so any changes that may be made can only be done by means of changes to the cocoa butter or milk fat. Both the EU and Codex standards allow the use of vegetable fats other than cocoa butter but differ in that the EU defines six base oils that can be used (see the previous section) while there is no restriction on the type of oil that can be used in the Codex standard. In both cases, however, the vegetable fat component is restricted to a maximum level of 5% of the chocolate.

Further restrictions in the EU legislation can also affect the level of vegetable fat that can be used and the absolute reduction in saturates that can be achieved. The EU legislation defines 'noble ingredients'. These are the cocoa, milk and sugar components. Vegetable fat is not classed as a 'noble ingredient'. The minimum total fat content in EU chocolate is 25% (23.5% for white chocolate). However, the vegetable fat does not count towards this; instead, there must be at least 25% fat from cocoa and milk (i.e. cocoa butter and milk fat). Only when this has been achieved can any vegetable fat be added. Therefore, for the full 5% of vegetable fat to be used the chocolate must contain at least 30% total fat. Plain chocolate can be made solely from cocoa butter or cocoa butter and vegetable fat (providing there is at least 25% cocoa butter present). The EU defines two types of milk chocolate – the so-called '14/25' milk chocolate and '20/20' milk chocolate. These numbers define the minimum levels of dry milk solids and dry cocoa solids respectively. Since full cream milk powders contain about 25% milk fat a chocolate made from 14% dry milk solids will contain 3.5% milk fat and one made from 20% dry milk solids will contain 5% milk fat. These are the minimum levels of milk fat defined in the EU legislation for the two types of milk chocolate.

© Woodhead Publishing Limited, 2011

Table 16.6   Base chocolate compositions (total fat 30%)

Component	Dark (%)	Milk (%)	Milk+CBE (%)
Cocoa mass (West African)	40.0	15.0	15.0
Cocoa butter (West African)	8.0	16.75	11.75
Sugar	51.6	47.85	47.85
Skimmed milk powder		15.0	15.0
Milk fat		5.0	5.0
CBE (vegetable fat)			5.0
Lecithin	0.4	0.4	0.4
% cocoa butter (fat phase)	100.0	83.3	66.6
% milk fat (fat phase)		16.7	16.7
% vegetable fat (fat phase)			16.7
Saturates from cocoa butter	64.0	53.3	42.6
Saturates from milk fat		10.7	10.7
Saturates from CBE			10.7
Total saturates (fat phase)	64.0	64.0	64.0
Total saturates (chocolate)	19.2	19.2	19.2

For the purposes of defining the reduction that can be made in the level of saturates in chocolate, three example chocolate recipes have been defined. These all contain a total fat content of 30% (to allow for the use of the full 5% vegetable fat) and are divided into a plain (dark) chocolate, a milk chocolate without CBE and one with CBE. The milk chocolates conform to both types of milk chocolate compositional legislation, i.e. the total dry cocoa solids is greater than 25% and the total dry milk solids is equal to 20%. Compositions that can be considered to be the starting point are shown in Table 16.6. In calculating the saturates contents it has been assumed that all three components contain 64% total saturates. In other words, each of the three base chocolates contains 64% saturates in the fat phase. As each chocolate contains 30% total fat, the level of saturates in each chocolate is 19.2%. The challenge, then, is what level of reduction can be achieved from this while staying within the legislation and what will be the effects of making these reductions. For the purposes of calculation the chocolate compositions considered will be limited by the EU Chocolate Directive. Use of the Codex standard may, under some circumstances, allow a greater reduction because some of the restrictions on the use of vegetable fat are not present. Use of the United States legislation would mean that none of the proposals that make use of changes to the vegetable fat part of the chocolate would be permitted.

16.2.2   Scope for and effects of reducing saturated fat in chocolate

In theory, there are four ways in which the level of saturates in chocolate can be reduced while staying within the scope of the EU Chocolate Directive:

- reduce total fat
- use a different type of cocoa butter

© Woodhead Publishing Limited, 2011

- use a softer (oleine) fraction of cocoa butter
- use a more unsaturated vegetable fat.

The Directive states that milk components in chocolate must be present in the ratios found in whole milk. This would suggest that any possibility of using a more unsaturated fraction of milk (i.e. milk fat oleine) would not be permitted.

Reduce total fat

Each of the basic chocolate compositions in Table 16.6 contains 30% total fat. The EU Directive, however, defines a minimum total fat content of 25%, giving some scope for reduction in total fat and, if the fat types do not change, then in saturated fat. The constraint that there shall be a minimum of 25% fat from 'noble ingredients' means that the composition containing CBE would no longer be legal. Therefore, the only two alternatives would be those shown in Table 16.7. Making such a change would result in a 16.7% reduction in saturates compared with the 30% fat product. On the face of it, this seems such a simple change to make that it might be questioned why the whole chocolate industry has not already made the change. The answer is that reducing the fat content of chocolate produces other changes which affect both processing and the sensory characteristics of chocolate. Kähkönen and Tuorila (1999) studied the consumer response to reduced and regular fat contents in a range of food products. They found that consumers rated 'pleasantness' higher in chocolate bars with a 'regular' level of fat compared with reduced-fat chocolate bars.

From a processing point of view, the main problem with reducing the fat content of chocolate is that such changes have a marked effect on the flow properties of chocolate. This is summarised in Fig. 16.2 (Wells, 2009), which demonstrates in the right-most line the relationship between the fat content of milk chocolate and its viscosity. As the fat content is reduced below 30% the viscosity of the chocolate increases exponentially. This can be reduced to some extent by changing the type

Table 16.7 Effect of reducing total fat from 30% to 25%

Composition	Dark (%)	Milk (%)
Cocoa mass	40.0	15.0
Cocoa butter	3.0	11.75
Sugar	56.6	52.85
Skimmed milk powder		15.0
Milk fat		5.0
Lecithin	0.4	0.4
% cocoa butter (fat phase)	100.0	80.0
% milk fat (fat phase)		20.0
Saturates from cocoa butter	64.0	51.2
Saturates from milk fat		12.8
Total saturates (fat phase)	64.0	64.0
Total saturates (chocolate)	16.0	16.0
% Reduction in saturates	16.7	16.7

© Woodhead Publishing Limited, 2011

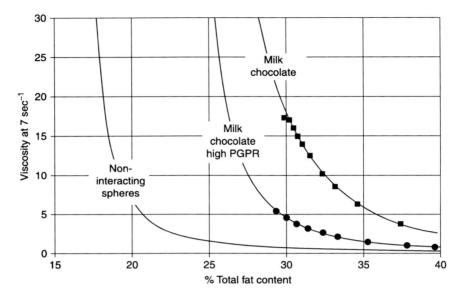

Fig. 16.2   Chocolate viscosity versus fat content (reproduced from Wells, 2009).

of emulsifier used in chocolate from one that is basically lecithin to an emulsifier cocktail in which polyglycerol polyricinoleate (PGPR) predominates. Even then, the increase in viscosity is such that 26 to 27% total fat would appear to be the minimum level to still be able to obtain 'workable' chocolate.

If it were possible to control and construct the shapes and sizes of the non-fat particles in chocolate such that they were non-interacting spheres, then it should, theoretically, be possible to reduce the total fat content to the minimum of 25% permitted in the EU Chocolate Directive without a substantial increase in viscosity. This, though, is a highly speculative procedure. Many of the patented procedures for producing low-fat chocolate and low-fat confectionery involve the use of water-in-oil emulsions (Rey *et al.*, 2007) or co-suspensions of the electrostatically charged particles (Rousset *et al.*, 2007).

Use a different type of cocoa butter
Table 16.2 showed that cocoa butters from different origins have different fatty acid distributions and different levels of total saturates. Cocoa butter from Ivory Coast, for example, contains about 64% saturates; cocoa butter from Brazil contains about 60% saturates. If we assume that West African (Ivory Coast-type) cocoa butter is used in the standard recipes shown in Table 16.6, then the levels of reduction in saturates that could be achieved by changing to a softer cocoa butter would range from 6.3% in dark chocolate to 4.2% in a milk chocolate containing CBE (Table 16.8). Although small, this would be a reduction worth having and would not contravene any EU Chocolate Directive (or, indeed, any other national chocolate regulations). There are two problems in going along this route. The first

Table 16.8   Use of softer cocoa butter and cocoa mass

Component	Dark (%)	Milk (%)	Milk+CBE (%)
Cocoa mass	40.0	15.0	15.0
Cocoa butter	8.0	16.75	11.75
Sugar	51.6	47.85	47.85
Skimmed milk powder		15.0	15.0
Milk fat		5.0	5.0
CBE (vegetable fat)			5.0
Lecithin	0.4	0.4	0.4
% cocoa butter (fat phase)	100.0	83.3	66.6
% milk fat (fat phase)		16.7	16.7
% vegetable fat (fat phase)			16.7
Saturates from cocoa butter	60.0	50.0	40.0
Saturates from milk fat		10.7	10.7
Saturates from CBE			10.7
Total saturates (fat phase)	60.0	60.7	61.4
Total saturates (chocolate)	18.0	18.2	18.4
% reduction in saturates	6.3	5.2	4.2

is that cocoas from different origins have different flavour profiles. This is a property that is being made a positive characteristic of some chocolates that are marketed as containing cocoa from a specific origin. Moving from a West African to a different origin cocoa butter could change the flavour profile of the chocolate – not making it worse, just making it different.

A potentially greater problem is that because such cocoa butters can contain lower levels of saturates they obviously also contain higher levels of unsaturates. This makes them softer than West African cocoa butters. Again, this is not an issue if a chocolate is designed originally to be based on such cocoa butters, but if a switch is suddenly made to a more unsaturated cocoa butter then consumers would notice a change and manufacturers would have to make some other changes to the product to redress this softening. The most obvious change to make would be to reduce the level of the softest component in chocolate, milk fat. It has been calculated (Talbot, 2009a) that the solid fat content of chocolate based on a fat phase of 83.3% West African cocoa butter and 16.7% milk fat is:

N20 63.5%
N25 53.1%
N30 23.2%

In order to get a close match to that melting profile using a softer, less saturated cocoa butter it would be necessary to reduce the level of milk fat in the fat phase from 16.7% down to 3.0%. Then the melting profile of the chocolate fat phase would be:

N20 62.6%
N25 53.3%
N30 25.1%

© Woodhead Publishing Limited, 2011

If the solid fat content at 30°C was considered to be of greatest importance then the reduction in milk fat could be less than this; if, though, the solid fat content at 20°C was considered to be more important then the reduction in milk fat may have to be even greater. Either way, the change is likely to move the level of milk fat in the chocolate from one conforming to a milk chocolate description to a composition that no longer conforms to this.

Use a softer fraction of cocoa butter
Just as palm oil and shea butter, for example, can be fractionated for use in CBEs so cocoa butter itself can also be fractionated in a similar way to separate a softer, more unsaturated fraction from a harder, more saturated fraction. This process has been described by Weyland (1992) as a means of producing a harder 'cocoa butter' for use in heat-resistant chocolate and a softer 'cocoa butter' for use in ice cream coatings. It could, however, also be a way of reducing saturates in chocolate because, although the difference in saturates between a full cocoa butter and its oleine fraction is not large, it could be enough to give a measurable reduction in saturates in the chocolate. Typically, cocoa butter oleine contains about 59% total saturates.

Cocoa butter oleine could be used in the standard recipes in Table 16.6 in two ways – either as a direct replacement of the added cocoa butter or, at a higher level, as a replacement of most of the cocoa butter in the cocoa mass, meaning that the non-fat cocoa solids in the recipe would need to come from added low-fat cocoa powder. Since cocoa butter oleine, because of the fractionation process it has undergone, needs to be fully refined and deodorised before use, these changes would certainly result in changes to the flavour profile of the chocolate, but these would be greater if the cocoa butter oleine replaced almost all of the original cocoa butter. This is not the only issue that relates to this option. Secondly, the cost of the oleine needs to be considered. Cocoa butter is already an expensive starting material. Fractionating it adds further costs. There is also the issue of what to do with the stearine fraction (potentially the most functional of the two fractions but also higher in saturates).

As with using a less saturated cocoa butter, the use of cocoa butter oleine will soften the chocolate and so the level of milk fat will need to be reduced to compensate for this. Talbot (2009a) calculated that not only would the level of milk fat need to be reduced to zero but, even then, not all of the cocoa butter could be replaced by cocoa butter oleine in order to match the melting profile of the standard milk chocolate (Table 16.9). Making such a change would (a) mean a change away from a milk chocolate declaration, (b) use more expensive components, (c) change the flavour profile of the chocolate, reducing the cocoa 'impact', and (d) reduce saturates by only 3.6%. This is also an option where it is imperative to check national chocolate regulations to ensure that cocoa butter oleine is considered to be cocoa butter and is not classed as part of the vegetable fat in the chocolate.

Use a more unsaturated vegetable fat
Apart from refining, the only process permitted by the EU Chocolate Directive with regard to the vegetable fat component is fractionation. Although the mid-

© Woodhead Publishing Limited, 2011

Table 16.9   Chocolates containing cocoa butter oleine (total fat 30%)

Component	Standard milk recipe (%)	Cocoa butter oleine recipe (%)
Cocoa mass	15.0	15.0
Cocoa butter	16.75	8.25
Cocoa butter oleine		13.5
Sugar	47.85	47.85
Skimmed milk powder	15.0	15.0
Milk fat	5.0	
CBE (vegetable fat)		
Lecithin	0.4	0.4
% cocoa butter (fat phase)	83.3	55.0
% cocoa butter oleine (fat phase)		45.0
% milk fat (fat phase)	16.7	
% vegetable fat (fat phase)		
Saturates from cocoa butter	53.3	35.2
Saturates from cocoa butter oleine		26.6
Saturates from milk fat	10.7	
Saturates from CBE		
Total saturates (fat phase)	64.0	61.8
Total saturates (chocolate)	19.2	18.5
% reduction in saturates		3.6
N20 of fat phase	63.5	63.6
N25 of fat phase	53.1	53.0
N30 of fat phase	23.2	20.0

fraction from palm oil usually forms the basis of many CBEs, the regulations would, in theory, permit the use of palm oleine, which contains a significantly lower level of saturates (43%) than does a conventional CBE (64%). It is worth mentioning, though, that the EU Directive also states that any vegetable fat used must be compatible and miscible with cocoa butter *at any level of use*, not just the maximum 5% permitted by the Directive. Depending on how compatibility and miscibility are defined, the use of only palm oleine as the vegetable fat component may be permitted – or not. This is another area where good legal advice would be necessary before considering such a change. From a purely technical point of view, though, it would be possible to make the changes shown in Table 16.10.

Making such a direct substitution would result in a reduction in saturates of 5.2%. It would, however, as with most of the other possible ways of reducing saturates, give a softer chocolate. In order to balance the melting profiles of a chocolate containing palm oleine as the vegetable fat with those of the standard milk chocolate it would be necessary to reduce the level of milk fat to 2% of the fat phase (see the right-most column of Table 16.10). This would still give a reduction in saturates of 5.2% but would no longer permit a milk chocolate declaration.

All of these possibilities have some drawback associated with them. Those that involve replacing part of the cocoa butter or CBE with a softer more unsaturated fat will result in softer chocolates or in chocolates that can no longer be labelled

© Woodhead Publishing Limited, 2011

Table 16.10 Use of palm oleine as the 'CBE' (total fat 30%)

Component	Milk chocolate Traditional CBE (%)	Milk chocolate Palm oleine (%)	Optimised chocolate Palm oleine (%)
Cocoa mass	15.0	15.0	15.0
Cocoa butter	11.75	11.75	16.15
Sugar	47.85	47.85	47.85
Skimmed milk powder	15.0	15.0	15.0
Milk fat	5.0	5.0	0.6
Traditional CBE	5.0		
Palm oleine		5.0	5.0
Lecithin	0.4	0.4	0.4
% cocoa butter (fat phase)	66.6	66.6	81.3
% milk fat (fat phase)	16.7	16.7	2.0
% vegetable fat (fat phase)	16.7	16.7	16.7
Saturates from cocoa butter	42.6	42.6	52.0
Saturates from milk fat	10.7	10.7	1.3
Saturates from CBE	10.7	7.2	7.2
Total saturates (fat phase)	64.0	60.5	60.5
Total saturates (chocolate)	19.2	18.2	18.2
% reduction in saturates		5.2	5.2
N20 of fat phase	63.5		62.2
N25 of fat phase	52.3		52.5
N30 of fat phase	20.7		23.3

'milk chocolate'. Reducing the total fat content may be the most feasible option but even this will involve a potential change in emulsifier in order to maintain the flow properties of the chocolate.

16.2.3   Stearic acid effects

Table 16.2 shows that the main saturated fatty acid in cocoa butter is stearic acid (well over 50% of the total saturates) with most of the rest being made up of palmitic acid. Various clinical nutrition studies have shown that stearic acid behaves differently from shorter chain-length saturates in terms of its effects on blood cholesterol levels. Mensink *et al.* (2003), in a meta-analysis of 60 controlled trials, found that, when used as a replacement for carbohydrate in a diet, stearic acid lowered total cholesterol and LDL cholesterol to greater extents than did shorter chain-length saturates. Grundy (1994) also reviews much of the literature on the effects of different fatty acids on blood lipids and concludes that 'stearic acid is essentially neutral in its effects on lipoproteins'. He suggests that this is because stearic acid is quickly converted in the body into oleic acid, only requiring desaturation at the omega-9 position of the chain. Palmitic acid, though, needs a chain elongation followed by desaturation in order to be metabolised into oleic acid, a process which is much slower.

However, Hoak (1994) describes how stearic acid is the most thrombogenic of all the saturated fatty acids. There is, though, contradicting evidence for this.

© Woodhead Publishing Limited, 2011

Tholstrup *et al.* (2003) describe the effects of stearic acid and other fatty acids on factor VIIa, an activated blood coagulant factor. They conclude that there is a lesser increase in factor VIIa after the consumption of saturated fats, especially stearic acid, than after consuming unsaturated fatty acids. On the other hand, a diet rich in stearic acid increased fibrinogen (another blood clotting factor) compared with a diet rich in myristic and lauric acids (Bladbjerg *et al.*, 1995). Baer *et al.* (2004) also found that consumption of about 38 g/day of stearic acid increased fibrinogen whereas consumption of 24 g/day had no effect. If we assume that cocoa butter contains 33% stearic acid and that chocolate contains 30% cocoa butter then the effect level would equate to consumption of 380 g of chocolate/day. However, since we also consume stearic acid from other sources in our diet then the point at which an effect may be seen will be at a lower chocolate consumption level than this.

A considerable amount of work has been published on the effects of stearic acid from cocoa butter and shea butter (one of the base oils permitted for use in cocoa butter equivalents) on blood lipids, factor VII and fibrinogen (Sanders *et al.*, 2001; Sanders and Berry, 2005; Berry and Sanders, 2005). Conclusions from much of this work were that stearic acid in cocoa butter resulted in similar postprandial lipemia and factor VII activation as did a meal containing high-oleic sunflower oil. Stearic acid from shea butter (which contains a higher level of stearic as a percentage of total saturates) decreased postprandial lipemia and activation of factor VII. As a result of this work Sanders (2009) concluded that 'chocolate confectionery fats do not have an adverse effect on the lipid profile' and 'are potentially less thrombogenic than high monounsaturated oils such as olive oil and high oleic sunflower oil'.

16.2.4   Other health benefits of chocolate
Although not specifically linked to the fat content of chocolate, other health benefits can be derived from the cocoa part of chocolate. These are particularly associated with the flavanols that are found in cocoa. These are antioxidants, similar to those found in red wine and green tea, that have positive effects on the cardiovascular system and also strengthen the immune system in case of oxidative stress (Yates, 2009). There is also evidence that they protect against the damaging effects that free radicals have on body cells. Chocolate, particularly dark chocolate, that is high in cocoa content contains the highest levels of flavanols although some chocolate manufacturers have also developed processes that retain these flavanols at higher levels during the processing (particularly during cocoa bean fermentation) of the chocolate (Yates, 2009).

16.3   Compound coatings

Not all confectionery or bakery products are coated in chocolate as defined by various national and international regulations. Some are covered in compound coatings. These are coatings which often look and taste like chocolate (although

© Woodhead Publishing Limited, 2011

white and pastel-coloured versions are also used) but whose compositions do not conform to chocolate regulations. They are generally based on one of three types of fat:

- Cocoa butter equivalents (CBEs) as described in section 16.2 but used at a much higher level than the 5% normally permitted in chocolate. Because they are chemically and physically similar to cocoa butter they are able to replace the whole of the added cocoa butter in Table 16.6 for example. When this occurs the resulting product can no longer be called 'chocolate' but is given the name 'supercoating'.
- Non-lauric cocoa butter replacers (CBRs). Historically these have been based on partially hydrogenated and fractionated oils such as palm, cottonseed, soyabean and rapeseed. More recently, non-hydrogenated alternatives based on palm fractions have been developed. These types of fat have a limited compatibility with cocoa butter, which means that some cocoa mass can be used in the recipe.
- Lauric cocoa butter substitutes (CBSs). These are based on oils rich in lauric (C12:0) acid. The most common of these are palm kernel oil and coconut oil and, indeed, most lauric CBS products are based on palm kernel oil. The processes used to generate the coating fats from palm kernel oil itself are hydrogenation and fractionation either together or singly. Coatings based on palm kernel oil (without fractionation or hydrogenation) are too soft for use on ambient products but are used on some coated ice cream products.

More detailed information on the fats used in compound coatings and the recipes and limitations of these are given by Talbot (2009b).

16.3.1   Effect of removing *trans* fats

In recent years there has been a move to replace partially hydrogenated vegetable oils which contain *trans* fatty acids by non-hydrogenated, *trans*-free alternatives. This is because *trans* fatty acids have been shown to have adverse effects on blood cholesterol (Mensink *et al.*, 2003) by increasing LDL cholesterol levels and lowering HDL cholesterol levels. These effects combine to increase the risk of cardiovascular disease. Some countries such as Denmark have put legislation in place to limit the amount of any artificially produced *trans* fatty acid in oils and fats to a maximum of 2%. The United States introduced in 2006 mandatory labelling of *trans* contents of more than 0.5 g per serving. The United Kingdom has not introduced either such restrictions or such labelling because the UK Food Standards Agency considers the current intake of *trans* fatty acids to be below the maximum recommended level of 2% of dietary energy. However, many retailers in the UK have prohibited the use of partially hydrogenated vegetable oils in their own-brand products.

Of the three types of compound coating fat, two have historically been hydrogenated. CBEs have never been hydrogenated as this would destroy their excellent compatibility and chemical and physical similarities with cocoa butter.

© Woodhead Publishing Limited, 2011

Lauric CBSs can be produced in a number of ways from palm kernel oil. The oil can be fractionated to give palm kernel stearine (PKS), which is a non-hydrogenated oil. It can also be hydrogenated to give hydrogenated palm kernel oil (HPKO) and the stearine, PKS, can also be hydrogenated after fractionation to give hydrogenated palm kernel stearine (HPKS). Each of these processes results in different levels of saturated and *trans* fatty acids in the end product. Typical fatty acid compositions of each of these types of fat are shown in Table 16.11.

Fractionation increases the saturated fatty acid content of the palm kernel oil from about 83% to about 87% in PKS. When PKS is then hydrogenated it is normally fully hydrogenated, i.e. beyond the stage at which any *trans* fatty acids remain. This means that HPKS contains a very high level of saturates, typically 99% or greater – but minimal *trans*. It does, though, still need to be labelled 'hydrogenated' despite the *trans* level being virtually zero. Hydrogenation of palm kernel oil gives different levels of *trans* and saturates depending on the degree to which the oil has been hydrogenated. Partial hydrogenation of the oil to a melting point of about 35°C results in about 5% *trans* fatty acid being formed while the saturates also increase by some 10% compared with the original palm kernel oil. Hydrogenation to a melting point of about 41°C is effectively a 'full' hydrogenation, which again means minimal *trans* remains and the saturates level is greater than 99%. Such a high melting point is above body temperature and so coatings made from HPKO41 will taste waxy. HPKO35, however, can be used to produce a compound coating that melts well in the mouth – but contains 5% *trans* fatty acid.

Because palm kernel oil itself is fairly limited in the level of unsaturated fatty acid it contains, when it is hydrogenated the amounts of *trans* fatty acids that are produced are relatively low (e.g. 5% *trans* in HPKO35). Nevertheless, even this low level combined with the necessity to still have to label the product 'hydrogenated' has meant that many users have moved to either non-hydrogenated versions or fully hydrogenated versions of lauric CBSs. Non-hydrogenated PKS

Table 16.11   Fatty acid compositions (%) of lauric CBS compound coating fats

Fatty acid	PKO	PKS	HPKS	HPKO35[a]	HPKO41[a]
C8:0	3.4	2.0	2.2	3.3	3.3
C10:0	3.4	2.9	3.2	3.4	3.4
C12:0	50.2	55.0	55.2	50.1	50.3
C14:0	15.9	20.9	20.6	16.0	15.7
C16:0	7.9	7.8	8.1	8.0	7.8
C18:0	2.2	2.1	9.6	12.0	18.7
C18:1 *cis*	14.5	7.8	1.1	2.0	0.7
C18:1 *trans*				5.0	
C18:2	2.1	0.5	0.0	0.0	0.0
Total saturates	83.0	86.7	98.9	92.8	99.2

[a] the number after HPKO (i.e. 35 and 41) denotes the slip melting point of the fat

Source: Hargreaves, 1988

© Woodhead Publishing Limited, 2011

contains about 87% saturates; fully hydrogenated HPKS contains about 99% saturates. Both then are rich in saturates and, predominantly, in lauric acid.

Non-lauric CBRs have historically been produced by first partially hydrogenating liquid oils such as soyabean oil, rapeseed oil, palm oil, cottonseed oil or blends of these to give a product with a high level of solid fat at 20°C. This has often also resulted in relatively high levels of solid fat at mouth temperature and above and so the material has been fractionated to remove much of the high-melting material and give a final product with a melting profile similar to that of cocoa butter. In fatty acid terms the end result was a fat containing, typically, 34% saturates but 53% *trans* fatty acids (Slager *et al.*, 2007). The health and consumer issues surrounding the use of *trans* fatty acids prompted many oils and fats processors to develop lower-*trans* versions of non-lauric CBRs and a number of products containing between 8% and 15% were launched. The drawback of these, however, was that they were still partially hydrogenated and still contained *trans* fatty acids.

In 2007, however, Loders Croklaan developed and launched the first non-lauric CBR that was also non-hydrogenated, Couva™ 850 NH. This was based on a blend of two main triglycerides, POP and PPO. By mixing these together a 1:1 compound is formed that has a stable polymorphic form and does not require tempering in the same way as cocoa butter does. The fat contains about 65% saturates and less than 1% *trans* (Slager *et al.*, 2007). The consequence, therefore, of moving from the partially hydrogenated traditional non-lauric CBRs to the new generation of non-hydrogenated non-lauric CBRs is that, while the *trans* level is reduced to virtually zero, the level of saturates doubles.

16.3.2   Scope for reductions in saturated fat in compound coatings

The question then arises: in terms of saturated fat content, which is the best confectionery coating system to use? This is not as simplistic a question as it sounds because saturated fat is not the whole story in making such a decision. There are manufacturing constraints to consider; there are consumer requirements to consider; there are sensory characteristics to consider. Table 16.12 summarises the level of saturates and *trans* in the main types of confectionery coating fat and also defines some of the advantages and disadvantages of using these.

The scope for reduction often depends on the starting point. If a manufacturer is already using cocoa butter (with or without CBE) to produce a 'real' chocolate then the scope for reducing saturates is very limited, especially if a 'chocolate' declaration is required. The only option (and this would result in many disadvantages, not least losing the 'chocolate' declaration) would be to switch to a traditional, hydrogenated, non-lauric CBR. This, however, while containing half the level of saturates of cocoa butter, would introduce more than 50% *trans* fatty acids into the product and would not, then, be seen as a nutritionally beneficial change to make.

If, however, a manufacturer is starting from, say, HPKO35, then the options for improvement are much greater both in terms of reducing saturates and in terms of improving the product in general. Moving from HPKO35 to PKS would allow a

© Woodhead Publishing Limited, 2011

Table 16.12 Comparison of confectionery coating fats

	Cocoa butter	CBE	Hydrog. non-lauric CBR	Non-hydrog. non-lauric CBR	PKS	HPKS	HPKO35
Saturates	64%	64%	34%	65%	87%	99%	93%
Trans	< 1%	< 1%	53%	< 1%	< 1%	< 1%	5%
Advantages	Can be labelled 'chocolate'. Good sensory properties. Good chocolate flavour.	Used at 5% in 'chocolate'. Used at higher levels in supercoatings. Fully compatible with cocoa butter. Good sensory and flavour properties.	Non-temper. Easy to use without complex processing equipment. Useful in bakeries where a soft, malleable coating is needed. Good flavour stability.	Non-hydrogenated. Non-temper. Easy to use without complex processing equipment. Useful in bakeries where a soft, malleable coating is needed. Good flavour stability.	Non-hydrogenated. Non-temper. Easy to use without complex processing equipment. Hardness and meltdown similar to that of chocolate.	Non-temper. Easy to use without complex processing equipment. Hardness and meltdown similar to that of chocolate.	Non-temper. Easy to use without complex processing equipment.
Disadvantages	Needs tempering.	Needs tempering. Supercoatings cannot be labelled 'chocolate'.	Hydrogenated. Cannot be labelled 'chocolate'. Limited compatibility with cocoa butter. Hardness and melting profile different from chocolate. Chocolate flavour not as intense as 'real' chocolate. Post-harden on storage giving inferior flavour release.	Cannot be labelled 'chocolate'. Limited compatibility with cocoa butter. Hardness and melting profile different from chocolate. Chocolate flavour not as intense as 'real' chocolate.	Cannot be labelled 'chocolate'. Incompatible with cocoa butter. Chocolate flavour limited by this incompatibility. Risks of soapy off-flavours and bloom.	Hydrogenated. Cannot be labelled 'chocolate'. Incompatible with cocoa butter. Chocolate flavour limited by this incompatibility. Risks of soapy off-flavours and bloom.	Hydrogenated. Cannot be labelled 'chocolate'. Incompatible with cocoa butter. Chocolate flavour limited by this incompatibility. Risks of soapy off-flavours and bloom.

© Woodhead Publishing Limited, 2011

small reduction in saturates from about 93% to 87% (probably not enough to make a significant difference) but would give a product with better sensory properties and would remove the 'hydrogenated' label. Staying within the lauric CBS group, moving from HPKO35 to HPKS would give a much better product in sensory terms but would increase the saturates from 93% to 99% and still need a 'hydrogenated' label.

To move away from the lauric CBS group of products totally to either a non-hydrogenated, non-lauric CBR, or to a CBE, or to cocoa butter itself would give a much greater reduction in saturates from about 93% in HPKO35 down to 64–65% in the other options. There would, however, be other implications. If the manufacturer is using HPKO35, for example, for ease of processing (no tempering, quick crystallisation) then some compromises would need to be made in moving away from this to one of the non-lauric options. Moving to a non-hydrogenated, non-lauric CBR would retain the ease of processing in terms of not having to temper but the speed of crystallisation would be reduced. This would mean that either a longer cooling tunnel for the products would be necessary or the existing cooling tunnel would need to be slowed down, resulting in a lower throughput. It is also likely that the texture (hardness, meltdown) of the coating would be different, although the flavour profile could be improved by the inclusion of cocoa mass, a component that would not be possible with the original HPKO35 coating fat.

The other options of moving to either cocoa butter or to a CBE (in combination with cocoa butter in chocolate or as a supercoating) would both require investment in tempering equipment. The costs of the fats would also be significantly higher than HPKO35, making this a more expensive option overall but one that would give a much improved product in the end, particularly in both sensory (flavour) terms and labelling.

16.3.3   Potential for novel compound coating compositions

In defining a suitable fat for a coating composition, be this chocolate or a compound coating, the melting profile is of paramount importance. For example, the non-lauric CBRs referred to above could be replaced by palm oil, or even by rapeseed oil in the same recipe to give greater reductions in saturated fat, but the 'coatings' produced would be liquid and would not crystallise and harden as confectionery coatings should. This would make them impossible to wrap and impossible for a consumer to hold without getting the coating on hands, clothing, etc. Is there scope, then, for producing novel compound coating compositions that have saturates levels even lower than those shown in Table 16.12?

To answer this we need to appreciate the link between fatty acid chain length and melting point and between the level of unsaturation and melting point. Taking the group of fatty acids normally found in food, for every two carbon atom increase in chain length the melting point increases and for every unsaturated double bond in the chain the melting point decreases (Table 16.13). The only exception to this is that the inclusion of a *trans* double bond increases the melting point relative to the corresponding *cis* double bond. When three fatty acids are

© Woodhead Publishing Limited, 2011

Table 16.13   Effect of chain length and unsaturation on fatty acid melting point

Fatty acid	Chain length	No. of double bonds	Melting point (°C)
Capric	10	0	31.6
Lauric	12	0	44.8
Myristic	14	0	54.4
Palmitic	16	0	62.9
Stearic	18	0	70.1
Arachidic	20	0	76.1
Oleic	18	1 – *cis*	16.0
Elaidic	18	1 – *trans*	44.0
Linoleic	18	2 – *cis*	−6.5
Linolenic	18	3 – *cis*	−12.8

Source: Talbot, 2006

combined together in a triglyceride molecule then the triglyceride takes on many of the melting characteristics of the individual fatty acids. This is the key to a potentially even greater reduction in saturates in compound coatings than has been seen previously.

If we start with HPKS, for example, this is a mix of triglycerides in which there is effectively no unsaturation and the fatty acids are predominantly lauric and myristic acids. The fat itself melts at around 35–36°C and is very high in solid fat at ambient temperatures, making it useful as a confectionery coating fat. If one of the saturated lauric and myristic acids on the triglyceride molecules in HPKS were replaced by an unsaturated oleic acid group then the overall melting profile would decrease and the fat would no longer be useful as a coating fat. If, however, as well as introducing this oleic acid group into the triglyceride molecule we were to increase the chain length of the saturates from 12–14 to 16–18 (i.e. from lauric and myristic to palmitic and stearic acids) then we would go from a triglyceride rich in LLL, LLM, MML, MMM to one rich in POP, POSt, StOSt.[2] This is cocoa butter and this also has the required physical characteristics for a coating fat but with a reduction in saturates of about 33% compared with the starting HPKS.

Taking this to the next logical step would be to add another oleic acid group to the triglyceride molecule and, at the same time, add another four carbon atoms to the saturated fatty acid. This would then give two oleic acid groups and one saturated fatty acid with a chain length of 20 or 22 carbon atoms. Would this also be a suitable confectionery coating fat? As far as the author is aware, such a fat has never been launched for this type of application. A product, BOB,[3] that contains two behenic acid (C22:0) groups and one oleic acid group was launched some years ago by Fuji Oil as a means of seeding the crystallisation of cocoa butter triglycerides in chocolate without the need for a full, formal tempering process. It was also used as an anti-bloom fat because, if chocolate melted, BOB would then

---

[2] L = lauric; M = myristic, P = palmitic, St = stearic, O = oleic.
[3] BOB = 1,3-dibehenyl-2-oleoylglycerol.

© Woodhead Publishing Limited, 2011

seed the crystallisation back into a stable crystal form as the chocolate cooled and resolidified without the formation of fat bloom (Koyano *et al.*, 1990). BOB, though, on its own is too high melting to form the basis of a new compound coating. The theory of increasing saturated fatty acid chain length at the same time as increasing the degree of unsaturation would require BOO[4] as the triglyceride system to examine. The preparation and properties of structured triglycerides containing behenic acid have been reported by Tanek and Ledochowska (2005). Behenic acid is most easily obtained by complete hydrogenation of high-erucic acid rapeseed oil. This was the original variety of rapeseed oil to be used. Erucic acid has 22 carbon atoms and one double bond and its use is restricted in foods because of concerns over its effects on heart health (Food Standards Australia New Zealand, 2003). Behenic acid is the saturated counterpart of erucic acid, i.e. 22 carbon atoms and no double bonds.

Tanek and Ledochowska (2005) interesterified olive oil (rich in oleic acid) with hydrogenated high erucic rapeseed oil (rich in behenic acid) and also carried out an acidolysis reaction between olive oil and behenic acid. The resulting fatty acid compositions are shown in Table 16.14. The acidolysis reaction gave the lower saturated fatty acid level in total and the resulting fat had a melting point of 37.5°C, suggesting its suitability for use in a compound coating. However, the solid fat content at 20°C was only about 30%, making it too soft for this use. Nevertheless, there may be some scope for improving these characteristics by blending with more 'mainstream' confectionery fat components such as those used in CBEs. This is presented here only as the theoretical basis of an idea. It would need much more research and development work to bring it to a commercial solution. This would need to (a) produce the appropriate melting profile for a compound coating, (b) answer questions about the heart-health implications (if

Table 16.14   Fatty acid compositions (%) of behenic-oleic-oleic triglycerides

Fatty acid	From interesterified olive oil and hydrogenated high-erucic rapeseed oil	From acidolysis of olive oil and behenic acid
C16:0	7.1	6.7
C18:0	17.2	3.6
C18:1	45.3	49.6
C18:2	3.4	4.0
C18:3	0.3	0.3
C20:0	4.9	
C22:0	20.9	34.6
Total saturates	53.5	44.9

Source: Tanek and Ledochowska, 2005

[4] BOO = 1-behenyl-2,3-dioleoylglycerol.

© Woodhead Publishing Limited, 2011

any) of using an erucic acid base, (c) overcome the labelling and consumer issues of the need to still use hydrogenation to generate the behenic acid from high erucic rapeseed oil, and (d) address availability issues of high-erucic rapeseed oil as almost all the rapeseed oil produced in the world today is now of the low-erucic (high-oleic) variety.

16.4   Filled confectionery products

In many ways, the fillings of confectionery products allow a much greater scope for saturates reduction than do the coatings. This is (a) because they are not subject to the same legislative constraints as is chocolate and (b) they are generally softer (and, therefore, more unsaturated) than chocolate and coatings. The softness and greater unsaturation of fillings is, though, the cause of perhaps one of the biggest problems in filled confectionery – oil migration from the filling to the coating causing softening and potentially fat bloom on the coating.

Just as coating fats conveniently fall into three main categories (polymorphic fats such as cocoa butter and CBEs; non-lauric CBRs; lauric CBSs), so many filling fats can be put into the same categories. The degree of hardness and the fatty acid compositions will, though, be different. Filling fats can therefore be produced from blends of fractions of palm oil and shea butter to give combinations that exhibit a degree of polymorphism and therefore need to ideally be tempered but, at the very least, precrystallised before use. These then equate to cocoa butter and CBEs in a coating context. Filling fats can also be made from hydrogenated or, more recently, non-hydrogenated but fractionated oils such as palm oil. These equate more closely to the non-lauric CBR category of coating fat. Fillings can also be produced from unhydrogenated and unfractionated palm kernel and coconut oils. These then equate to the lauric CBS type of coating. To these (although, more usually, to the non-lauric types) other oils can be added in a filling such as nut oils from nut pastes (hazelnut paste, peanut butter, etc). These are highly unsaturated oils and so their inclusion, as well as adding flavour, also reduces saturates. Unfortunately, their inclusion also increases the rate and extent of oil migration. More detailed descriptions of the fats used in confectionery fillings are given by Talbot (2006, chapter 6) and Birkett (2009).

Taking a simple filled chocolate shell as may be found in many chocolate assortments as an example, these products generally contain more filling than coating and the filling generally has a higher total fat content than the coating. In suggesting ways of reducing saturates in filled confectionery products, various calculations will be made of total fat and saturated fat in the combined coating/ filling. Unless otherwise indicated the assumptions have been made that the product is composed of 40% coating (shell) and 60% filling and that the coating contains 30% total fat while the filling contains 40% total fat. Indeed, to simplify the systems further, only chocolate will be considered as the coating, partly because this is the system that is generally used and partly because this will have the lowest saturated fat content of the various coating systems that could be considered.

© Woodhead Publishing Limited, 2011

16.4.1   Scope for and effects of reducing saturated fat in filled confectionery products

As has already been mentioned, confectionery fillings vary widely in their textures, hardnesses, nut oil contents and so on, so it is difficult to give all the examples of filling fats that are used. To exemplify what may be possible in confectionery fillings a range of filling systems from the highly saturated palm kernel oil to the very unsaturated hazelnut oil will be considered. The fatty acids compositions of these are shown in Table 16.15. Using the example structure of a filled chocolate product (in terms of chocolate:filling ratio and chocolate and filling total fat contents) highlighted in section 16.4 it is then possible to calculate the contribution of saturates from both phases of the product and hence of the total product (Table 16.16). The total saturates range from 9.1% with a hazelnut oil filling up to 27.1%, i.e. three times as much, with a palm kernel oil filling.

Table 16.15   Fatty acid compositions (%) of a range of typical filling fats

	Palm kernel oil	Fractionated palm oil	Hazelnut oil	60/40 hazelnut oil/ cocoa butter	80/20 hazelnut oil/ cocoa butter
C8:0	3.4				
C10:0	3.4				
C12:0	50.2	0.1			
C14:0	15.9	0.9		0.3	0.1
C16:0	7.9	46.4	4.7	12.9	8.8
C18:0	2.2	5.1	1.6	15.2	8.4
C18:1	14.5	38.4	76.4	59.9	68.2
C18:2	2.1	7.8	16.3	11.1	13.7
C18:3		0.2	0.1	0.1	0.1
C20:0		0.4	0.1	0.1	0.1
Total saturates	83.0	52.9	6.4	28.5	17.4

Table 16.16   Saturated fat contents (%) of a range of filled chocolates

Filling fat	Saturates from chocolate	Saturates from filling	Total saturates
Palm kernel oil	7.4	19.7	27.1
Fractionated palm oil	7.4	13.0	20.4
Hazelnut oil	7.4	1.7	9.1
60/40 hazelnut oil/cocoa butter	7.4	7.0	14.4
80/20 hazelnut oil/cocoa butter	7.4	4.3	11.7

© Woodhead Publishing Limited, 2011

The problem of oil migration from filling to coating has already been mentioned. This is discussed in much greater detail by Ziegler (2009), but for present purposes it is sufficient to highlight that the main issues associated with oil migration are a softening of the chocolate coating, which makes it difficult to unwrap and hold, and the possible formation of fat bloom on the surface of the chocolate as a result of such softening. The softening is a result of two factors (which can sometimes occur together): (a) eutectic formation and (b) dilution with liquid oil. Eutectics are formed when two fats that are incompatible in terms of the triglyceride composition and crystal structure mix together. The prime example of this in confectionery products is when lauric fats mix with cocoa butter. This results in solid fat contents that are lower than those of either of the two components. The dilution effect is much more obvious – if an oil such as hazelnut oil or peanut oil migrates into a cocoa butter coating then it is clearly going to soften the coating because the amount of liquid oil present in the coating is higher.

To show the effects of eutectic formation, a filling containing palm kernel oil and one containing a fractionated palm oil-based filling fat were stored in a model cell system – the 'washer test' (Talbot, 1996) – in such a way that there was complete contact between the two phases. These systems were held for four weeks at 25°C. At the end of this storage period the softness of the chocolate coating was measured by texture analysis (penetrometry). Samples were taken of the chocolate phase and these were (a) analysed for filling fat to determine the degree of migration that had occurred and (b) analysed for solid fat content to determine the change in this from the original chocolate. These results are shown in Table 16.17. Both filling fats have very similar solid fat contents in themselves and so they migrate to fairly similar degrees (40% with palm kernel oil and 33% with fractionated palm oil). They differ, however, significantly in the effect they have on the chocolate. Palm kernel softens the chocolate considerably. This can be seen in both the huge increase in softness measured by penetrometry and the large

Table 16.17 Comparison of effects of oil migration from lauric and non-lauric filling fats (after four weeks at 25°C)

Filling fat	Degree of migration (%)	Softness of chocolate[a] (0.1mm)	Solid fat content of chocolate (%)			Total saturates (%)
(0.1 mm)			20°C	25°C	30°C	
None (control)	0	~4	76.0	70.7	51.8	
Palm kernel oil	40	66	36.1	18.3	8.8	27.1
Fractionated palm oil	33	21	56.1	47.7	24.7	20.4

[a] Measured by penetrometry of a 9° angled cone into the chocolate in units if 0.1 mm

Source: Talbot, 2009a

© Woodhead Publishing Limited, 2011

decrease in the solid fat contents of the chocolate. A solid fat content at 20°C of 36.1% would make the chocolate very soft and difficult to unwrap and consume. The fractionated palm oil, on the other hand, softens the chocolate to a much lesser degree with a softness measurement of only 21 compared with 66 with palm kernel oil and a solid fat content in the chocolate at 20°C of 56.1%. This would still be high enough for the chocolate to be unwrapped and consumed without sticking to either the wrapper or the fingers. In addition to this the total saturates level is 20.4% with the fractionated palm oil filling compared to 27.1% with the palm kernel oil filling. Thus, if palm kernel oil in a filling is replaced by a fractionated palm oil filling fat then not only can a 25% reduction in saturates be achieved but a better product will also result.

Using a filling containing a highly unsaturated oil such as hazelnut oil will, of course, allow an even greater reduction in saturates but, potentially, suffer from an even greater degree of oil migration and softening. Ziegler and Szlachetka (2005) studied this problem and found, not surprisingly, that if squares of chocolate were laid on filter paper saturated with hazelnut oil, significant migration of oil into the chocolate occurs. However, if the hazelnut oil were saturated with cocoa butter (which equates to about 20% cocoa butter in the oil), then migration was significantly reduced. This effect is shown in Fig. 16.3, in which cumulative weight gain in the chocolate squares is plotted against a function of time. The circles show the effect when the filter paper is saturated with hazelnut oil – the chocolate increases in weight as time goes on. If the filter paper is saturated with cocoa butter (squares in Fig. 16.3) then no increase in weight of the chocolate and

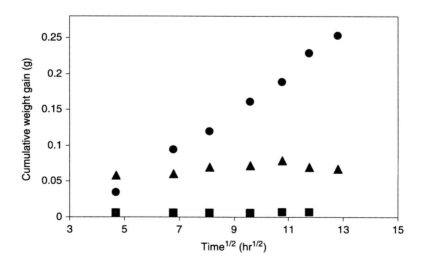

Fig. 16.3 Net migration of hazelnut oil into a 3 g sample of chocolate (38 mm × 38 mm × 1.4 mm). ●: hazelnut oil alone; ■: liquid phase of cocoa butter: ▲: 80:20 hazelnut oil:cocoa butter blend (Ziegler and Szlachetka, 2005; reproduced from Ziegler, 2009).

© Woodhead Publishing Limited, 2011

hence no migration occurs. If, though, the filter paper is saturated with 80% hazelnut oil and 20% cocoa butter (triangles in Fig. 16.3) then some migration takes place initially but this quickly reaches an equilibrium and no further migration occurs. A filling fat phase of 80% hazelnut oil/20% cocoa butter would result in a filled chocolate containing 11.7% saturates in total. This would allow a reduction in saturates of 43% compared to a filling based on fractionated palm oil and a reduction in saturates of 57% compared to one based on palm kernel oil. Even using a filling containing 60% hazelnut oil and 40% cocoa butter (for added security against oil migration) would give a reduction in saturates of 29% compared to one based on fractionated palm oil and of 47% compared to one based on palm kernel oil. Because of the chemical and physical similarity between cocoa butter and CBEs it would be expected that CBEs could be used as alternatives to cocoa butter in such filling compositions.

16.4.2   Potential for novel filling compositions

In response to the demands of consumers, retailers and governments for reductions in saturated fat in food products the major oils and fats suppliers have developed and are continuing to develop confectionery filling fats with lower levels of saturated fat. Varying technologies are being used to achieve these, including the use of specifically structured triglycerides and the use of hardstock technology. This is the technology used particularly by the margarines and spreads industry to allow a structure to be achieved in what is essentially a fairly liquid system. Because developments along these lines are likely to continue, no specific brand names will be mentioned here as these are likely to be superseded as time goes on.

The effects of chain length and degree of unsaturation on melting point and functionality was described earlier in connection with compound coatings. The same arguments can also apply to fillings. Vereecken et al. (2009) studied a number of model systems based on either palm mid-fraction (rich in POP) or shea stearine (rich in StOSt) in blends with high-oleic sunflower oil (HOSF). Blends were made such that the total saturates level in the blend was 30%. They measured melting profiles (by nuclear magnetic resonance) and crystallisation rates (by differential scanning calorimetry) and found that the solid fat contents at any given temperature of the shea stearine/HOSF were significantly higher than those of the palm mid-fraction/HOSF blend. Not only that, but the crystallisation of the shea stearine/HOSF blend was faster than that of the palm mid-fraction/HOSF blend. Both of these results would suggest that it ought to be possible to reduce the level of shea stearine and increase the level of HOSF in this system to a point where (a) it matches the melting profile and crystallisation of the palm mid-fraction/HOSF blend and, at the same time, (b) reduce the total level of saturates. One drawback to this (other than the potential for a greater degree of oil migration) was that the shea stearine/HOSF system showed a greater instability in storage than did the palm mid-fraction/HOSF system with respect to the microstructure of the fat phase. After one month's storage very large fat crystals were found in the shea stearine/HOSF blend which would adversely affect the sensory characteristics of a filling based on this system.

© Woodhead Publishing Limited, 2011

The same researchers also looked at the effects of trisaturated triglycerides on these two systems and found that PPP (from the high-melting fraction of palm oil) was better at seeding a stable crystal structure than was StStSt. Although including trisaturated triglycerides in a filling composition will increase rather than decrease saturates, their functionality may be such that, at low levels of use, they can impart sufficient structure and stability to allow an overall reduction in saturates. As far as the author is aware no work has been published on this particular aspect and so this is still currently in the realms of speculation.

16.5   Future trends

In some ways, one of the major areas where reduction in saturates in chocolate confectionery would be facilitated would be to make changes in the legislation and regulations regarding the composition of chocolate (particularly in the EU and USA). However, realistically this is unlikely to happen (in the short to medium term, at least) so what are likely to be the trends in other areas?

The area with the greatest potential is that of filling fats. Each of the products shortlisted for the Food Ingredients Excellence Awards of 2009 (Food Ingredients Europe, 2009) in the category of 'Confectionery Innovation of the Year' is, to a large extent, a product that will contribute to reduced saturates in a confectionery filling. Biscuitine™ 580 from Loders Croklaan achieves this through the use of a specific combination of designed triglycerides. Deliair™ NH from AAK has the ability to incorporate large amounts of air into a filling, thus reducing total fat levels. Redusat from Fuji Oil Europe crystallises in a network structure that allows high levels of liquid oil to be captured within this to reduce saturates (Vanderlinden, 2009). The use of each of these technologies is likely to expand into future examples of confectionery filling fats.

In the longer term the manipulation of fatty acid chain lengths to give more functionality at lower saturates levels may well be used to produce fats for these applications. Various issues would need to be solved or overcome first. As has been mentioned, in terms of filling fats some of the longer chain (but less saturated) systems may not crystallise in a stable configuration and either fat 'seeds' (which potentially would be higher in saturates) would need to be used or changes would need to be made to processing to enable a stable crystal structure to form. In other cases, the structure could be so different from anything used in food thus far that Novel Foods clearance would be needed.

The technology behind the use of longer-chain-length systems is that it is possible to obtain higher melting and higher solid fat systems at the same level of saturates, thus allowing scope for dilution with unsaturated liquid oils to then lower the saturates. An alternative way of approaching this is the use of partial glycerides. Diacylglycerol (DAG) oils are essentially rich in diglycerides (as opposed to the triglycerides which are the predominant components of vegetable and animal fats). These have a higher melting point than the corresponding triglyceride and could therefore be used as a means of reducing saturates. DAG oils are considered in

© Woodhead Publishing Limited, 2011

more detail in Chapter 8. Taking this one stage further, monoglycerides have even higher melting points than the corresponding diglycerides and triglycerides (Vereecken, 2008) and could also be used to structure more unsaturated fat systems for use in fillings.

Finally, a further area likely to be exploited in the reduction of total fat in confectionery fillings is that of emulsion technology. Water in a filling will attack the chocolate shell, dissolving out the sugar and thus weakening the shell structure. Encapsulating that water in a water-in-oil emulsion, however, protects the chocolate shell against such attack and reduces the amount of oil present in the filling. This is also an area that is being investigated in terms of coatings. Norton *et al.* (2009) have already produced a tempered cocoa butter emulsion containing up to 60% water.

16.6   Sources of further information and advice

The following books contain more detailed discussions and background on chocolate, compound coatings and confectionery fillings:

Application of Fats in Confectionery by G. Talbot, published by Kennedy's Publications Ltd, London, UK, 2006. ISBN 0-904725-11-1

Industrial Chocolate Manufacture and Use, 4th Edition, edited by S. T. Beckett, published by Wiley-Blackwell, Oxford, 2009. ISBN 978-1-4051-3949-6

Science and technology of enrobed and filled chocolate, confectionery and bakery products edited by G. Talbot, published by Woodhead Publishing Ltd, Cambridge, 2009. ISBN 978-1-84569-390-9

Further information and advice can be obtained from the author (geoff@thefatconsultant. co.uk; www.thefatconsultant.co.uk) and from the main producers of speciality fats for the confectionery industry: Loders Croklaan (http://www.croklaan.com), AAK (http:// www.aak.com) and Fuji Oil Europe (http://www.fujioileurope.com).

16.7   References

Baer DJ, Judd JT, Clevidence BA, Tracy RP (2004). 'Dietary fatty acids affect plasma markers of inflammation in healthy men fed controlled diets: a randomised crossover study'. *Am. J. Clin. Nutr.* **79**, 969–73.

Berry SEE, Sanders TAB (2005). 'Influence of triacylglycerol structure of stearic acid-rich fats on postprandial lipaemia'. *Proc. Nutrition Soc.* **64**, 205–12.

Bhattacharyya S, Bhattacharyya DK (1991). 'Enzymatic acidolysis of sal fat and its fractions'. *Oléagineux* **46**, 509–13.

Birkett J (2009). 'Fat-based centres and fillings' in *Science and technology of enrobed and filled chocolate, confectionery and bakery products*, ed. Talbot G. Woodhead Publishing, Cambridge, Chapter 6, pp 101–22.

Bladbjerg EM, Tholstrup T, Marckmann P, Sandstrom B, Jespersen J (1995). 'Dietary changes in fasting levels of factor VII coagulant activity (FVII:C) are accompanied by changes in Factor VII protein and other vitamin K-dependent proteins'. *Thromb. Haemost.* **73**, 239–42.

Bracco U, Rostagno W, Egli EH (1970). 'A Study of cocoa butter – illipé butter mixtures'. *International Chocolate Review* **25**, 41–8.

CAOBISCO (2009). Consumption Trends and Ranking of Consumption of Chocolate Confectionery. www.caobisco.com (accessed 23 July 2009).

© Woodhead Publishing Limited, 2011

Chaiseri S, Dimick P (1989). 'Lipid and hardness characteristics of cocoa butter from different geographical areas', *J. Amer. Oil Chem. Soc.* **66**, 1771–6.

DEFRA (2002, 2003, 2005, 2007). *Family Food – Report on the Expenditure and Food Survey*. Department of Environment, Food and Rural Affairs, London, United Kingdom.

European Union (2000). European Parliament and Council Directive 2000/36/EC (23 June 2000) relating to cocoa and chocolate products intended for human consumption. *Official Journal of the European Communities* **43**(L197), 19.

Food Ingredients Europe (2009). Food Ingredients Excellence Awards 2009. http://fieurope.ingredientsnetwork.com/awards (accessed 16 September 2009).

Food Standards Australia New Zealand (2003). 'Erucic acid in food: A toxicological review and risk assessment'. *Technical Report Series No. 21*, page 4 paragraph 1; ISBN 0 642 34526 0; ISSN 1448-3017.

German JB, Dillard CJ (2004). 'Saturated fats: what dietary intake?', *Am. J. Clin. Nutr.* **80**(3), 550–9.

Grundy SM (1994). 'Influence of stearic acid on cholesterol metabolism relative to other long-chain fatty acids'. *Am. J. Clin Nutr.* **60(Suppl)**, 986S–990S.

Hargreaves NG (1988). 'Chemical and physical properties of cocoa butter alternatives'. Lecture given at the German Confectionery School, ZDS, Solingen, Germany.

Henderson L, Gregory J, Swan G (2002). *The National Diet and Nutrition Survey: Types and Quantities of Food Consumed v. 1: Adults Aged 19 to 64 Years*. Office for National Statistics, London.

Hoak JC (1994). 'Stearic acid, clotting and thrombosis'. *Am. J. Clin. Nutr.* **60(Suppl)**, 1050S–1053S.

Jensen RG, Gander GW, Sampugna J (1962). 'Fatty acid composition of the lipids from pooled raw milk'. *J. Dairy Sci.* **45**, 329–31.

Jurriens G (1968). 'Analysis of Triglycerides' in *Analysis and Characteristics of Oils and Fats and Fat Products*, Vol. 2, Boekenoogen HA (ed.). Interscience Publications, London.

Kähkönen P, Tuorila H (1999). 'Consumer responses to reduced and regular fat content in different products: effects of gender, involvement and health concern'. *Food Quality and Preference.* **10**(2), 83–91.

Koyano T, Hachiya I, Sato K (1990). 'Fat polymorphism and crystal seeding effects on fat bloom stability of dark chocolate'. *Food Structure* **9**, 231–40.

Lambert J (2008). The Role of CAOBISCO Products in the Diet of the European Union. http://www.caobisco.com/caobisco_invites/docs/2008-5-28_02-Janet_Lambert.pps (accessed 13 December 2010).

Lipp M, Anklam E (1998). 'Review of cocoa butter and alternative fats for use in chocolate – Part A. Compositional data'. *Food Chem.* **62**, 73–97.

Mensink RP, Zock PL, Kester ADM, Katan MB (2003). 'Effects of dietary fatty acids and carbohydrates on the ratio of serum total to HDL cholesterol and on serum lipids and apolipoproteins: a meta-analysis of 60 controlled trials'. *Am. J. Clin. Nutr.* **77**, 1146–55.

Norton JE, Fryer PJ, Parkinson J, Cox PW (2009). 'Development and characterisation of tempered cocoa butter emulsions containing up to 60% water' *J. Food Eng.* **95**(1), 172–8.

Rey B, Rossi-Vauthey P, Rousset P, Schafer O (2007). 'Low-fat confectionery product being a water-in-oil emulsion'. *WO Patent 2007/025756 A1*.

Rousset P, Sandoz L, Schmitt CJE (2007). 'Low-fat confectionery product'. *WO Patent 2007/025757 A1*.

Sanders TAB, Oakley FR, Cooper JA, Miller GJ (2001). 'Influence of a stearic acid-rich structured triacylglycerol on postprandial lipemia, factor VII concentrations and fibrinolytic activity in healthy subjects'. *Am. J. Clin. Nutr.* **73**, 715–21.

Sanders TAB, Berry SEE (2005). 'Influence of stearic acid on postprandial lipemia and hemostatic function', *Lipids* **40**(12), 1221–7.

Sanders TAB (2009). 'Nutritional aspects of chocolate confectionery fats'. Lecture at *56th Technology Conference of the Biscuit, Cake, Chocolate and Confectionery Sector of the Food and Drink Federation*. Ettington Chase, UK, 26–27 March 2009.

© Woodhead Publishing Limited, 2011

Sawadogo K, Bézard J (1982). 'Étude de la structure glyceridique du beurre de karité'. *Oléagineux* **37**, 69–74.

Seligson FH, Krummel DA, Apgar JL (1994). 'Patterns of chocolate consumption'. *Am. J. Clin. Nutr.* **60**(6 Suppl), 1060S–1064S.

Shukla VKS (1994). 'Milkfat in Sugar and Chocolate Confectionery' in *Fats in Food Products*, ed Moran DPJ and Rajah KK, Chapter 7, pp 257–8.

Slager H, Favre L, Talbot G (2007). 'The Ultimate Confectionery Coating'. *Food Marketing and Technology*, December, 12–14.

Sridhar R, Lakshminarayana G (1991). 'Triacylglycerol compositions of some vegetable oils with potential for preparation of cocoa butter equivalents by high performance liquid chromatography'. *J. Oil Technology Assoc. of India* **23**, 42–3.

Talbot G (1996). 'The "washer test" – a method for monitoring fat migration'. *Manufacturing Confectioner* **76**(9), 87–90.

Talbot G (2006). *Applications of Fats in Confectionery*. Kennedy's Publications, London.

Talbot G (2009a). 'Technical Difficulties of Reducing Saturated Fat in Filled Chocolate Confectionery'. Lecture at *56th Technology Conference of the Biscuit, Cake, Chocolate and Confectionery Sector of the Food and Drink Federation*. Ettington Chase, UK, 26–27 March 2009.

Talbot G (2009b). 'Compound coatings' in *Science and technology of enrobed and filled chocolate, confectionery and bakery products*, ed. Talbot G. Woodhead Publishing, Cambridge, Chapter 5, pp 80–100.

Tan BK, Oh FCH (1981). 'Malaysian palm oil: chemical and physical characteristics'. *PORIM Technology*, **3**.

Tanek M, Ledochowska E (2005). 'Structured triacylglycerols containing behenic acid: Preparation and properties'. *J. Food Lipids.* **12**, 77–89.

Tholstrup T, Miller GJ, Bysted A, Sandström B (2003). 'Effect of individual dietary fatty acids on postprandial activation of blood coagulation factor VII and fibrinolysis in healthy young men'. *Am. J. Clin. Nutr.* **77**, 1125–32.

Vanderlinden B (2009). 'Op weg naar confectionery fats met verbeterde functionaliteit en nutritionele waarde'. Lecture given at *VLAZ Seminarie*, University of Ghent, Belgium, 2 June 2009. http://www.fte.ugent.be/vlaz/VLAZ_chocolade2009_Fuji.pdf (accessed 13 December 2010).

Vereecken J (2008). 'Fat structuring with partial glycerides: effect on solid fat profiles'. Lecture given at conference on 'Crystallisation and Physical Properties of Fats: from Molecules to Market', University of Ghent, Belgium, 18–19 June 2008.

Vereecken J, Foubert I, Smith KW, Dewettinck K (2009). 'Effect of SatSatSat and SatOSat on crystallization of model fat blends'. *Eur. J. Lipid Sci. and Technol.* **111**(3), 243–58.

Wells MA (2009). 'Controlling the rheology of chocolate and fillings' in *Science and technology of enrobed and filled chocolate, confectionery and bakery products*, ed. Talbot G. Woodhead Publishing, Cambridge, Chapter 13, pp 255–84.

Weyland M (1992). 'Cocoabutter fractions: A novel way of optimising chocolate performance'. Lecture given at *Pennsylvania Manufacturing Confectioners Association 46th Annual Production Conference*. Hershey, PA, USA.

Wong Soon (1991). *Speciality Fats Versus Cocoa Butter*. Wong Soon, Malaysia.

Yates P (2009). 'Formulation of chocolate for industrial applications' in *Science and technology of enrobed and filled chocolate, confectionery and bakery products* ed. Talbot G. Woodhead Publishing, Cambridge, Chapter 3, p 50.

Ziegler G (2009). 'Product design and shelf-life issues: oil migration and fat bloom' in *Science and technology of enrobed and filled chocolate, confectionery and bakery products*, ed. Talbot G. Woodhead Publishing, Cambridge, Chapter 10, pp 185–210.

Ziegler GR, Szlachetka K (2005). Where is the nut oil in chocolate? New Food, **8**(3), 45–52.

© Woodhead Publishing Limited, 2011

17

Saturated fat reduction in ice cream

J. Underdown and P. J. Quail, Unilever R&D, UK and K. W. Smith, Fat Science Consulting Ltd, UK

Abstract: Ice cream is made and eaten in almost every country in the world and the total global production is around 15 billion litres annually with a market value of around £35 billion. The challenge in reducing saturated fat (SFA) is to retain the desirable eating qualities of the ice cream, to which fat contributes a great deal. This chapter will explore the reduction of fat level, the option of fat replacers, the use of fats containing lower SFA and the application of novel processing to enable reformulation.

Key words: low fat, fat replacer, emulsion, crystallisation, creaminess, iciness, frozen, flavour delivery, processing.

17.1 Introduction

17.1.1 Historical context

There are many early references to the consumption of products containing ice that date back more than a thousand years, although it is not possible to attribute the invention of ice cream to a specific period in history or to any particular group of individuals. Ice cream as we know it today has been in existence for at least 300 years but the first ice cream making machine that froze the ice cream mix and also whipped in air at the same time was not invented until the 1840s. Thus, it was not until the second half of the nineteenth century that ice cream consumption progressed from the dining table to the street and ice cream was produced on a commercial scale. Products became available in reusable glass containers or served in paper to be taken away and eaten directly from the wrapper. These were the early forerunners of the now ubiquitous ice cream cone that first appeared around the turn of the twentieth century in America.

Around this time, the US Federal Department of Agriculture proposed a standard milk fat content of 14% for ice cream. The manufacturers thought this

© Woodhead Publishing Limited, 2011

was too high and advocated a lower fat content. It was not until 1960 that the minimum milkfat content for dairy ice cream was fixed at 10%.

In the UK, it was during the 1920s that grocers and restaurant owners started to sell factory-produced ice cream in their outlets. Wall's ice cream was advertised as being made in precisely the same way as American ice cream, using pure cream and ripe fruit juices. However, this changed during and after the Second World War when there were global food shortages. Important raw materials for ice cream production such as butter and sugar were rationed and the use of cream in the making of ice cream was forbidden. This prompted manufacturers to try using different vegetable fats and even certain types of animal fats to produce ice cream. These early experiments with alternative fats had different degrees of success. The more liquid oils (e.g. rapeseed) were found to be unsuitable whereas the more solid fats (e.g. palm and coconut oils) were used successfully to make good-quality ice cream. Most food rationing ended in the UK in 1953 but a lot of standard ice cream continued to be made with vegetable fat and this practice was also adopted in some other European countries and continues to the present day.

17.1.2   Defining ice cream

The term 'ice cream' covers a broad range of different types of frozen desserts with the common link that they are all sweet tasting, distinctively flavoured, contain particles of ice and, unlike any other food, are consumed directly from the frozen state. There is no universal definition of ice cream and legislation varies from country to country and often prescribes a minimum quantity of fat and the sole use of milkfat in order to use the descriptor *dairy ice cream*. It is often categorised as premium, standard or economy and in more recent years a new segment of light or fat-reduced ice creams has appeared.

17.1.3   Ice cream consumption and dietary impact

Ice cream is made and eaten in almost every country in the world and the total global production is around 15 billion litres annually with a market value of around £35 billion (Clarke, 2004). The USA is the largest producer of ice cream and has a per capita annual consumption of about 22 litres. European consumption is lower, and typically ranges between 4 litres (Portugal) and 12 litres (Sweden).

At these relatively low annual consumption levels, ice cream plays only a small part in the overall diet, contributing typically 1–3% of the recommended annual energy intake for an adult (assuming average consumption of a regular vanilla ice cream providing 1000 kcal per litre). However, when considered on an individual portion basis, fat can generate more than half of the total product energy content and saturated fat normally provides a significant proportion of this. For example, a 100 ml portion of premium vanilla ice cream can provide up to 50% of an adult's Guideline Daily Amount (GDA) for saturated fat and about 20% of an adult's GDA for total fat but only contributes about 10% of GDA for total energy. Thus technical options to reduce the fat and saturated fat in ice cream

© Woodhead Publishing Limited, 2011

and its associated components have received a great deal of attention in recent years and many examples of light, reduced-fat and even fat-free ice cream products have appeared on the market around the world.

17.2   Basic components and processing of ice cream

17.2.1   Basic elements of ice cream

Ice cream in its simplest form can be considered as a four-phase system where the product typically consists of (by volume) 50% air, 30% ice, 15% 'matrix' (which contains the sugars, milk proteins and unfrozen water) and only 5% fat (Clarke, 2004). The relative proportions of these components can vary depending on the type of ice cream produced. However, if these same basic components are considered on an energy, or calorific basis, the picture is very different and the role of fat (and hence saturated fat) provides a much more significant contribution to the overall product, around 50% (Table 17.1).

Table 17.1   Contribution of calories from ice cream ingredients

Ingredient	% v/v	% w/w	% calories
Air	50.0	0	0
Water/ice	32.5	65	0
Sugars/proteins	12.5	25	53
Fat	5.0	10	47

Ice cream comes in an almost bewildering array of different colours and flavours but in many countries the most popular flavours are the very traditional ones of vanilla, chocolate and strawberry (Thomas, 2009). Almost all of these basic ice creams contain either milkfat (i.e. derived from milk, cream or butter) or a limited number of vegetable fats, primarily coconut oil, palm kernel oil (PKO) or palm oil. Very rarely are ice creams made with a combination of dairy and vegetable fats, since labelling regulations often limit the fat to purely dairy origin. Thus the sources of fat used in almost all ice creams around the globe come from either dairy or coconut- or palm-based oils.

17.2.2   Processing of ice cream

Industrially manufactured ice cream is normally produced via a semi-continuous process that is made up of a number of unit operations. Firstly, all of the major ingredients are mixed together in hot water to produce a liquid emulsion of oil droplets dispersed in a continuous aqueous phase. In addition to the basic ingredients mentioned above, emulsifiers (typically mono-/diglycerides) are also added at a level of around 0.3% by weight. This liquid emulsion is usually homogenised to produce very small oil droplets (mean diameter typically less

© Woodhead Publishing Limited, 2011

than 1 μm) and pasteurised under prescribed time/temperature conditions for microbiological quality reasons. The mix is then rapidly cooled to a temperature of 5°C or under and held in a vessel for a period of hours to 'age' prior to freezing.

During this ageing operation, a number of important changes occur to the mix. A key mechanism at this point in the manufacturing process is fat crystallisation, where the liquid oil droplets start to form solid fat crystals at a rate and extent which is dependent on the fat type selected. Fats with higher saturated contents tend to crystallise faster and to a greater extent than less saturated fats.

After ageing, the mix is pumped though a continuous ice cream freezer where it is rapidly cooled from a temperature of 5°C to typically −5°C via contact with a scraped surface heat exchanger with a wall temperature of −30°C or below. As the temperature of the mix is reduced, ice is formed on the inner wall of the cold barrel, which is scraped off by the scraper blades and mixed back into the bulk. Air is normally introduced into the freezer so that the mix is simultaneously frozen and aerated. On exiting the ice cream freezer the partially frozen ice cream can be shaped, portioned and optionally combined with other ingredients before packaging and hardening in a blast freezer to temperatures of −25°C or below. The products are then stored in a cold store prior to distribution to the various outlets.

17.3   Sources of fat and saturated fat in ice cream products

In addition to the basic ice cream, many products contain other components to generate visual, texture and flavour contrasts. The most commonly used examples are chocolate, cereal wafers and cones, biscuits, fruit pieces, sauces and nuts.

All of these can contribute to the overall fat and saturated fatty acid (SFA) content associated with a particular product and in many cases the fat and SFA contribution from the added components actually exceeds that from the basic ice cream.

Table 17.2 gives the typical nutritional breakdown for some of the components commonly used to make many ice cream products around the world (on a % w/w basis). A typical pre-packaged ice cream cone product (100 g total weight) would comprise approximately 62 g of ice cream, 16 g of wafer, 12 g of chocolate, 5 g of chocolate sauce and 5 g of hazelnuts. Based on these weight percentages and the data given in Table 17.2, the product breakdown in terms of fat, SFA and energy is given in Table 17.3.

Table 17.2   Typical nutritional breakdown for common components used in ice cream products

	Dairy ice cream	Dry wafer	Milk chocolate	Chocolate sauce	Hazelnut
Energy (kcal/100g)	207	500	625	220	650
% fat (w/w)	10.0	23.0	50.0	5.0	62.0
% SFA (w/w)	6.5	20.0	30.0	3.5	5.0

© Woodhead Publishing Limited, 2011

Table 17.3   Breakdown showing energy contribution in a multi-component ice cream product

	Weight (g)	Fat (g)	SFA (g)	Energy (kcal)
Ice cream	62	6.0	3.9	124
Wafer	16	3.7	3.2	80
Chocolate	12	5.5	3.3	69
Sauce	5	0.3	0.2	11
Nuts	5	2.5	0.2	26
Total	100	18.0	10.8	310

So in this example, although the ice cream by weight is by far the most significant component it contributes only one-third of the total SFA content, compared to the other components, which combined provide almost twice the amount of SFA. The technical challenges associated with SFA reduction in these other components will not be addressed in this chapter of the book but detailed consideration is now given to the issues pertaining to ice cream.

17.4   The function of fat in ice cream

Fat fulfils a number of important roles in ice cream. While zero-fat and low-fat ice cream-type products are known, these lack many of the distinguishing characteristics of typical ice creams. The contribution of fat to the structure and properties of ice cream is discussed to provide a basis for understanding the implications of reducing saturated fat, which are then addressed in section 17.6.

17.4.1   Emulsion properties

Ice cream can be considered as an oil-in-water emulsion in which the fat droplets are dispersed within a continuous aqueous matrix phase. The other main components of ice crystals and air bubbles also contribute to the ice cream structure and properties. The liquid fat droplets are initially formed during homogenisation of the hot ice cream mix. After homogenisation the droplets are stabilised by some of the milk proteins present in the mix, which readily adsorb onto the fat droplet surface (Clarke, 2004; Goff, 2008).

17.4.2   Fat destabilisation

After homogenisation and pasteurisation the mix is cooled to around 5°C and held at this temperature with gentle stirring for a period of a few hours. This step is known as ageing and allows time for certain processes to take place that aid in the subsequent formation of the ice cream microstructure when the mix is aerated and frozen in the scraped surface heat exchanger.

© Woodhead Publishing Limited, 2011

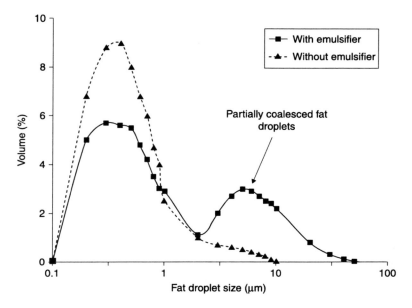

Fig. 17.1   Fat particle size distributions in ice cream made with and without emulsifier.

The first process that occurs is that the emulsifiers replace some of the proteins adsorbed at the fat droplet interface (Clarke, 2004; Zhang and Goff, 2005; Gelin *et al.*, 1994; Goff and Jordan, 1989). The second process is fat crystallisation – of some of the fat inside the droplets and also of the mono-/diglyceride emulsifiers (Clarke, 2004; Gelin *et al.*, 1994). These processes have the effect of making the emulsion less stable under shear, resulting in fat partial coalescence, i.e. an irreversible agglomeration of fat globules, held together by a combination of fat crystals and liquid fat (Goff *et al.*, 1999). Partially crystalline fat droplets are necessary for optimal fat structure formation to occur during freezing (Marshall *et al.*, 2003). The optimal formation of fat structure in ice cream is responsible for many desirable properties, including dryness and shape retention at extrusion from an ice cream freezer and slowness of meltdown and smooth-eating textural properties after hardening (Goff, 2002).

The effect of the emulsifier on the distribution of fat droplet sizes in (melted) ice cream is shown in Fig. 17.1. The main peak without emulsifier is due to homogenised discrete fat droplets; whereas when emulsifier is present some of the fat droplets are partially coalesced, resulting in a second peak at larger particle size.

17.4.3   Foam stabilisation
The ice cream texture is a result of its structure, as contributed by the various phases present – namely ice crystals, air bubbles, partially coalesced fat globules, and the continuous serum phase of dissolved and suspended solutes and macromolecules – that are formed during the many stages of manufacture, especially homogenisation, ageing and whipping/freezing (Goff, 1997).

© Woodhead Publishing Limited, 2011

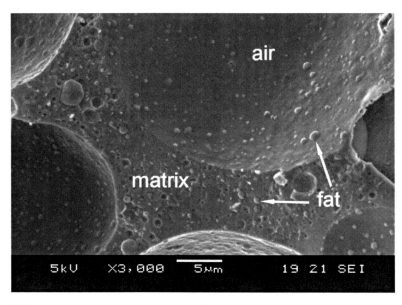

Fig. 17.2 Scanning electron micrograph of a typical ice cream microstructure showing fat droplets adsorbed at the air bubble surface and also present in the matrix phase.

Fat plays a critical role in stabilising the air structure in ice cream (Koxholt *et al.*, 2001; Clarke, 2004). The aged ice cream mix is passed through a scraped surface heat exchanger (ice cream freezer) to aerate and freeze the ice cream. As the mix is sheared and air is incorporated, the fat droplets (coated in protein/emulsifier) and milk proteins adsorb onto the surface of the air bubbles, forming a boundary between them and the surrounding matrix phase (Goff *et al.*, 1999). This helps to stabilise the air bubbles against coalescence (Clarke, 2004).

It is possible to form aerated ice creams without the air being stabilised by fat droplets, but the resulting structures are less stable and more prone to form channelled air structures. This occurs particularly during the temperature fluctuations typically experienced during storage and distribution, which can result in shrinkage of the product and loss of eating quality.

A scanning electron micrograph of a typical ice cream microstructure is shown in Fig. 17.2. The fat droplets are adsorbed at the air bubble surface and are also distributed in the matrix phase. The fat droplets that are present throughout the matrix phase also contribute to air phase stability by increasing the matrix viscosity and so making it more difficult for air bubbles to come together and coalesce (Clarke, 2004).

17.4.4 Structural stability of the frozen product

As discussed above, there are many steps involved in the formation of the ice cream microstructure, and fat plays a key role at each stage. During ageing at 5°C

© Woodhead Publishing Limited, 2011

the nature of the interfaces and the state of the fat begin to change. These changes continue as the mix is processed through an ice cream freezer at around −5°C, then hardened and stored below −25°C. As the mix temperature is lowered, more of the fat in the droplets crystallises and the amount of solid fat present in the final product has an impact on the product properties such as rate of melt and creamy texture. The fat type and the fat level both determine the amount of solid fat present. Ice cream that melts too rapidly is normally an indication of an unstable structure, which will lead to poor quality and stability throughout the product life cycle, whereas ice cream with a slower melting profile has the opposite tendency, giving products that can maintain their structural stability for long periods.

17.4.5   Creaminess

Fat contributes to the sensory properties of ice cream. One main attribute is creaminess or creamy texture. Fat with a high content of solid fat at ice cream storage temperatures will melt slowly in the mouth during consumption, coating the tongue and giving the perception of a thicker and creamier product. Products with higher contents of liquid fat or reduced fat contents (Fig. 17.3) are less likely to be perceived as creamy.

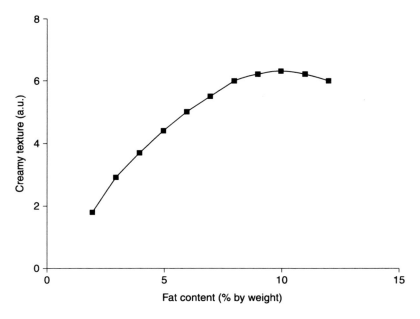

Fig. 17.3   Creamy texture as a function of fat content of ice cream.

17.4.6   Flavour delivery

Many flavour cocktails that are added to ice cream contain both oil-soluble and water-soluble components. These complex flavour cocktails partition between the oil and aqueous phases of the product and are released in the mouth as the product warms up during mastication. The presence of at least some fat in the product thus plays a key part in solubilising some of the flavour components and distributing them throughout the product. In the absence of fat, the oil-soluble components associated with the flavour cocktail are not delivered in a controlled way, giving an unbalanced flavour profile evident in many reduced-fat and fat-free products.

17.5   Properties of fats used in current ice cream products

The sources of fat in ice cream products were discussed in section 17.3 with a focus on the individual components within a complete ice cream product. Here we take a look in more detail at the fats used for the ice cream component and how they impact on the ice cream properties.

17.5.1   Fat composition

Traditionally ice cream was made with dairy fat in the form of milkfat or cream. More recently, many products are made using vegetable fats such as coconut oil, palm oil or palm kernel oil. Fats are composed of a range of triacylglycerols (TAGs), which give rise to their physical and nutritional properties. Each TAG contains three fatty acid groups and each of these can be saturated, monounsaturated or polyunsaturated. The fatty acid composition of the common ice cream fats is given in Table 17.4. Clearly the SFA level in the four common ice cream fats varies widely from about 50% to almost 100%. On this basis, in order to have a lower SFA content in the ice cream, of these four, palm oil would be the preferred fat.

Table 17.4   Fatty acid compositions (%) of typical ice cream fats

Fatty acid class	Coconut	Palm	Palm kernel	Milk fat	Sunflower
SFA*	92	51	82	69	11
MUFA*	6	39	16	28	25
PUFA*	2	10	2	3	64

* SFA = saturated fatty acid, MUFA = monounsaturated fatty acid, PUFA = polyunsaturated fatty acid

17.5.2   Fat crystallisation

The TAG composition of fats gives rise to their physical properties. Certain TAGs will be liquid at a given temperature and some will be solid (crystalline). Thus fats typically contain a mixture of solid and liquid phases at any given temperature and melt over a range of temperatures rather than at a single point.

The solid fat contents for the common ice cream fats are compared between 35°C and −10°C in Table 17.5. It should be noted that these values are for bulk fats and the extent of crystallisation can be lower in the ice cream emulsion due to

© Woodhead Publishing Limited, 2011

Table 17.5 Typical solid fat contents (%) for different fat types determined by pNMR (IUPAC 2.150a)

Temp. (°C)	Coconut	Palm	Palm kernel	Milk fat	Sunflower
−10	94	79	87	72	3
−5	92	73	83	70	1
0	90	66	81	66	1
5	87	60	76	61	1
10	82	50	72	52	1
15	66	40	62	40	1
20	37	26	44	21	0
25	1	16	17	13	0
30	0	11	0	8	0
35	0	7	0	1	0

the requirement for each droplet to nucleate and crystallise. It is evident from these data that milk fat, coconut oil, palm kernel oil and palm oil are predominantly crystalline at the characteristic 'production' temperatures (5°C and below) as is conventionally required of an ice cream fat.

When eating ice cream, the mouth temperature can be reduced by 5–10°C from its normal value of 37°C. This being so, palm oil, having some residual solid fat at 35°C, may not melt completely and may give rise to a slightly waxy sensation in the mouth. So from an organoleptic point of view, palm oil may not be the best ice cream fat despite its better nutritional properties.

As described in section 17.2, the fat is molten at the start of the ice cream making process and during the ageing step the fat starts to crystallise. Different fats will crystallise at different rates and to different extents. Therefore the time the ice cream mix needs to be aged is in part dependent on the rate of crystallisation of the fat. Figure 17.4 gives the isothermal crystallisation profiles at 5°C (measured by NMR) for the same four common ice cream fats. It is evident that coconut and palm kernel oil (PKO) crystallise most rapidly, with milkfat and particularly palm oil crystallising more slowly and to a lesser extent. Despite the differences in crystallisation profiles over 60 minutes, all four ice cream fats will have crystallised sufficiently during typical ageing times of four hours or more. However, the rapid crystallisation of coconut and PKO could allow shorter ageing times should this be required.

17.6   Challenges associated with saturated fatty acid (SFA) reduction

There are two basic approaches to reducing the saturated fat content of ice cream products. Each has its own merits but it is unlikely that a single approach will deliver the solution with no compromises to quality or stability; rather, a carefully optimised combination of technical approaches could lead to a new generation of lower SFA products.

© Woodhead Publishing Limited, 2011

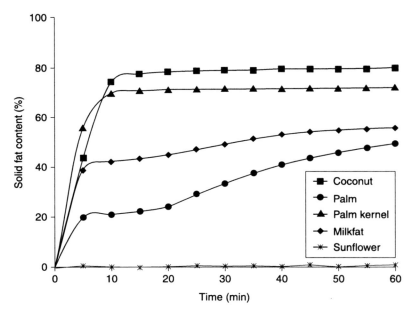

Fig. 17.4   Isothermal crystallisation profiles at 5°C (measured by pNMR).

Before discussing the approaches in detail it is useful to mention the legal and regulatory constraints in some countries that constrain reformulation of ice cream products to improve nutritional profiles. In the European Union, a Euroglaces (EG) code (Euroglaces, 2006) exists that attempts to define certain compositional criteria for different classifications of edible ices (e.g. water ice, ice cream, milk ice, dairy ice cream, fruit ice, sorbet). For example, the descriptor 'dairy ice cream' is reserved for a product containing at least 5% of dairy fat with the exclusion of any fat and/or protein other than of dairy origin. The term 'milk ice' is reserved for a product containing at least 2.5% of exclusively dairy fat and at least 6% of non-fat milk solids. This is only a code, but it contains guidelines that have been implemented in some countries. Most EU countries have some form of local edible ice legislation and these often contain prescribed minima for fat levels in dairy ice cream, ice cream and milk ice products. However, these are not harmonised and the legislation varies from country to country, although some member states are lobbying to change their ice cream legislation and align with the EG code. One of the arguments for doing this is related to saturated fat reduction.

In the USA, standards of identity (USA CFR, 2010) exist which define compositional criteria for different classifications of frozen desserts (e.g. ice cream, frozen custard, goat's milk ice cream, mellorine, sherbert and water ice). Ice cream should not contain less than 10% milkfat and not less than 20% total milk solids (including the fat component). Mellorine products should not contain

© Woodhead Publishing Limited, 2011

less than 6% fat and this includes, but is not limited to, milk-derived non-fat solids and animal or vegetable fat, or both, only part of which may be milkfat.

Ice cream legislation thus varies from country to country, and this needs to be taken into consideration before any product reformulation can take place. There is more scope for reformulation with some product classifications than others and, as many dairy ice cream products are already on the prescribed lower limit for fat content, options to significantly reduce SFA content are limited.

The first approach that can be taken to reduce SFA is to reduce the overall fat content of the product. On a per serving basis, this reduces the intake of saturated fat. There are several ways in which this reduction of fat may be achieved, and these will be elucidated below.

The second approach is to alter the fat composition, reducing the level of saturates in the fat itself. Again, there are several ways in which this can be accomplished, which will be described below.

17.6.1   Fat reduction and replacement

The challenge for manufacturers of low-fat ice cream products is to replace the fat with ingredients that can mimic, at least to some extent, the properties of the fat. In a typical ice cream, the fat plays a key role in the microstructure that is built up during the ageing, freezing and aeration steps, as discussed in section 17.4 above. In addition, the fat plays a part in flavour release and acts as a carrier for lipid-soluble flavours.

If the fat level is to be reduced, the first consideration is what should be used to replace it. The obvious first thought is to replace fat with water, without any reformulation or alteration of the amounts of the other ingredients. However, although it is possible to effect a modest level of fat reduction, it results in an icier, colder-eating and less creamy ice cream due to the increased ice content (see e.g. Roland, et al., 1999a). In addition, the flavour profile of the ice cream is altered since the lipophilic compounds are released differently during eating (Schirle-keller et al., 1994; Guinard et al., 1996; 1997; Li et al., 1997; Roland et al., 1999a; Chung et al., 2003; Hyvönen et al., 2003). The processing of the ice cream mix and the storage stability are also affected by a reduction in the level of fat, since there is less stabilisation of the air cells.

In order to maintain product quality, reformulation routes may be adopted, with the most common being to elevate the amounts of the other ingredients present in the formulation, such as the simple sugars, or include glucose syrups. While these may act to maintain the ice content of the product at the same level as the full fat version, these ingredients do not fulfil the same functions as small fat droplets. As fat plays a key role in stabilising the air phase, simple substitution of fat with sugars can result in detrimental effects on product quality during storage and distribution, ultimately leading to product shrinkage (overrun loss) and less creamy products. Further, the nutritional benefits of reducing fat and saturated fat are in part compromised by the higher sugar levels required to equalise the overall ice content. Thus although this is an obvious approach to achieve fat-reduced products it cannot be the definitive solution on either quality or nutritional grounds.

© Woodhead Publishing Limited, 2011

Selection of the level and type of emulsifier can improve the body and texture, and reduce the size of ice crystals in low-fat ice cream (Baer *et al.*, 1997), but such products still suffer with respect to flavour profile. However, it should be noted that saturated fatty acids in a lipid-based emulsifier will also be counted in the total SFA.

An alternative approach is to use specialist fat replacers, which have been designed to fulfil some of the properties of fat. These ingredients fall into two categories: those of a lipid nature (containing fatty acyl groups) and those based on proteins or carbohydrates. The latter come in many different forms including gel particles, structure-forming hydrocolloids, modified proteins, specialist starches and maltodextrins. Lipid fat replacers include surface active ingredients (emulsifiers) and acyl substituted polyols (e.g. sucrose, sorbitol). Many of these fat replacers were developed initially for non-frozen applications and some remain unproven in ice cream applications. In addition, they are invariably more expensive than the fat they replace, are not always familiar to the consumer and do not fulfil all of the functions of fat in ice cream.

In most cases of non-lipid fat replacement, the resulting ice cream quality does not measure up to consumers' expectations. Ice creams formulated with low fat have poorer flavour and worse texture than a comparable full fat product. As far as acceptability to the average consumer is concerned, texture can be more important than flavour (Devereux *et al.*, 2003). Without fat, the ice cream exhibits textural defects like coarseness, iciness, crumbliness, shrinkage on storage and reduced flavour release (Marshall and Arbuckle, 1996; Berger, 1990). Non-lipid fat replacers include whey protein and inulin – a source of dietary fibre extracted from non-starchy plants (Marshall *et al.*, 2003; Sangeetha *et al.*, 2005).

Several studies have looked at the effects of various commercial whey protein-based fat replacers in ice cream (e.g. Ohmes *et al.*, 1998; Prindiville *et al.*, 2000; El-Nagar *et al.*, 2002; Schaller-Povolny and Smith, 1999 and 2001). Welty *et al.* (2001) compared Simplesse®, Dairy-Lo™ and Oatrim, finding that they increased the level of certain volatile components in the headspace, i.e. would impact the flavour profile. Kailasapathy and Songvanich (1998) looked at N-Lite D®, Slendid™ and Paselli® SA2 (all carbohydrate based) and Simplesse® (protein based), concluding that the latter was best from the iciness perspective but that Slendid™ was best with respect to viscosity and foaming. A comparison of whey protein isolate with inulin found that both produced a harder ice cream (Akalin *et al.*, 2008), although the use of inulin in a low-fat probiotic ice cream improved the texture (Akalin and Erisir, 2008). Inulin reportedly increases the viscosity and decreases the freezing point of reduced-fat ice cream and yields an improvement in the sensory properties (Schaller-Povolny and Smith, 1999 and 2001).

One issue that needs to be addressed is the iciness of the ice cream when the fat content is reduced. Ice-structuring proteins can be used in ice cream to inhibit the crystallisation of ice (Bramley *et al.*, 2006, 2007; Byass *et al.*, 1998; Regand and Goff, 2006). This can allow a reduction in the level of fat below 5% without increasing the apparent iciness.

The function of fat in ice cream has already been described, above, and reduction or removal of fat from the formulation can necessitate a change in the processing.

© Woodhead Publishing Limited, 2011

For example, Asher *et al.* (1993) describe a process adapted to permit the use of whey protein as a substitute for fat. The general observation for all ice creams formulated with current non-lipid fat replacers is that the impact on texture and/or flavour leads to an inferior ice cream compared to that formulated with fat (Roland *et al.*, 1999b). Thus the fat level (and so also the saturated fat level) can be reduced to zero, but since the fat is a main component of an ice cream, these are generally very different products. However, even a small level of fat can aid in stabilising the microstructure.

There are a few fat replacers of a lipid nature, which might, therefore, be expected to perform better due to their closer similarity to fat. Caprenin® and Benefat® are both composed of triacylglycerols, like natural fats, but both have reduced calories due to the specific types of triacylglycerol present. However, both are high in saturated fatty acids and have not, in any case, been evaluated in ice cream. Olestra® (or Olean®) is composed of sucrose polyesters of fatty acids, with at least four, but preferably seven or more, fatty acids per molecule. Such molecules are not digested, leading to a zero-calorie material. However, they have similar properties to the triacylglycerols of which natural fats are composed. Thus ice cream can be prepared using Olestra® (Whelan *et al.*, 2000). The fact that Olestra® is not digested can lead to problems. The principal drawback here is that product labels must contain the warning 'This product contains Olestra. Olestra may cause abdominal cramping and loose stools. Olestra inhibits the absorption of some vitamins and other nutrients. Vitamins A, D, E, and K have been added' (Akoh, 1998).

Lipsch *et al.* (1996) describe a whipped frozen dessert that contains no fat, using monoglyceride emulsifiers to create a smooth, aerated texture. However, this has its own character and is an alternative to ice cream.

17.6.2 Alternative oils and fats for ice cream

There is an alternative to reducing the fat level, or removing it altogether, to reduce the SFA content: utilise a fat that contains less SFA. If it is required to use milkfat in the ice cream (e.g. due to labelling regulations), then it is necessary to seek methods for altering the composition of milkfat. There are two approaches that may be followed. Firstly, the milkfat can be fractionated to remove a stearin with a high level of SFA, leaving an olein with reduced SFA. Secondly, the composition of the milk as produced by the cow can be altered. There are two ways in which to achieve this: diet and genetics.

Fractionation of milkfat involves cooling the molten fat until some part of it crystallises (the stearin), which can then be removed by filtration to leave a liquid oil (olein) with reduced SFA. In this way the SFA can be reduced from about 70% to around 52–58% (Van Aken *et al.*, 1999). However, the yields of such fractions are relatively low and they tend to be quite liquid/soft. Ice cream produced using such lower SFA fractions is not rated as highly as unfractionated milkfat (Abd El-Rahman *et al.*, 1997).

Milk composition varies, to a certain degree, by genetics or breed (Soyeurt and Gengler, 2008). However, the prospect of maintaining separate herds for different end products has been considered impractical (Gibson, 1991). As demand for healthier food products increases, the desirability of low SFA milk may tip the balance of practicality. Much more pragmatic is the approach of feeding cows a diet rich in MUFA or PUFA. In this way, SFA levels in milkfat can be reduced from about 65% to around 50% (Ashes *et al.*, 1997; Fearon *et al.*, 2004). As with the other methods mentioned above, this results in a modest reduction in SFA. Nevertheless, some milk producers have pursued this approach and now market milk with higher levels of unsaturated fatty acids (e.g. Campina, 2010).

With the reduction in SFA and the increase in unsaturated fatty acids, there is a potential problem of greater oxidative degradation. In ice cream, however, Gonzalez *et al.* (2003) showed that two months' storage did not lead to significant differences in the degree of oxidation or hydrolytic rancidity.

The next step to consider is the dilution of milkfat with a liquid oil. Tong *et al.* (1984) have shown that an acceptable overrun can be achieved with high levels (40%) of safflower oil in the fat phase, provided the emulsifier concentration and processing are adjusted. If milkfat can be dispensed with, the obvious first option is to use a liquid oil, such as sunflower oil, in place of the vegetable fats typically used (coconut oil, palm kernel oil, palm oil). However, simply replacing the fat with liquid oil has a detrimental effect on the ice cream properties, such as the rate of melt. The ability of products to resist melting and serum leakage when exposed to ambient temperatures for an extended period of time can be measured by recording the mass loss as a function of time for ice cream blocks placed on a wire mesh positioned over a balance in a temperature controlled cabinet at 20°C. Figure 17.5 shows that an ice cream made with sunflower oil has a much faster

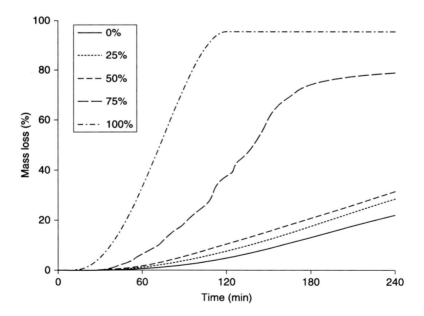

Fig. 17.5   Meltdown profiles for 9% fat ice cream with varying percentages of sunflower oil in a sunflower oil/coconut oil blend.

© Woodhead Publishing Limited, 2011

Table 17.6 Effect of replacing coconut oil with sunflower oil in a 9% fat ice cream on key sensory properties (as scored by a trained taste panel)

Sensory property	Coconut oil	Sunflower oil
Firmness	5.45	4.75
Rate of melt	4.29	4.80
Thickness	4.21	3.58
Creamy flavour	3.07	2.68

meltdown than one made with coconut oil. Table 17.6 shows that it also has an undesirable impact on sensory properties.

As Fig. 17.5 indicates, however, there is some potential for reducing the SFA in the fat phase by using blends of liquid oil and harder fat (in this case, sunflower oil and coconut oil). A blend of 50% coconut oil and 50% sunflower oil shows a slow rate of melt similar to that for 100% coconut oil, indicating that up to half of the coconut oil can be replaced by sunflower oil without significantly affecting the meltdown properties of the ice cream, and reducing the SFA content to 52%, instead of 92%.

The amount of solid fat in an oil globule can influence the amount of adsorbed protein and impact the droplet size, destabilisation and meltdown. Blends of palm kernel oil with 30–50% high-oleic sunflower oil appear to yield optimum properties in this regard (Sung and Goff, 2010). Similarly, blends of palm oil fractions and sunflower oil reportedly are suitable for use in ice cream (Talbot and Slager, 2007; Dilley et al., 2006; Nilsson and Persson, 2009). Blends of similar composition but including coconut oil are also suitable for ice cream (Noor and De Ruiter, 2008). All of these fat blends permit the reduction of SFA, some to as low as around 30–35%. This is about half the level in milkfat and one third that of coconut oil.

As will be clear from the above discussion, there are a variety of ways in which to produce an ice cream having lower SFA. Since the characteristics of the product can vary somewhat from a standard full-fat milkfat or vegetable oil ice cream, it is necessary to choose the option or options that, in the selector's view, compromises the least on product quality.

Ice cream consumption is primarily about fun and enjoyment. Most consumers will not compromise product quality or enjoyment for the sake of improved nutrition. Therefore it is necessary for manufacturers to offer a wide range of products from the highly indulgent, intended for infrequent consumption, through to lower fat/lower calorie/lower SFA products, which are, perhaps, more suited to regular consumption.

17.7   Future trends

There is little doubt that reducing SFA in the diet will remain high on the nutrition agenda. While the immediate focus is on frequently consumed foods, it is also

© Woodhead Publishing Limited, 2011

apparent that ice cream, in many guises, can be seen as one such food. In order to achieve a significant reduction in SFA with minimal compromise on product quality, it is likely that a combination of approaches will be needed. Thus selection of a low SFA fat blend, with some adjustment of the other ingredients (emulsifiers, fat replacers), alongside a change in processing will be required.

There are several examples that illustrate this approach. Some properties (overrun, shape and aeration) of an ice cream made with liquid oil can be improved by excluding emulsifier from the formulation (Quail and Underdown, 2008). By reducing the ageing temperature, certain oils with a reduced level of saturated fat, for example olive oil, can be induced to crystallise, thus enabling optimal fat structure formation during freezing (Bartkowska and Underdown, 2005). A change in the typical ice cream process may also help at low fat levels. According to Burmester *et al.* (2005), 'Low temperature extrusion of ice cream can improve the ice cream quality, compared to that achieved conventionally, or may allow reduction of levels of ingredients such as fat, without loss of quality.' Applying high shear after freezing the ice cream mix can have benefits (Windhab and Tapfer, 2005), apparently restoring the creamy mouthfeel. Advances in homogeniser technology should enable very small fat droplets to be created (Hayes *et al.*, 2003), which could permit the manufacture of lower fat healthier products with similar textural properties to a higher fat ice cream.

One potential route to fat (and SFA) reduction not mentioned above is to increase the overrun of the ice cream, i.e. increase the amount of air! This would work since ice cream is served on a volume, rather than weight, basis. However, overruns can already be very high (e.g. up to 130%), so the challenge exists to incorporate even higher levels of air without compromising product quality and stability.

While there is pressure to produce low-fat, low-SFA ice cream, where it is intended as an everyday food item, the pressure will be less, for the moment, on indulgent treat products, such as chocolate-coated bar/stick products. However, it is likely that attention will eventually fall on these, too.

Finally, it should be noted that the relative health benefits of specific fat types is still a matter of debate. Some researchers question the negative health aspects of SFA (e.g. Siri-Tarino *et al.*, 2010). However, the general consensus remains that individuals should reduce fat, especially saturated fat, in their diet. Consequently there will continue to be a drive to reduce dietary SFA from the current high levels and, thus, there will be a consumer demand for foods, including ice cream, with lower saturated fat content.

17.8   References

Abd El-Rahman A M, Shalabi S I, Hollender R and Kilara A (1997), 'Effect of milk fat fractions on the sensory evaluation of frozen desserts', *J Dairy Sci*, 80, 1936–40.
Akalin A S and Erisir D (2008), 'Effects of inulin and oligofructose on the rheological characterisitics and probiotic culture survival in low-fat probiotic ice cream', *J Food Sci*, 73(4), M184–8.

Akalin A S, Karagözlü C and Ünal G (2008), 'Rheological properties of reduced-fat and low-fat ice cream containing whey protein isolate and inulin', *Eur Food Res Technol*, 227, 889–95.

Akoh C. (1998), 'Fat replacers', *Food Technol*, 52(3) 47–53.

Asher Y J, Mollard M A, Maurice T J and Caldwell K B (1993), 'Process for producing low or non fat ice cream', Patent US 5215777.

Ashes J R, Gulati S K and Scott T W (1997), 'Potential to alter the content and composition of milk fat through nutrition', *J Dairy Sci*, 80, 2204–12.

Baer R J, Wolkow M D and Kasperson K M (1997), 'Effect of emulsifiers on the body and texture of low fat ice cream', *J Dairy Sci*, 80, 3123–32.

Bartkowska B and Underdown J (2005), 'Frozen aerated products and methods for preparation thereof', Patent application US 2005/0042333.

Berger K G (1990), 'Ice cream in food emulsions', in Larsson K and Friberg S E, *Food emulsions, 2nd edn.*, New York, Marcel Dekker, Inc., pp 367–444.

Bramley A S, Gray S J, Turan S M, Spors D D and Frisch S M (2007), 'Low fat frozen confectionery product', Patent application US 2007/0014908.

Bramley A S, Lacy I, Lindner N M and Quail P J (2006), 'Low fat frozen confectionery product', Patent application WO 2006/042632.

Burmester S, Russell A and Cebula D (2005), 'The evolution of ice cream technology', *New Food*, 8(2), 42–5.

Byass L J, Darling D F, Doucet C J and Fenn R A (1998), 'Frozen confectionery products', Patent application WO 98/04148.

Campina (2010), 'Campina milk – the difference starts at the farm gate', Available from: http://www.frieslandcampina.com/english/innovation/innovations/drinks-and-desserts/campina-milk-unsaturated-fatty-acids-outdoor-grazing-selected-farmers.aspx [accessed June 2010].

Chung S-J, Heymann H and Grün I U (2003), 'Temporal release of flavor compounds from low-fat and high-fat ice cream during eating', *J Food Sci*, 68, 2150–6.

Clarke C (2004), *The science of ice cream*, Cambridge, The Royal Society of Chemistry.

Devereux H M, Jones G P, McCormack L and Hunter W C (2003), 'Consumer acceptability of low fat foods containing inulin and oligofructose', *J Food Sci*, 68, 1850–4.

Dilley K M, Greenacre J. Smith K W and Underdown J (2006) 'Frozen aerated confections', Patent application WO 2006/066979.

El-Nagar G, Clowes G, Tudoriĉ C M, Kuri V and Brennan C S (2002), 'Rheological quality and stability of yog-ice cream with added inulin', *Int J Dairy Technol*, 55, 89–93.

Euroglaces (2006), 'Code for Edible Ices', European Association of the Edible Ices Industry vzw, Available from: http://euroglaces.eu/en/upload/docs/Edible%20ices%20codes/English%20-%20Code%20for%20Edible%20Ices%202006.pdf [accessed 16 July 2010].

Fearon A M, Mayne C S, Beattie J A M and Bruce D W (2004), 'Effect of level of oil inclusion in the diet of dairy cows at pasture on animal performance and milk composition and properties', *J Sci Food Agric*, 84, 497–504.

Gelin J L, Poyen L, Courthaudon J L, Le Meste M and Lorient D (1994), 'Structural changes in oil-in-water emulsions during the manufacture of ice cream', *Food Hydrocolloids*, 8, 299–308.

Gibson J P (1991), 'The potential for genetic change in milk fat composition', *J Dairy Sci*, 74, 3258–66.

Goff H D (1997), 'Colloidal aspects of ice cream – a review', *Int Dairy J*, 7, 363–73.

Goff H D (2002), 'Formation and stabilisation of structure in ice-cream and related products', *Current Opinion in Colloid and Interface Sci*, 7, 432–7.

Goff H D (2008), '65 Years of ice cream science', *Int Dairy J*, 18, 754–8.

Goff H D and Jordan W K (1989), 'Action of emulsifiers in promoting fat destabilization during the manufacture of ice cream', *J Dairy Sci*, 72, 18–29.

Goff H D, Verespej E and Smith A K (1999), 'A study of fat and air structures in ice cream', *Int Dairy J*, 9, 817–29.

Gonzalez S, Duncan S E, O'Keefe S F, Sumner S S and Herbein J H (2003), 'Oxidation and textural characteristics of butter and ice cream with modified fatty acid profiles', *J Dairy Sci*, 86, 70–7.

Guinard J-X, Zoumas-morse C, Mori L, Panyam D and Kilara A (1996), 'Effect of sugar and fat on the acceptability of vanilla ice cream', *J Dairy Sci*, 79, 1922–7.

Guinard J-X, Zoumas-Morse C, Mori L, Panyam D and Kilara A (1997), 'Sugar and fat effects on sensory properties of ice cream', *J Food Sci*, 62, 1087–94.

Hayes, M G, Lefrancois, A C, Waldron, D S, Goff H D and Kelly A L (2003) 'Influence of high pressure homogenisation on some characteristics of ice cream', *Milchwissenschaft*, 58, 519–23.

Hyvönen L, Linna M, Tuorila H and Dijksterhuis G (2003), 'Perception of melting and flavour release of ice cream containing different types and contents of fat', *J Dairy Sci*, 86, 1130–8.

Kailasapathy K and Songvanich W (1998), 'Effects of replacing fat in ice cream with fat mimetics', *Food Australia* 50(4), 169–73.

Koxholt M M R, Eisenmann B and Hinrichs J (2001), 'Effect of the fat globule sizes on the meltdown of ice cream', *J Dairy Sci*, 84, 31–7.

Li Z, Marshall R, Heymann H and Fernando L (1997), 'Effect of milk fat content on flavor perception of vanilla ice cream', *J Dairy Sci*, 80, 3133–41.

Lipsch M H, Van Beek M J and Fung Kon Yin J S (1996), 'Zero fat whipped frozen dessert', Patent US 5547697.

Marshall R T and Arbuckle W S (1996), *Ice cream, 5th edn.*, New York, Chapman & Hall.

Marshall R T, Goff H D and Hartel R W (2003), *Ice cream, 6th edn.*, New York, Kluwer/Plenum Publishers.

Nilsson D and Persson M (2009), 'Glyceride mixture for frozen confection', Patent application WO 2009/067069.

Noor A and De Ruiter G A (2008), 'Aerated food product and method of manufacturing such product', Patent application WO 2008/026920.

Ohmes R L, Marshall R T and Heymann H (1998), 'Sensory and physical properties of ice creams containing milk fat or fat replacers', *J Dairy Sci*, 81, 1222–8.

Prindiville E A, Marshall R T and Heymann H (2000) 'Effect of milk fat, cocoa butter, and whey protein fat replacers on the sensory properties of lowfat and nonfat chocolate ice cream', *J Dairy Sci*, 83, 2216–23.

Quail P J and Underdown J (2008), 'Frozen aerated confections and methods for production thereof', Patent application US 2008/0220141.

Regand A and Goff H D (2006), 'Ice recrystallization inhibition in ice cream as affected by ice structuring proteins from winter wheat grass', *J Dairy Sci*, 89, 49–57.

Roland A M, Phillips L G and Boor K J (1999a), 'Effects of fat content on the sensory properties, melting, color and hardness of ice cream', *J Dairy Sci*, 82, 32–8.

Roland A M, Phillips L G and Boor K J (1999b), 'Effects of fat replacers on the sensory properties, color, melting and hardness of ice cream', *J Dairy Sci*, 82, 2094–2100.

Sangeetha P T, Ramesh M N and Prapulla S G (2005), 'Recent trends in the microbial production, analysis and application of fructooligosaccharides', *Trends Food Sci Technol*, 16(10), 442–57.

Schaller-Povolny L A and Smith D E (1999), 'Sensory attributes and storage life of reduced fat ice cream as related to inulin content', *J Food Sci*, 64, 555–9.

Schaller-Povolny L A and Smith D E (2001), 'Viscosity and freezing point of a reduced fat ice cream mix as related to inulin content', *Milchwissenschaft* 56, 25–29.

Schirle-Keller J P, Reineccius G A and Hatchwell L C (1994), 'Flavor interactions with fat replacers: effect of oil level', *J Food Sci*, 59, 813–15.

Siri-Tarino P W, Sun Q, Hu F B and Krauss R M (2010), 'Meta-analysis of prospective cohort studies evaluating the association of saturated fat with cardiovascular disease', *Am J Clin Nutr*, 91(3), 535–46.

© Woodhead Publishing Limited, 2011

Soyeurt H and Gengler N (2008), 'Genetic variability of fatty acids in bovine milk', *Biotechnol Agron Soc Environ*, 12(2), 203–10.

Sung K K and Goff H D (2010), 'Effect of solid fat content on structure in ice creams containing palm kernel oil and high oleic sunflower oil', *J Food Sci*, 75, C274–9.

Talbot G and Slager H (2007), 'Oil alternative in ice cream', *The World of Food Ingredients*, March, 62–3.

Tapfer U and Austin M (1996), 'Ice cream confection', Patent US 5482728.

Thomas J (2009), 'Clouds on the horizon', *Frozen Food Europe*, 21(2), 32–5.

Tong P S, Jordan W K and Houghton G (1984), 'Response surface methodology to study fat destabilization and development of overrun in ice creams produced with polyunsaturated safflower oil and milk fat blends', *J Dairy Sci* 67, 779–93.

USA CFR (2010), 'Frozen Desserts', Code of Federal Regulations (1 April 2010 Edition), Title 21, Ch. I, Part 135, 402–9.

Van Aken G A, Ten Grotenhuis W, Van Langevelde A J and Schenk H (1999), 'Composition and crystallization of milk fat fractions', *J Am Oil Chem Soc*, 76, 1323–31.

Welty W M, Marshall R T, Grün I U and Ellersieck M R (2001), 'Effects of milk fat, cocoa butter, or selected fat replacers on flavor volatiles of chocolate ice cream', *J Dairy Sci*, 84, 21–30.

Whelan R H, Rudolph M J and Petrossian V D (2000), 'Low calorie fat-containing frozen dessert products having smooth, creamy, nongritty mouthfeel', Patent US 6010734.

Windhab E J and Tapfer U (2005), 'Aerated frozen suspension with adjusted creaminess and scoop ability based on stress-controlled generation of superfine microstructures', Patent application US 2005/0037110.

Zhang Z and Goff H D (2005), 'On fat destabilization and composition of the air interface in ice cream containing saturated and unsaturated monoglyceride', *Int Dairy J*, 15, 495–500.

© Woodhead Publishing Limited, 2011

18

Saturated fat reduction in sauces

P. Smith, Cargill R&D Centre Europe, Belgium

Abstract: The reduction of fat in sauces can be a complex issue. This is because the attributes of a sauce are often determined by the fat content. In order to reduce the overall and saturated fat, careful control of the emulsion structure and the role of thickeners must be undertaken. Choice of ingredients is critical for an optimal product. This extends particularly to the emulsifiers and thickeners that will manipulate the structure to give the desired performance. As well as considering the structure of a sauce, its lifetime and breakdown of a product is important. Consideration of the oxidation, flavour development and microbiology of a system is critical. Reduction of saturated fat will mean that more sophisticated techniques may be needed in order to provide a product with a long lifetime. The way in which a system breaks down in the mouth will then determine how it is perceived on eating. As such, the emulsion breakdown and the flavour delivery must be considered.

Key words: sauces and dressings, emulsion science, hydrocolloids, emulsifiers, oxidation, microbiology.

18.1   Introduction

There is a growing desire to produce lower calorie and lower fat – especially lower saturated fat – products. Sauces are a particular target for the food manufacturer because they are typically chosen by the consumer because of their texture, mouthfeel and taste. Fat plays a large role in all of these attributes. We can envisage many sauces from the ketchup and mayonnaise type of cold condiments through to hot cooking sauces. However, in all cases we can think of the same kind of properties and behaviour that are required. Generally the sauces are emulsions and so it is necessary to understand and control the emulsion science and microstructure in order to deliver the sensory properties that are desirable. Also, as well as the sensory properties other factors must come into play in the design of a sauce. The lifetime of a food product must be considered and undesirable changes in physical properties eliminated; also there must be strong consideration of the microbiological behaviour. Nevertheless, it is presumably the sensory performance of the product that is its

© Woodhead Publishing Limited, 2011

major importance. Thus a good grounding in emulsion science is necessary to design a good product. More and more natural and healthy products are desired by the customer. Therefore there will be an increasing drive to deliver these.

18.2   Sensory properties of sauces

18.2.1   Fat content

Creaminess and mouthfeel are the primary attributes of sauces. It is generally desirable to have a thick sauce, implying a high level of fat. The richness of the fat is generally the overriding pleasure from a sauce. However, the creaminess of a food is not actually very dependent upon the fatty content of the food. As long ago as 1977 Kokini *et al..* demonstrated that creaminess could be predicted from perceived thickness, smoothness and slipperiness. Other researchers have expanded on this work and Richardson and Booth (1993) have shown that the role of dairy fat globules or emulsion droplets is critically important. Thus delivering the creaminess is a job for the emulsion scientist rather than his colleague, the fat scientist and it should be possible to deliver the required mouthfeel with any selected fat. An even density of small globules in homogenised milks gives a creamier, smoother and thicker sensation. Also sensations vary from one person to another, suggesting that this knowledge must be learned. Of course one could expect that the amount of fat present in an emulsion could have an effect. Indeed Elmore *et al.* (1999) have shown that in chocolate ice cream higher fat contents of 6% and 9% were creamier than ones of 1.3% or 3.5%. However, Frost *et al.* (2001) revealed that certain increases in fat enhance creaminess more than others, showing that the effect of fat content is not linear.

Furthermore, it has been shown that the four factors that affect the creaminess (Clegg *et al.*, 2003) are oil droplet size, fat content, air bubble size and air content. Thus it can be seen that it is the number and size of the particles in the system that are the most important factor in controlling the mouthfeel of a product. The choice of the components of the particles should not be too important. Thus in order to control the fat level in a system it is necessary to create droplets that can behave in a similar way to the fat. It is necessary to consider how to do this.

There is much more detailed information about the relationship between the different components and their effect on the sensory field that has recently been developed. It is clear that the actual role of creaminess must also depend on the nature of the system in the mouth. Therefore interactions of the emulsion system with the saliva are important and the rate and manner of the breakdown of the system in the mouth should play a significant role. Therefore one needs to consider the way in which the emulsion interacts with saliva, more particularly with the enzymes such as saliva in the mouth. The way in which the broken-down fat lubricates the mouth is then important (De Wijk *et al.*, 2003). Of course the fat is not the only important factor in this kind of system. Other factors such as thickener type must also be considered in the lubricating behaviour. We should consider the rheological and tribological (friction) effects of a system in order to be able to predict its behaviour (Le Reverend *et al.*, 2010).

© Woodhead Publishing Limited, 2011

The manner in which a food is processed in the mouth also plays a role. Chewing, etc can be thought to be important. Perceived creaminess may increase by up to 75% with increasingly complex movements of the mouth (De Wijk *et al.*, 2006).

18.2.2   Texturising systems

If we desire to get away from a very high fat system then we need to carefully structure a sauce emulsion. In order to fully understand a sauce we need to consider the role of thickeners.

18.2.3   Hydrocolloids

Hydrocolloids are the most common thickeners. We can think of a wide range such as locust bean gum (LBG), carageenan, guar, starches, etc. The structure of a system is usually made and controlled by use of thickening and gelling agents. Most commonly polysaccharides and protein hydrocolloids are used. They can be natural or chemically modified and may come from a wide range of different sources, usually from seaweed, plants, algae or insects. The most important properties are summarised below.

Aqueous solubility
It is necessary for the thickener to be present in the aqueous phase.

Thickening
The hydrocolloids form suspensions, solutions and colloidal suspensions that are non-Newtonian fluids. Polysaccharide hydrocolloids are very effective at this and thus are preferentially used.

Gelling ability
The chains of the hydrocolloids can interact, forming a network. By means of this the overall structure of the system can be controlled. It may be possible to have a system that contains 1% polymer and 99% water in a strong gel (Whistler and BeMiller, 1977). Thus careful control is needed for the correct properties of the system desired. The gelling can be influenced and controlled by different factors (thermal, chemical or thermo-chemical) (Glicksmann, 1982).

Morris (1991) investigated how, by using two different polysaccharides, mixed gels could be created. These can give much more complex and subtle behaviours. It is possible to have independent or interlocked systems. Depending upon how the thickeners interact the properties can be enhanced or we can have two different networks breaking separately and so providing a complex texture upon eating. The nature of the network will depend upon the specific interactions and behaviours of the two systems. Chemical consideration will need to be undertaken in order to see how they will behave. The colloid chemist will be ideally placed to develop new systems with specific requirements.

© Woodhead Publishing Limited, 2011

18.2.4   Emulsion behaviour

As well as thickening and gelling, hydrocolloids can stabilise emulsions and foams by means of their amphiphilic and film forming nature (Morris *et al.*, 1980). The role and application of polysaccharide thickeners in these cases is relevant in controlling the properties.

Solubility

Solubility is of course important for a thickener but 100% solubility is not necessarily required (Liao and Mangino, 1987). Solubility is based on many factors, such as molecular size and charge and specific interactions. Generally, higher charge density and lower hydrophobicity are required for good solubilisation.

Viscosity

The viscosity is important in determining the behaviour of a system. Generally larger molecular weight, flexible hydrophilic biopolymers will give higher viscosities.

Emulsification properties

Amphiphilic molecules will act as emulsifiers and so it is clear that this will be a property of thickeners. A study of the effect of corn starch with treated corn starch (Singhal and Kulkarni, 2000) showed that breakdown occurred much earlier for the untreated system as it had much worse emulsification properties.

18.2.5   Choice of polymeric emulsifiers

Carbohydrates

Different carbohydrates can be used as emulsifiers. The systems are well described in the literature. Modified hydrocolloids can be used to enhance the properties as well as emulsifiers made out of non-emulsifying starting material (Stewart and Mazza, 2000).

Proteins

The emulsifying power of a protein depends on the solubility and surface activity (Bergenstahl and Claesson, 1990). Effective emulsifiers are soluble and denature at the interface to form a surface film. Commonly used proteins are milk proteins and whey proteins.

18.3   Product lifetime

The lifetime of a product will be critically important to its use. Therefore, as well as considering how we can build up structures without help from solid, saturated fats, we also need to see how they are damaged and destroyed and how the new ingredients in a system may decay over time. By doing this, great-tasting products with longer lives can be developed.

© Woodhead Publishing Limited, 2011

18.3.1   Oxidation

Oxidative stability of an emulsion will tend to be a critical factor in considering its lifetime. This will become more and more important as the drive to include healthier oils in a system is increased. To prevent oxidation, free radicals must not come into contact with the oil. There are different ways of helping to achieve this. Higher pHs and lower storage temperatures (Mistry and Min, 1992) lead to lower amounts of oxygen in an oil. Chemical antioxidants such as butylated hydroxyanisole (BHA), butylated hydroxytoluene (BHT) and tertiary butylhydroquinone (TBHQ) may also be used. As well as antioxidants it may be necessary to prevent metal ions from entering the oils at all. Therefore materials can be added to the aqueous phase as well. An example of such a commonly used metal sequestrant is ethylenediaminetetraacetic acid (EDTA). Many of these materials are more or less controversial due to their possible health implications and so more natural products are desirable. Different natural extracts of products such as sage, rosemary and oregano (Abdalla and Roozen, 2001) can be used as antioxidants. However, these may naturally have taste implications for a milder tasting product.

Light can catalyse the reactions that lead to oxidation. This may be wavelength dependent. For example, blue light encourages oxidation in mayonnaise (Lennertsen and Lignert, 2000). Oxidation caused by light is also accelerated when photosensitising agents such as carotenoids are present. The cool fluorescent lights that are commonly found in supermarkets are particularly strong emitters of this 'blue' wavelength. This means that serious packaging considerations are needed.

18.3.2   Emulsion breakdown

Interaction between droplets and then the breakdown of an emulsion is affected by very many different factors. Polyvalent ions can promote interactions which can lead to droplet clumping and breakdown. Thus the presence of salt may affect the system significantly. Also sucrose may weaken interactions and certain hydrocolloids and proteins form cross links between the droplets, so effectively encouraging breakdown as shown by Yang and Cotterill (1989) as well as Kiosseoglu and Sherman (1983).

18.3.3   Flavour stability

The flavour delivery of a sauce will depend upon the components in the aqueous and the fat phases. As the sauce is diluted by saliva and warmed, the rates of delivery from the different phases will be different. In the first instance the flavours in the aqueous phase will be detected and longer flavours will come from the fat phase (McClements and Demetriades, 1998). Any interactions in storage may of course affect this and lead to a much less desirable product for the consumer.

18.3.4   Microbiology

The microbiological behaviour of oil-in-water systems presents a certain risk. This is because the water phase is continuous and so pathogens can easily be well

© Woodhead Publishing Limited, 2011

distributed throughout the entire system. Therefore it is necessary to carefully consider the pathogen route and possibility of attack of a specific product. The nature of the nutrients contained in a product may also lead to a system with more or less risk.

Often vinegar is added to dressings. The pH was the most significant factor in destroying bacteria (Smittle and Cirigliano, 1992), and keeping a pH of below around 4.4 gives products with acceptable lifetimes of 9 to 12 months. Salad dressings and mayonnaises can be particularly vulnerable because of the presence of egg in the system. Many fast-food restaurant and street-vended sauces can contain high amounts of pathogens. Estrada-Garcia *et al.* (2002) found very high contamination for chilli sauces in Mexico. Consequently significant and special care must be taken by a manufacturer to reduce risk in these areas. Salt can also play an important role. However, there is currently a very strong drive to reduce the amount of salt in the diet. Thus alternatives must be considered. However, these may not be as effective, or may potentially have off flavours and so cannot necessarily be easily added to a pre-designed product. Packaging can also be expected to play a role. It should be clear that the pathogens must be kept away from the product. This leads to the application of specific impermeable packaging for critical performance.

18.4   Conclusions

We can see that the behaviour of sauces is extremely complex. Many different factors are necessary in order for the development of a new system. In particular we should consider the mouthfeel that we wish to have and then work out how this can be designed by the correct control of the microstructure. Thereafter the thickness and gelling of a system becomes important. Correct choice of hydrocolloid will be required to give desirable and expected properties. However, as well as the physical and chemical aspects of building the sauce the ways in which it can be damaged also need to be taken into account. In particular, factors such as microbiology and oxidative stability can be very important if we are to produce a system with any lifetime whatsoever. Finally, and most importantly, the effect of the sauce to delight the customer must be the ultimate goal of any such product.

18.5   Future trends

Overall in the food industry there is a strong drive to manufacture healthier products. In sauces this can lead to the use of healthier, more unsaturated oils (that are more susceptible to oxidation), the elimination of effective chemical antioxidants and preservatives, the shortening of the ingredients list and a shift to kitchen ingredients. Sauce developers currently have an armoury of different materials to use. The above-mentioned drives are reducing the choice of weapons

© Woodhead Publishing Limited, 2011

for the sauce designer. As such, careful consideration of the use of natural products and the application and control of systems by natural means is necessary. It can only be imagined that this drive will continue at an ever-increasing rate and so the search for new ways of control and possibilities for property manipulation must continue as the drive for new products progresses. In particular we should look at removing calorific ingredients such as fat and potentially replacing them with air bubbles that can give a 'fatty' performance. In order to do this the colloidal structure of foods must be well understood and utilised (Le Reverend *et al.*, 2010).

As well as the desire for healthy foods, more indulgent products are also demanded. In order to achieve this it will be necessary to further optimise and control the thickener and develop emulsion properties that can give the expected products. This will be particularly the case for low-fat products.

Looking into a crystal ball it seems that, certainly for the upcoming decade, these will be the most important drivers for the product developer to consider. There will be a corresponding push back from the developer to the ingredient manufacturer in order to provide him with new products that can be utilised in these novel systems. Non-chemical treatment and 'natural' will be the watchwords.

18.6   Sources of further information and advice

Food Emulsifiers and their Applications, eds. Hasenhuettl GL and Hartel RW, 2008, Springer, New York, USA.
Food Stabilizers, Thickeners and Gelling Agents, ed. Imeson A, 2009, Wiley Blackwell, Chichester, UK.
Cargill Texturizing Solutions: http://www.cargilltexturising.com

18.7   References

Abdalla AE and Roozen JP, 2001, The effects of stabilized extracts of sage and oregano on the oxidation of salad dressings *Eur. Food Res Technol.* 212: 551–60.
Bergenstahl BA and Claesson PM, 1990, Surface Forces in Emulsions in *Food Emulsions* ed. Larsson K. and Friberg SE, Marcel Dekker Inc, New York, USA, pp 41–96.
Clegg S, Kilcast D and Arazi S, 2003, The structural and compositional basis of creaminess in food emulsion gels in *Proceedings of the third international symposium on food rheology*, pp 373–7.
De Wijk RA, Prinz JF and Engelen L, 2003, The role of intra-oral manipulation in the perception of sensory attributes, *Appetite* 40: 1–7.
De Wijk RA, Terpstra MEJ, Janssen AM and Prinz JF, 2006, Perceived creaminess of semi-solid foods, *Trends Food Sci. Technol.* 17: 412–22.
Elmore JR, Heymann H, Johnson J and Hewett JE, 1999, Preference mapping, relating acceptance of creaminess to a descriptive model of a semi-solid, *Food Qual. Pref.* 10: 465–75.
Estrada-Garcia T, Cerna JF, Thompson MR and Lopez-Saucedo C, 2002, Faecal contamination and enterotoxigenic Eschericha *coli* in street vended chilli sauces in Mexico and its public health relevance *Epidemiology Infect* 129: 223–36.
Frost MB, Dijksterhuis C and Martens M, 2001, Sensory Perception of Milk, *Food Qual. Pref.* 12: 327–36.

LIBRARY, UNIVERSITY OF CHESTER

Glicksmann M, 1982, *Food Hydrocolloids* vol. 1, CRC Press, Boca Raton, Florida, USA.

Kiosseoglu VD and Sherman P, 1983, Influence of egg yolk lipoproteins on the rheology and stability of oil/water emulsions and mayonnaise 1. Viscoelasticity of groundnut oil-in-water emulsions and mayonnaise, *J. Text. Studies* 14: 397–417.

Kokini JL, Kadane J and Cussler EL, 1977, Liquid texture perceived in the mouth, *J. Texture Studies 8*: 195–218.

Lennertsen M and Lignert H, 2000, Influence of wavelength and packaging material on lipid oxidation and colour change in low-fat mayonnaise, *Lebens. Wiss. Technol.* 33: 253–60.

Le Reverend BJD, Norton IT, Cox PW and Spyropoulos F, 2010, Colloidal aspects of eating, *Current Op. Coll. Interf. Sci.* 15: 84–9.

Liao SY and Mangino ME, 1987, Characterisation of the composition, physiochemical and functional properties of acid whey protein concentrates, *J. Food Sci. 52*: 1033–7.

McClements DJ and Demetriades K, 1998, An integrated approach to the development of reduced fat food emulsions *Crit. Rev. Food Sci. Nut.* 38: 511–36.

Mistry B and Min DB, 1992, Reduction of dissolved oxygen in model salad dressing by glucose oxidase-catalase dependent on pH and temperature *J. Food Sci.* 57: 196–9.

Morris ER, Rees DA and Robinson G, 1980, Cation-specific aggregation helices: domain model of polymer: polymer gel structure *J. Mol. Biol.* 138: 196–9.

Morris V.J, 1991, Weak and strong polysaccharide gels pp 310–321 in *Food Polymers and Colloids* ed. Dickenson E, RSC, London, UK.

Richardson NJ and Booth DA, 1993, Effect of homogenization and fat content on oral perception of low and high viscosity model creams *J Sens. Studies* 8: 133–43.

Singhal RS and Kulkarni PR, 2000, Utilisation of Rajgeera starch in salad dressing *Starch/ Sterke*, 42: 52–3.

Smittle RB and Cirigliano MC, 1992, Salad Dressings pp 975–983 in *Compendium of Methods for Microbiological Examination of Foods*, eds Vanderzant C and Spittstoesser DF, American Public Health Association, Washington DC, USA.

Stewart S and Mazza G, 2000, Effect of flaxseed gum on quality and stability of a model salad dressing, J. *Food Qual.* 24: 373–90.

Whistler RL and BeMiller JN, 1977, *Carbohydrate chemistry for food scientists*, Eagen Press, St Paul, Minnesota, USA., pp 63–217.

Yang S and Cotterill OJ, 1989, Physical and functional properties of 10% salted egg yolk in mayonnaise, *J. Food Sci.* 54: 210–13.

© Woodhead Publishing Limited, 2011

Index

α-tending emulsifiers, 141
acetic acid esters, 141
acrylamide, 271–2
aerated products, 151–2
African palm oil *see Elaeis guineensis*
American Heart Association, 90–1
American palm oil *see Elaeis olifera*
analogue milk *see* filled milk
anhydrous milk fat, 64, 188
animal bone, 196
animal carcass fats, 65–6
    fatty acid compositions, 66
    lard, beef tallow, sheep and deer fats,
      65–6
      saturated fat contents of fats from pig
        and beef carcasses, 65
animal fats, 210
animal feeds, 134
animal production, 196–203
APcI-MS *see* atmospheric pressure
    chemical ionisation-mass
    spectrometry
apolipoproteins, 78
asparaginase, 272
atherogenesis, 78–9
    lipid hypothesis, 78, 79
      total energy percentage from SFA in
        the diets, 79
    lipoproteins, 78–9
      characteristics, 79
atmospheric pressure chemical
    ionisation-mass spectrometry, 37

β-carotene, 120, 121
bacon, 215

bad cholesterol *see* low-density lipoproteins
barley-β-glucan, 217
beef dripping, 66
beef patties, 212–15
beef tallow *see* beef dripping
behenic acid, 340
Benefat, 363
beta-glucan, 147
BHA *see* butylated hydroxyanisole
BHT *see* butylated hydroxytoluene
Biscuitine 580, 346
biscuits
    fat replacers, 295–8
      effect of emulsifiers on fat coating of
        gluten, 297
      emulsifiers, 296–7
      fibres, 297–8
      hydrocolloids, 297
      starches, 296
    fat substitutes, 298–9
      change the backbone of the fat, 298
      change the fatty acids, 298
      reduce the number of fatty acids, 299
    saturated fat reduction, 283–99
      future trends, 299
      saturated fat content of McVitie's
        plain biscuits, 293
      techniques for saturates reduction,
        289–99
      use of fats with lower levels of
        saturates, 293–5
    technology of biscuits, 285–9
      coated biscuits, 288–9
      crackers, 285–7
      hard sweet and semi-sweet biscuits, 287

© Woodhead Publishing Limited, 2011

sandwich/filled biscuits, 288
short dough biscuits, 287–8
wafers, 288
total fat content reduction, 289–93
coating fat, 292
cryo-crystallisation, 291
dough fat, 289–91
influence of fat content on viscosity
of chocolate, 292
laminating fat, 291–2
spray oils, 293
types of fat used, 284–5
saturated fat content as percentage of
total fat, 285
solid fat content of typical dough
fat, 284
BOB, 339–40
bologna, 218–25, 224
Book of the Pig, 195–6
bovine milk, 182–4, 252, 254
breakfast sausage, 215–18
Bruker Avance 300, 306
burgers, 212–15
butchered meat
animal production, 196–203
animal growth and selection for
slaughter, 196–7
carcass composition assessment, 197–9
beef and lamb carcasses, 198–9
instruments approved for pig carcass
classification, 198
pig carcasses, 197–8
carcass fatness changes over time,
199–202
carcass quality of cattle and sheep,
200–1
changes in average carcass
characteristics of pigs, 199
changes in fat available for
consumption, 201–2
fat class distribution for lamb
carcasses, 201
fat class distribution for prime beef
carcasses, 201
reduction in fat content of pig
carcasses, 199–200
cooking and plate waste, 204–5
effect of cooking on fat content, 204
trimming on the plate, 205
current carcass composition, 202–3
estimated physical composition of
beef carcasses, 202
fatty acid composition, 203
overall carcass composition, 202

fat reduction on meat quality, 205–6
fat in meat and juiciness, 206
fatness and flavour, 206
role of fat in meat tenderness, 205–6
preparation of cuts, 203–4
changes to butchery, 203–4
mince, 204
saturated fat reduction, 195–207
future trends, 207
butter, 64, 134, 187–9
composition, 187
butterfat, 13, 14
consumption, 14
butylated hydroxyanisole, 374
butylated hydroxytoluene, 374
butyric acid, 99

cakes, 22–3
cancer, 90
canola oil, 115
CAOBISCO, 319, 321
caprenin, 363
carbohydrates, 91, 92, 102
carboxymethyl cellulose, 217, 224–5
cardiovascular diseases, 77, 100, 113
carrageenan, 225
carrageenan gum, 213
carrageenan patties, 213
CBE *see* cocoa butter equivalents
CHD *see* coronary heart disease
Cheddar, 186, 190
cheddaring time, 186
cheese, 33, 34, 184–7
see also specific types
fat contents of certain varieties, 185
processed cheese, 186–7
Cheeses in Brine, 185
chocolate, 137, 319
base composition (total fat 30%), 326
containing cocoa butter oleine (total fat
30%), 331
EU chocolate
basic vegetable oils triglyceride
composition, 323
fatty acid composition of cocoa butter
and vegetable oils and fractions,
324
triglyceride composition of vegetable
fats and fractions used, 323
fatty acid composition of cocoa butter
from different origins, 322
legislative constraints, 325–6
other health benefits of chocolate, 333
saturated fat reduction, 321–33

© Woodhead Publishing Limited, 2011

future trends, 346–7
scope for and effects of saturated fat
    reduction, 326–32
    chocolate viscosity vs fat content, 328
    different type of cocoa butter, 328–30
    effect of reducing total fat from 30%
        to 25%, 327
    more saturated vegetable fat, 330–2
    palm oleine as the CBE, 332
    reduce total fat, 327–8
    softer cocoa butter and cocoa
        mass, 329
    softer fraction of cocoa butter, 330
    stearic acid effects, 332–3
choux pastry, 304–5
chronic disease
    associated with different dietary
        saturated fatty acids, 98–108
    chronic disease risk differences
        between different SFA, 100–5
    chronic disease risk effects of stearic
        acid, 105–6, 107
    future trends, 106, 108
    key dietary saturated fatty acids,
        99–100
chylomicrons, 78
cis configuration, 7
cis fatty acids, 67, 68
    structures, 67
cis unsaturated fatty acids, 18–19
Citri-fi, 214
CLA *see* conjugated linoleic acid
coagulation, 184
coarse-ground sausages, 215–18
coated biscuits, 288–9
coated meat products, 227–9
cocoa *see* Theobroma cacao
cocoa butter, 57–61, 137, 321, 328–9
    fatty acid composition, 324
cocoa butter equivalents, 57–61, 323, 334
    base oils SOS triglyceride
        compositions, 60
    fatty acid composition of base oils, 60
    triglyceride composition, 61
cocoa butter oleine, 330
coconut milk, 134
coconut oil, 12–13, 53–6, 352, 359
    carbon number triglyceride
        compositions, 54
    consumption, 13
    fatty acid compositions, 54
    melting profiles, 55
Code of Federal Regulations, 325
Code of Practice for Yoghurt, 183

Codex Alimentarius Commission, 181, 325
Codex General Standard for Cheese, 184
Codex General Standard for the Use of
    Dairy Terms, 181
CODEX STAN 243–2003, 183
CODEX STAN 253–2006, 188–9
CODEX STAN 253–2007, 189
CODEX STAN 263–1966, 185
Codex Standard for Fermented Milks, 183
cold shortening, 206
cold water swelling, 214
collagen hydrolysate, 149
Commission Decision 2004/370/EC, 197
Commission Directive 2000/36/EC, 289
Commission Directive 2001/101/EC, 195
Common Agricultural Policy, 200
compound coatings, 319
    comparison of confectionery coating
        fats, 337
    effect of removing *trans* fats, 334–6
    fatty acid composition of lauric CBS
        compound coating fats, 335
    potential for novel compound coating
        compositions, 338–41
    behenic-oleic triglycerides fatty acid
        composition, 340
    effect of chain length and
        unsaturation on fatty acid
        melting, 339
    saturated fat reduction, 333–41
    future trends, 346–7
    scope, 336–8
confounders, 86
conjugated linoleic acid, 257, 259
cooked salami, 215–18
coronary heart disease, 17, 77, 98, 113
coronary vascular disease, 17
cottage cheese, 137
Council Regulation (EC) 1234/2007,
    181, 197
Couva 850 NH, 336
cow's milk *see* bovine milk
crackers, 285–7
    cream crackers, 285–6
    puff biscuits, 286
    savoury crackers, 286
cream, 134
cream crackers, 285–6
cream fats, 288
croissants, 302
cross-modal interaction, 32
crude palm oil, 49, 120, 122
cryo-crystallisation, 151, 153, 290, 291
CVD *see* cardiovascular diseases

© Woodhead Publishing Limited, 2011

DAG oils *see* diacylglycerol oils
dairy ice cream, 351, 360
Dairy-Lo, 362
dairy products, 179–90
Danish pastry, 302, 307–8
DATEM *see* diacetyl tartaric ester of
    monoglyceride
de-oiling process, 276
Deliair NH, 346
Delyte, 296
denatured whey protein isolate, 228
DGAT *see* diacylglycerol acyltransferase
diacetyl tartaric ester of monoglyceride,
    141, 145, 150, 297
diacylglycerol, 299
diacylglycerol acyltransferase, 162
diacylglycerol oils, 21–2, 159, 299
    chemistry, 159–61
        crystal arrangement, 161
        structures of various isoforms, 160
    digestion, absorption and metabolism,
        161–4
    health benefits, 162–4
    nutritional aspects and applications in
        foods, 158–74
    future trends, 173–4
    product application patents, 167–72
        DAG containing-foods, 171
        frying applications, 171
        ice-cream coating fats, 171–2
        oil composition containing
            phytosterols, 170
        oil composition for physiological
            benefits, 167–9
        oil-in-water type emulsion foods, 169
        shortenings, 170–1
        water-in-oil type emulsion foods,
            169–70
    production process patents, 164–7
        process parameters on DAG and TAG
            yields, 166
    regulatory status, 172–3
    safety, 172–3
dietary fats, 32, 99
    sources, 47–73
        animal carcass fats, 65–6
        future trends, 73
        hydrogenated fats, 67–9
        mammalian milk fats, 61–4
        trans effect, 69–73
        vegetable oils rich in saturated fats,
            48–61
Directive 2000/36/EC, 325
domestic disappearance, 10, 71

double emulsions, 133
doughnuts, 22–3
dressings, 375
droplet attractive interactions, 315
dry fermented sausages, 225–7
dry fractionation, 51
dry salami, 225–7
duplex emulsions, 20, 133
DWPI *see* denatured whey protein isolate

Eatwell Plate, 179–80
EBLEX Better Returns Programme, 197
EBV *see* Estimated Breeding Values
EDTA *see* ethylenediaminetetraacetic acid
Elaeis guineensis, 48, 112
Elaeis olifera, 48
elaidic acid, 82
emulsifiers, 132, 135–6
    fat phase structuring, 141–2
emulsion, 131–53
    applications, 151–2
        aerated products, 151–2
        cryo-scanning electron micrograph of
            a whipped cream, 151
        frozen products, 152
    droplets, 138–41
        aggregation, 138–40
        size changes, 140–1
    emulsifiers, 132
    fat composition, 134–8
        changes, 134–6
        cheese products, 135
        fat level changes, 136–8
        food emulsions, 136
    fat replacers, 146–50
        examples, 148
        ingredients, 147–9
        structures, 149–50
    future trends, 152–3
        controlled aggregation of O/W
            emulsions, 153
        cryo-crystallisation, 153
        fat replacers, 152–3
        W/O/W multiple emulsions, 153
    multiple emulsions, 133
    oil and water in foods, 131
    oil-in-water emulsions, 132
        mayonnaise-type product, 132
    phase structuring and emulsions,
        141–6
        fat phase structuring, 141–2
        oil-in-water-in-oil multiple
            emulsions, 145
        oil-in-water-in-water emulsions, 146

© Woodhead Publishing Limited, 2011

water-in-oil-in-water multiple
    emulsions, 142–5
water phase structuring, 146
processing, 150–1
    cryo-crystallisation, 151
    interesterification, 150
water-in-oil emulsions, 132–3
    spread-type products, 133
water-in-oil-in-water emulsion, 133
emulsion droplets, 32, 33, 34, 138–41
    aggregation, 138–40
        characterisation of aggregated
            structures, 139–40
        ingredients for controlled
            aggregation, 138–9
        processing for controlled
            aggregation, 139
emulsion technology, 20
emulsion-type sausages, 218–25
energy intake, 100, 105
English method, 306
Enova, 299
enzyme-catalysed interesterification, 21
erucic acid, 340
Estimated Breeding Values, 200
Etenia, 296
ethnic dishes, 24
ethylenediaminetetraacetic acid, 374
EU Chocolate Directive, 326–32
EU Regulation 1234/2007, 189
Euroglaces code, 360
EUROP, 198
European Community Scale, 198–9
European Community Scale for beef
    carcass, 198
European Union Chocolate Directive,
    59, 61
eutectic formation, 343
Expert Consultation on Fats and Fatty
    Acids in Human Nutrition, 190
extensible dough, 302

Factor VII, 85
Factor VIIa, 333
familial hypercholesterolemia, 86
fat carcasses, 196
fat composition, 134–8
    changes, 134–6
        alternative oils and blends, 135, 136
        animal feeds, 134
        cheese products, 135
        emulsifiers, 135–6
        filled emulsions, 134–5
        food emulsions, 136

fat level changes, 136–8
    oil-in-water emulsions, 137
    water-in-oil emulsions, 137–8
fat fraction, 188
fat phase structuring, 141–2
fat replacement, 146–50
fat replacers, 19–20, 146–50, 152–3,
    295–8
fat sparing, 296
fats, 5
    aroma carrier, 35–8, 39
        aroma solvent, 36–7
        differences of retro-nasal aroma
            release during consumption, 39
        fat affecting aroma release, 37–8, 39
        yoghurts average *in vivo* flavour
            release curves, 37
    consequences for strategies to reduce
        fat, 41–2
    engineering fat to tailor appetite, 38,
        40–1
        change in satiation VAS rating after
            stimulation with aroma, 41
    functional attributes in foods,
        29–43
    future trends, 42–3
    perception, 30–2
        hearing, 30
        smell, 30–1
        taste, 31–2
        touch, 30
    role in foods texture, 33–8, 39
        friction coefficient for commercial
            dairy products varying in fat
            content, 35
        lubricant, 34–5
        texturiser, 33–4
fattening, 195
fatty acids
    chemistry and structure, 5–10
    saturated fats consumption in EU, US
        and UK, 10–15
        butterfat, 13
        coconut oil, 12–13
        lard, 13–15
        palm kernel oil, 12
        palm oil, 10–12
    triglycerides chemistry and structure
        food groups contributions to total and
            saturated fat intake, 6–7
feed, 189, 190
fermented milk, 183–4
fibrinogen, 85
filled confectionery products, 319

potential for novel filling compositions, 345–6
saturated fat reduction, 341–6
    future trends, 346–7
    scope for and effects of saturated fat reduction, 342–5
        effects of oil migration from lauric and non-lauric filling fats, 343
        fatty acid composition of typical filling fats, 342
        net migration of hazelnut oil into a chocolate, 344
        saturated fat contents of filled chocolates, 342
filled emulsions, 134–5
filled milk, 183
filling, 288
filling fats, 341
finishing, 195
fish sausage, 222
fluid shortenings, 294
foam cells, 80
Food for Specified Health Use, 172
foods
    fats functional attributes, 29–43
        consequences for strategies to reduce fat, 41–2
        engineering fat to tailor appetite, 38, 40–1
        future trends, 42–3
        perception, 30–2
        role in foods texture, 33–8, 39
    saturated fats and their replacement strategies, 3–26
        fatty acids and triglycerides chemistry and structure, 5–10
        future trends, 25–6
        need to reduce saturated fats, 3–5
        replacements for saturates, 18–22
        saturated fat and fatty acid consumption in EU, US and UK, 10–15
        saturates effects on cardiovascular disease, 15–17
FOSHU see Food for Specified Health Use
fractionation, 21, 50, 54, 55, 59, 112, 188
    see also specific fractionation
frankfurters, 218–25
French method, 306
fresh cheese, 184
friable mixtures, 302
fried foods
    effects of frying oils and frying parameters on quality, 268–74

acrylamide content, 271–3
fat uptake, 268–70
quality of frying oil and its effect on storage stability, 273–4
texture, 270–1
fatty acid composition of frying oils, 268
frying oils, 267–8
innovating technologies in frying and their impact on quality, 274–7
    microwave frying, 277
    vacuum frying, 275–7
saturated fat reduction, 266–79
    future trends, 279
frozen products, 152
frying oils, 267–8
    fatty acid composition, 268
    quality and its effect on storage stability of fried foods, 273–4
furaneol, 35

Garibaldi, 287
GDL see glucono-δ–lactone
GEFI test, 307
gelation, 152
generally recognised as safe, 159, 172
ghee, 64
glucono-δ–lactone, 152
good cholesterol see high-density lipoproteins
Good fry oil, 268
GRAS see generally recognised as safe
ground meat products, 212–15
guar gum, 147

'half-fat-to-flour' ratio, 302
hard palm stearin, 51
hard sweet biscuits, 287
hardening see hydrogenation
HD-WPI see heat-denatured whey protein isolate
HDL see high-density lipoproteins
health aspects
    saturated fatty acids, 77–93
        atherosclerosis as the basis for cardiovascular diseases, 78–81
        cancer, 90
        dietary recommendations, 90–2
        effects on disease states related to cardiovascular disease, 88–90
        evidence linking LDL to atherosclerosis and CHD development, 85–8

fatty acids effects on other biomarkers related to coronary heart disease, 84–5
individual fatty acids effects on plasma total cholesterol, LDL, HDL and VLDL, 81–4
trends in consumption as related to CVD mortality and incidence, 92
'Healthy Econa Cooking Oil,' 159
heat-denatured whey protein isolate, 146
HeatWave fryers, 275
high-density lipoproteins, 15, 68, 79, 80, 100, 101, 102, 113, 134, 164, 219
high oleic sunflower oil, 114
HLB see hydrophilic-lipophilic balance
HobNobs, 293
homozygous apoE4, 103
HPKO see hydrogenated palm kernel oil
HPKO35, 336, 338
HPKS see hydrogenated palm kernel stearin
hydrocolloid gums, 221
hydrogenated fats, 67–9
    cis and trans fatty acids structures, 67
hydrogenated palm kernel oil, 335
hydrogenated palm kernel stearin, 335
hydrogenated soybean oil, 114
hydrogenation, 20–1, 50, 52, 54, 67, 312
hydrophilic-lipophilic balance, 170
hypercholesterolemia, 85, 86

ice cream
    basic components and processing, 352–3
        basic elements, 352
        contribution of calories from ice cream ingredients, 352
        processing, 352–3
    challenges associated with saturated fat reduction, 359–65
        alternative oils and fats, 363–5
        effect of replacing coconut oil with sunflower oil, 365
        fat reduction and replacement, 361–3
        meltdown profiles for 9% fat ice cream, 364
    consumption and dietary impact, 351–2
    definition, 351
    function of fat, 354–8
        creaminess, 357
        creamy texture as function of fat content, 357
        emulsion properties, 354
        fat destabilisation, 354–5

fat droplets absorbed at the air bubble surface, 356
fat particle size distribution, 355
flavour delivery, 357–8
foam stabilisation, 355–6
frozen product structural stability, 356–7
future trends, 365–6
historical context, 350–1
properties of fats used in current products, 358–9, 360
    fat composition, 358
    fat crystallisation, 358–9
    fatty acid compositions, 358
    isothermal crystallisation profiles, 360
    solid fat contents for different fat types, 359
saturated fat reduction, 350–66
sources of fat and saturated fat, 353–4
    energy contribution in multi-component ice cream, 354
    nutritional breakdown for common components used, 353
ice-cream coating fats, 171–2
ice cups, 56
IHD see ischemic heart disease
insulin sensitivity, 90
interesterification, 50, 52–3, 54, 150, 313
intramuscular fat, 237
inulin, 137, 225
ionic coemulsifiers, 141
ionophores, 255
iota carrageenan, 213, 216, 221
ischemic heart disease, 77–8
Italian 'cornetto,' 302
Italian salami, 226

Japanese breadcrumb patties, 228

Kettle Chips, 278
konjac flour, 216
konjac gels, 216–17
Kozeny-Carman's equation, 165–6
kung-wans, 219, 221

lactic acid esters, 141
lard, 13–15, 65–6
    consumption, 14
lauric acid, 82, 100, 101, 334
lauric cocoa butter substitutes, 334
lauric fat, 53, 288
LDL see low-density lipoproteins
lecithin, 297
lemon albedo, 222–3

© Woodhead Publishing Limited, 2011

lingual lipase, 32
linoleic acid, 8
linolenic acid, 8
lipid fat replacers, 362
lipid hypothesis, 77, 78, 79, 258
lipoproteins, 78–9, 81
    characteristics, 79
long-mixing time method, 307
low-density lipoproteins, 15, 68, 78, 80,
    100, 101, 102, 113, 180
low-fat milks, 183
lubrication theory, 310

MAG see monoacylglycerols
Maillard browning reactions, 271,
    276, 277
maltodextrin, 213, 222
mammalian milk fats, 61–4
marbling, 205, 237
margarine, 303, 311–14
Marie, 287
mayonnaise, 33, 374, 375
McLean Delux hamburger, 213
MCT see medium chain triglycerides
McVitie's Light Digestives, 290, 293–4
    saturated fat content of McVitie's plain
        biscuits, 293
meat, 195
    see also butchered meat
    additives on saturated fatty acids, 255–8
        selected micronutrients on fatty acid
            composition, 256
    altering animal diet to reduce saturated
        fat, 234–59
        dietary effects on the fat content and
            fatty acid composition of milk,
            249–55
        future trends, 258–9
    contribution to saturated fatty acid
        consumption, 236
    dietary effects on fat content and fatty
        acid composition, 238–49
        fat content, 238
        saturated fatty acids in beef, 238–45
        saturated fatty acids in other meat,
            245–9
    fat content, 237
    saturated fatty acid composition, 235
medium chain triglycerides, 56
mellorine products, 360–1
metabolic syndrome, 89–90, 106
microcrystalline cellulose, 224
microparticulated protein particles, 149
microwave frying, 277

milk, 62, 134, 182–4
    see also specific types
    additives on saturated fatty acids, 255–8
        selected micronutrients on fatty acid
            composition, 256
    altering animal diet to reduce saturated
        fat, 234–59
        future trends, 258–9
    contribution to saturated fatty acid
        consumption, 236
    dietary effects on the fat content and
        fatty acid composition, 249–55
        influence on non-dietary factors, 249
        saturated fatty acids, 249–55
    drinking milk, 182–3
    fat content, 237
    saturated fat reduction, 179–90
    saturated fatty acid composition, 235
    yoghurts and fermented milk, 183–4
'14/25' milk chocolate, 325
'20/20' milk chocolate, 325
milk fat, 189, 321
'milk ice,' 360
milk products, 181
modified potato starch, 222
MONICA study, 92
monoacylglycerols, 159
monounsaturated fatty acids, 81–3, 98,
    113, 219, 234
Morning Coffee, 287
mortadella, 225
MPPP see microparticulated protein
    particles
MPS see modified potato starch
MUFA see monounsaturated fatty acids
multiple emulsions, 133
myristic acid, 82, 100, 101

N-Dulge, 296
N-Dulge FR, 22
N-Lite, 296
N-Lite D, 362
nickel, 67
'noble ingredients,' 325, 327
non-chocolate confectionery, 25
non-digestible lipids, 147
non-lauric cocoa butter replacers, 334
non-lipid fat replacers, 362
nuggets, 227–9

oat bran, 147, 214
oat fibre, 214, 225
Oatrim, 298, 362
obesity, 88–9

© Woodhead Publishing Limited, 2011

oil curtains, 275
oil-in-water emulsion, 20, 36, 132, 137, 153
oil-in-water-in-oil emulsion, 133, 145
oil-in-water-in-water emulsions, 146
oil-in-water type emulsion foods, 169
oils
    see also specific oils
    sources, 59
Olean, 363
oleic acid, 8, 15, 100
Olestra, 211, 298, 363
olive oil, 340
omega-3 fatty acid, 8
omega-6 fatty acid, 8
omega nomenclature, 8
Orafti, 298
OSET index, 274
Oslo Diet, 88

PAI-1 see plasminogen activator inhibitor-1
palm kernel oil, 12, 21, 53–6, 112, 335, 352, 359
    carbon number triglyceride compositions, 54
    consumption, 12
    fatty acid compositions, 54
    melting profiles, 55
palm kernel stearin, 335
palm mid-fraction, 51
palm oil, 10–12, 21, 48–53, 83
    African and Asian palm oils triglyceride compositions, 50
    consumption, 11
    dietary fatty acids on LDL-C/HDL-C ratios, 117–20
        trans fatty acids on plasma lipids and CHD, 118–20
    minor components, 120–2
        palm tocotrienols, 122
    nutritional characteristics, 112–24
        future trends, 122–4
        serum cholesterol, lipoproteins and dietary fatty acids, 113–15
    palm fractions
        fatty acid compositions, 52
        melting profiles, 52
    palm olein as part of low-fat healthy diet, 115–17
        vs oleic rich oils, 115–16
        vs saturated fats, 116–17
    risk of replacing carbohydrates amounts

effects on CHD and type II diabetes, 119
    effects on TC/HDL-C ratio, 118
vitamin A, 121–2
    deficiency, 121
    status in pregnant and lactating women, 121–2
palm olein, 51, 115
palm stearin, 51
palm top-fraction, 51
palmitic acid, 15, 82, 83, 90, 100, 101, 332
partially hydrogenated vegetable oil, 118
partition coefficient, 36
Paselli SA2, 296, 362
pasta, 24
pastry, 301
    classification, 302–3
        according to fat/dough matching process and ingredients, 303
    dough/fat matching process, 304–8
        commercial puff pastry NMR image analysis, 307
        extruder-cooking equipment for cereal goods, 305
        fourfold pastry production, 308
        lamination, 306–8
        mixing, 304
        mixing/extrusion, 304–5
        threefold pastry production, 306
    general definitions, 301–2
    ingredients, 303–4
    margarine and shortenings for reducing saturated fats, 311–14
    olive oils shortenings in various markets, 314
    process rheological modelling, 308–11
        bubble expansion in viscoelastic matter, 308–10
        lamination process modelling, 310–11
        sketch of gas bubble immersed in infinite medium, 309
        sketch of sheeting, 311
    saturated fat reduction, 301–15
        future trends, 315
pâte feuilletage see puff pastry
pâte feuilletée see puff pastry
PCT see pork skin connective tissue
pellets, 266
PGPR see polyglycerol polyricinoleate
PHVO see partially hydrogenated vegetable oil
pies, 227–9
pig carcasses, 197–8
pizzas, 24

© Woodhead Publishing Limited, 2011

PKO *see* palm kernel oil
PKS *see* palm kernel stearin
plasma cholesterol, 78, 81, 86
plasminogen activator inhibitor-1, 85
plate waste, 205
Polydextrose, 211
polyglycerol polyricinoleate, 137, 328
polymer network formation, 315
polyphosphates, 187
polysaccharides, 41
polyunsaturated fatty acids, 81–3, 103, 113, 234
pork skin connective tissue, 218
potato crisps, 266, 270–1
poultry fats, 65
poyunsaturated fatty acids, 219
premier jus, 66
prepared sandwiches, 25
pressurisation, 276
primed pressed cocoa butter, 58
processed cheese, 186–7
'Processed Emmental cheese,' 187
processed meat
    dry fermented sausages, 225–7
        fat replacement effect on chemical composition, 227
    emulsion type sausages, 218–25
        fat and fluid losses from meat batters, 220
        sensory evaluation results, 223
    ground meat products, 212–15
        fat level on composition, sensory, texture and yield parameters, 212
    saturated fat reduction, 210–29
        coarse ground sausages, 215–18
        future trends, 229
        prepared and coated meat products, 227–9
propylene glycol esters, 141
proteins, 41
PUFA *see* polyunsaturated fatty acids
puff biscuits, 286
puff pastry, 302, 306–7

quiches, 25

ready meals, 23–5
red meat, 196
red palm oil, 121
reduced fat cheddar, 186
reduced fat yoghurt, 184
Redusat, 346
remnant-like lipoprotein particles, 164
REPLACE, 257

reverse cholesterol transport, 79
Rich Tea, 287, 293
ripened cheese, 184, 186
Ritz, 285
RLP *see* remnant-like lipoprotein particles
Roncal cheese, 137
rumen fermentation modifiers, 255

salami, 226
Salatrim, 298
salt, 186
sandwich/filled biscuits, 288
Saturated Fat and Energy Intake Programme, 3
saturated fat reduction
    altering animal diet for meat and milk, 234–59
        additives on saturated fatty acids in meat and milk, 255–8
        dietary effects on fat content and fatty acid composition of meat, 238–49
        dietary effects on the fat content and fatty acid composition of milk, 249–55
        fat content of meat and milk, 237
        future trends, 258–9
    biscuits, 283–99
        future trends, 299
        techniques for saturates reduction, 289–99
        technology of biscuits, 285–9
        types of fat used, 284–5
    butchered meat, 195–207
        animal production, 196–203
        cooking and consumption, 204–5
        effect on meat quality, 205–6
        future trends, 207
        preparation of cuts, 203–4
    chocolate, compound coatings and filled confectionery products, 318–47
        chocolate, 321–33
        chocolate confectionery consumption trends 2005–2007, 319
        compound coatings, 333–41
        filled confectionery products, 341–6
        future trends, 346–7
        household purchases of chocolate confectionery in the UK, 320
    emulsion technology, 131–53
        applications, 151–2
        emulsifiers, 132
        emulsion droplets, 138–41
        fat composition, 134–8
        fat replacers, 146–50

© Woodhead Publishing Limited, 2011

future trends, 152–3
multiple emulsions, 133
oil and water in foods, 131
oil-in-water emulsions, 132
phase structuring and emulsions,
    141–6
processing, 150–1
water-in-oil emulsions, 132–3
ice cream, 350–66
associated challenges, 359–65
basic components and processing,
    352–3
function of fat, 354–8
future trends, 365–6
properties of fats used in current
    products, 358–9
sources of fat and saturated fat, 353–4
milk and dairy products, 179–90
butter and spreadable fats, 187–9
cheese, 184–7
future trends, 190
legislative background, 181
milk, 182–4
milk fat through feed, 189
pastry, 301–15
classification, 302–3
dough/fat matching process, 304–8
future trends, 315
general definitions, 301–2
ingredients, 303–4
margarine and shortenings for
    reducing saturated fats, 311–14
process rheological modelling,
    308–11
processed meat, 210–29
coarse ground sausages, 215–18
dry fermented sausages, 225–7
emulsion type sausages,
    218–25
future trends, 229
ground meat products, 212–15
prepared and coated meat products,
    227–9
sauces, 370–6
future trends, 375–6
product lifetime, 373–5
sensory properties, 371–3
savoury snacks and fried foods,
    266–79
changes in savoury snacks, 277–8
frying oils, 267–8
frying oils and frying parameters on
    fried foods quality, 268–74
future trends, 279

innovating technologies in frying and
    their impact on fried foods quality,
    274–7
new product introductions in France,
    Germany, Italy, Netherlands, Spain
    and UK, 279
saturated fats
animal carcass fats, 65–6
    lard, beef tallow, sheep and deer fats,
        65–6
    saturated fat contents of fats from pig
        and beef carcasses, 65
changes in fatty acid consumption
    UK (1992–2008), 72
    US (1992–2008), 72
cocoa butter and cocoa butter equivalent
    fats, 57–61
    cocoa beans world production
        (2006–2009), 57
consumption in EU, US and UK, 10–15
    butterfat, 13
    coconut oil, 12–13
    lard, 13–15
    palm kernel oil, 12
    palm oil, 10–12
fatty acid compositions
    animal carcass fats, 66
    base oils used in cocoa butter equiva-
        lents, 60
    cocoa butters, 57
    milk fats, 62
    palm fractions, 52
    palm kernel and coconut oil, 54
    palm oils, 49
fatty acids and triglycerides chemistry
    and structure, 5–10
    food groups contributions to total and
        saturated fat intake, 6–7
    saturated fatty acids structures, 7
    triglyceride structure, 10
    unsaturated fatty acids structures, 8
hydrogenated fats, 67–9
    cis and trans fatty acids structures, 67
mammalian milk fats, 61–4
melting profiles
    cocoa butters, 58
    hydrogenated and fractionated palm
        kernel oil and coconut oil, 56
    palm fractions, 52
    palm kernel and coconut
        oil, 55
    spring and summer milk fats, 63
    stearin and oleine milk fat, 64
need to reduce saturated fats, 3–5

© Woodhead Publishing Limited, 2011

changes in UK energy intake from
fat, 5
fatty acids effect on changing total
cholesterol levels, 4
replacement strategies in foods, 3–26
future trends, 25–6
replacements for saturates, 18–22
diacylglycerol oils, 21–2
emulsion technology, 20
fat replacers, 19–20
other fatty acids, 18–19
structured triglycerides, 20–1
saturates effects on cardiovascular
disease, 15–17
total energy from saturates vs death
rates from CHD in men aged under
65, 17
saturates effects opposing views on
cardiovascular disease
fatty acids effect on changing total
HDL cholesterol ratio, 16
sources, 47–73
fatty acid contents of fats and oils, 48
future trends, 73
trans effect, 69–73
UK biscuits changes in total and
saturated fat contents, 70
triglyceride compositions
African and Asian palm oils, 50
cocoa butter, 58
cocoa butter equivalent
components, 61
palm kernel oil and coconut oil
carbon number, 54
vegetable oils rich in saturated fats,
48–61
palm kernel and coconut oils, 53–6
palm oil, 48–53
saturated fatty acids, 189
associated chronic disease risk, 98–108
future trends, 106, 108
atherosclerosis as the basis for
cardiovascular diseases, 78–81
HDL protective role, 80
LDL as the pathogenetic factor, 80
lipid hypothesis in atherogenesis,
78, 79
lipoproteins and their role in
atherogenesis, 78–9
lipoproteins characteristics, 79
roles of other lipoproteins, 81
total energy percentage from SFA in
the diets, 79
beef, 238–45

composition of intramuscular lipids
from *M. longissimus dorsi*, 239
influence of pasture on fatty acid
composition, 241
pasture or forage, 240–2
supplementation with protected lipids,
242, 244, 245
supplementation with unprotected
lipids, 242, 243
chicken, 247–9
chronic disease risk differences between
different SFA, 100–5
changes in ratio of serum total to
HDL cholesterol and in LDL- and
HDL-cholesterol concentrations,
103
diets on serum cholesterol
concentrations, 101
effect of replacing dietary
carbohydrates with SFA, 102
effects on disease outcome, 104–5
effects on serum lipids and
lipoproteins, 100–3
hazard ratios for selected fatty acids,
105
chronic disease risk effects of stearic
acid, 105–6, 107
vs other dietary fatty acids and other
factors, 107
dietary recommendations, 90–2
effects on disease states related to
cardiovascular disease, 88–90
criteria for diagnosis of metabolic
syndrome, 89
insulin sensitivity and type 2 diabetes,
90
metabolic syndrome, 89–90
obesity, 88–9
epidemiological studies, 86–7
associations between dietary
fatty acids and coronary heart
disease, 86–7
mean saturated fat intake and CHD
deaths in Seven Countries
study, 87
risk factors identification, 86
evidence linking LDL to atherosclerosis
and CHD development, 85–8
animal experiments, 85–6
clinical observations, 86
fatty acids effects on other biomarkers
related to CHD
haemostatic factors, 85
inflammation markers, 85

© Woodhead Publishing Limited, 2011

fatty acids on other biomarkers related
    to coronary heart disease, 84–5
health aspects, 77–93
    cancer, 90
    trends in consumption as related to
        CVD mortality and incidence, 92
individual fatty acids effects on plasma
        total cholesterol, LDL, HDL and
        VLDL, 81–4
    common SAFA in food fats and
        oils, 83
    individual cholesterol-increasing fatty
        acids coefficients, 82
    lauric, myristic and palmitic acid in
        Norwegian diet, 84
    palmitic acid in Western diet, 83–4
    SFA, MUFA, PUFA and TFA effects,
        81–3
    SFA distributions in US diet, 84
intakes by men in 11 EU member states,
    100
intervention studies, 87–8
    dietary interventions, 87–8
    interventions at national level, 88
    interventions with cholesterol
        reducing drugs, 88
key dietary saturated fatty acids, 99–100
lipid sources on fatty acid composition
    bovine milk: oils and oilseeds, 252
    bovine milk: protected lipids, 254
    bovine muscle: oils and oilseeds, 243
    bovine muscle: protected lipids, 244
    chicken muscle, 248
    pig muscle, 246
milk, 249–55
    forage on fatty acid composition, 251
    pasture or forage, 250, 251
    supplementation with protected lipids,
        253–5
    supplementation with unprotected
        lipids, 250, 252–3
milk and meat contribution to SFA
        consumption by European
        consumers, 236
pigmeat, 245–7
saturated-oleic-saturated triglycerides,
    322–3
saturates see saturated fats
sauces
    choice of polymeric emulsifiers
        carbohydrates, 373
        proteins, 373
    emulsion behaviour
        emulsification properties, 373

solubility, 373
viscosity, 373
hydrocolloids
    aqueous solubility, 372
    gelling ability, 372
    thickening, 372
product lifetime, 373–5
    emulsion breakdown, 374
    flavour stability, 374
    microbiology, 374–5
    oxidation, 374
saturated fat reduction, 370–6
    future trends, 375–6
sensory properties, 371–3
    fat content, 371–2
    texturising systems, 372
sausages, 215–27
savoury crackers, 286
savoury snacks
    changes, 277–8
    saturated fat reduction, 266–79
    future trends, 279
scald temperature, 186
Scottish method, 306
semi-skimmed milk, 182, 183
semisweet biscuits, 287
Seven Countries Study, 98
SFA see saturated fatty acids
short dough biscuits, 287–8
short-mixing time method, 307
short-path distillation, 167
shortcrust pastry, 302, 304
shortenings, 170–1
Simplesse, 362
Single Farm Payment, 200
skimmed milk, 182, 183
skimmed milk powder, 182
Slendid, 362
SLS see sodium lauryl sulphate
small amplitude oscillatory test, 304
small molecule surfactants, 33
Smoking Study, 88
sodium chloride, 187
sodium citrate, 187
sodium lauryl sulphate, 150
sodium stearoyl lactylate, 141, 297
soya bean flour, 147
SPD see short-path distillation
species flavour, 206
'sponge effect,' 276
spreadable fats, 187–9
'Spreadable Processed Emmental Cheese,'
    187
SSL see sodium stearoyl lactylate

© Woodhead Publishing Limited, 2011

STAN 87–1981, Rev. 1–2003, 325
starches, 213
statins, 88
stearic acid, 15, 82, 332–3
'stearic acid' effect, 105–6, 107
stearin fraction, 323, 330
striploin, 237
structured triglycerides, 20–1
subcutaneous fat, 237
sulphated butyl oleate, 150
summer sausage, 225–7
'supercoating,' 334
surfactant, 33
Surimi, 215

TAG see triacylglycerols
tertiary butylhydroquinone, 374
TFA see trans fatty acids
Theobroma cacao, 57
thermo-oxidation, 267
threshold hypothesis, 117
tiger nut fibre, 215
'time cure test,' 305
tocopherols, 120
tocotrienols, 113, 120, 122
toffees, 25
total cholesterol, 113
trans effect, 69–73
    UK biscuits changes in total and
        saturated fat contents, 70
trans fats, 334–6
trans fatty acids, 8–9, 12, 16, 18, 20, 67,
        68, 69, 81–3, 105, 106, 303, 312
    structures, 67
trans isomers, 267
trans MUFA, 118
TRANSFACT Study, 9
triacylglycerols, 5, 358
tribometer, 34
triglycerides, 5, 9, 78, 80, 81, 303, 312
    chemistry and structure, 5–10
    structure, 10
tropical oils, 69

Tuc crackers, 285
type 2 diabetes, 90

Unripened Cheese, 184, 185
unsaturated fatty acids, 7, 180
    structures, 8

'vacuum effect,' 269
vacuum frying, 275–7
vegetable fat, 325
very low-density lipoproteins, 78, 117
Vitacel, 298
vitamin A, 121–2
vitamin E, 113, 120
VLDL see very low-density lipoproteins

wafers, 288
'washer test,' 343
water-in-oil emulsion, 18, 20, 132–3,
        137–8
water-in-oil-in-water emulsion, 20, 133,
        142–5, 153
    alternatives to polyglycerol
        polyricinoleate, 144
    characterisation, 144–5
    stability, 143–4
water-in-oil type emulsion foods, 169–70
wet fractionation, 51
WFC see white fresh cheese
whey protein isolate, 228
white fresh cheese, 145
whole milk, 182
    fat content, 180
World Cancer Research Fund, 90
WPI see whey protein isolate

xanthan gum, 147, 216, 221, 227

yoghurt, 33, 34, 183–4
    average in vivo flavour release
        curves, 37

Z Trim, 298

© Woodhead Publishing Limited, 2011

Lightning Source UK Ltd.
Milton Keynes UK
UKOW030812100312

188645UK00002B/14/P